Arteriogenesis

Arteriogenesis—Molecular Regulation, Pathophysiology and Therapeutics II

Special Issue Editors

Elisabeth Deindl
Paul Quax

MDPI • Basel • Beijing • Wuhan • Barcelona • Belgrade

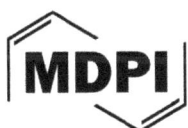

Special Issue Editors

Elisabeth Deindl
Walter-Brendel-Centre of
Exp. Medicine
Germany

Paul Quax
Department of Surgery,
Leiden University
Medical Center
The Netherlands

Editorial Office
MDPI
St. Alban-Anlage 66
4052 Basel, Switzerland

This is a reprint of articles from the Special Issue published online in the open access journal *International Journal of Molecular Sciences* (ISSN 1422-0067) from 2019 to 2020 (available at: https://www.mdpi.com/journal/ijms/special_issues/arteriogenesis).

For citation purposes, cite each article independently as indicated on the article page online and as indicated below:

LastName, A.A.; LastName, B.B.; LastName, C.C. Article Title. *Journal Name* **Year**, *Article Number*, Page Range.

ISBN 978-3-03936-435-0 (Hbk)
ISBN 978-3-03936-436-7 (PDF)

Cover image courtesy of Elisabeth Deindl (Artist Xenia Deindl).

© 2020 by the authors. Articles in this book are Open Access and distributed under the Creative Commons Attribution (CC BY) license, which allows users to download, copy and build upon published articles, as long as the author and publisher are properly credited, which ensures maximum dissemination and a wider impact of our publications.

The book as a whole is distributed by MDPI under the terms and conditions of the Creative Commons license CC BY-NC-ND.

Contents

About the Special Issue Editors vii

Elisabeth Deindl and Paul H. A. Quax
From Increased Fluid Shear Stress to Natural Bypass Growth
Reprinted from: *Int. J. Mol. Sci.* **2020**, *21*, 3707, doi:10.3390/ijms21103707 1

Zeen Aref, Margreet R. de Vries and Paul H.A. Quax
Variations in Surgical Procedures for Inducing Hind Limb Ischemia in Mice and the Impact of These Variations on Neovascularization Assessment
Reprinted from: *Int. J. Mol. Sci.* **2019**, *20*, 3704, doi:10.3390/ijms20153704 4

Hua Zhang, Dan Chalothorn and James E Faber
Collateral Vessels Have Unique Endothelial and Smooth Muscle Cell Phenotypes
Reprinted from: *Int. J. Mol. Sci.* **2019**, *20*, 3608, doi:10.3390/ijms20153608 18

Anna-Kristina Kluever, Anna Braumandl, Silvia Fischer, Klaus T. Preissner and Elisabeth Deindl
The Extraordinary Role of Extracellular RNA in Arteriogenesis, the Growth of Collateral Arteries
Reprinted from: *Int. J. Mol. Sci.* **2019**, *20*, 6177, doi:10.3390/ijms20246177 38

Konda Kumaraswami, Natallia Salei, Sebastian Beck, Stephan Rambichler, Anna-Kristina Kluever, Manuel Lasch, Lisa Richter, Barbara U. Schraml and Elisabeth Deindl
A Simple and Effective Flow Cytometry-Based Method for Identification and Quantification of Tissue Infiltrated Leukocyte Subpopulations in a Mouse Model of Peripheral Arterial Disease
Reprinted from: *Int. J. Mol. Sci.* **2020**, *21*, 3593, doi:10.3390/ijms21103593 55

Alexander M. Götze, Christian Schubert, Georg Jung, Oliver Dörr, Christoph Liebetrau, Christian W. Hamm, Thomas Schmitz-Rixen, Christian Troidl and Kerstin Troidl
IL10 Alters Peri-Collateral Macrophage Polarization and Hind-Limb Reperfusion in Mice after Femoral Artery Ligation
Reprinted from: *Int. J. Mol. Sci.* **2020**, *21*, 2821, doi:10.3390/ijms21082821 63

Yvonn Heun, Katharina Grundler Groterhorst, Kristin Pogoda, Bjoern F Kraemer, Alexander Pfeifer, Ulrich Pohl and Hanna Mannell
The Phosphatase SHP-2 Activates HIF-1α in Wounds In Vivo by Inhibition of 26S Proteasome Activity
Reprinted from: *Int. J. Mol. Sci.* **2019**, *20*, 4404, doi:10.3390/ijms20184404 74

Senthilkumar Thulasingam, Sundar Krishnasamy, David Raj C., Manuel Lasch, Srinivasan Vedantham and Elisabeth Deindl
Insulin Treatment Forces Arteriogenesis in Diabetes Mellitus by Upregulation of the Early Growth Response-1 (Egr-1) Pathway in Mice
Reprinted from: *Int. J. Mol. Sci.* **2019**, *20*, 3320, doi:10.3390/ijms20133320 87

Catherine M. Gorick, John C. Chappell and Richard J. Price
Applications of Ultrasound to Stimulate Therapeutic Revascularization
Reprinted from: *Int. J. Mol. Sci.* **2019**, *20*, 3081, doi:10.3390/ijms20123081 99

Ayko Bresler, Johanna Vogel, Daniel Niederer, Daphne Gray, Thomas Schmitz-Rixen and Kerstin Troidl
Development of an Exercise Training Protocol to Investigate Arteriogenesis in a Murine Model of Peripheral Artery Disease
Reprinted from: *Int. J. Mol. Sci.* **2019**, *20*, 3956, doi:10.3390/ijms20163956 117

Johanna Vogel, Daniel Niederer, Tobias Engeroff, Lutz Vogt, Christian Troidl, Thomas Schmitz-Rixen, Winfried Banzer and Kerstin Troidl
Effects on the Profile of Circulating miRNAs after Single Bouts of Resistance Training with and without Blood Flow Restriction—A Three-Arm, Randomized Crossover Trial
Reprinted from: *Int. J. Mol. Sci.* **2019**, *20*, 3249, doi:10.3390/ijms20133249 129

Bigler Marius Reto and Christian Seiler
The Human Coronary Collateral Circulation, Its Extracardiac Anastomoses and Their Therapeutic Promotion
Reprinted from: *Int. J. Mol. Sci.* **2019**, *20*, 3726, doi:10.3390/ijms20153726 146

About the Special Issue Editors

Elisabeth Deindl graduated from the ZMBH in Heidelberg, Germany, where she worked on hepatitis B viruses. Thereafter, she joined the lab of Wolfgang Schaper at the Max-Planck-Institute in Bad Nauheim, where she started to decipher the molecular mechanisms of arteriogenesis. After a short detour to study stem cells, she again focused on arteriogenesis, and became a leading expert in her field. By using a peripheral model of arteriogenesis, she demonstrated that collateral artery growth is a matter of innate immunity and presents a blueprint for sterile inflammation, which is locally triggered by extracellular RNA.

Paul Quax completed his PhD at the University of Leiden, the Netherlands, on the role of plasminogen activators in tissue remodeling. He continued to work on this topic in relation to vascular remodeling, first at the Gaubius Laboratory TNO, and later at the Leiden University Medical Center, as a professor in experimental vascular medicine. His interest in arteriogenesis has been driven by the lack of therapeutic options for patients with peripheral arterial disease. The topics of his research are therapeutic arteriogenesis and angiogenesis induced by gene therapy, growth factors, modulation of inflammatory and immune response, the modulation of microRNAs, and other noncoding RNAs in small animal models.

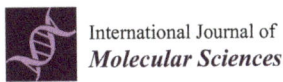

Editorial

From Increased Fluid Shear Stress to Natural Bypass Growth

Elisabeth Deindl [1],* and Paul H. A. Quax [2],*

1. Walter-Brendel-Centre of Experimental Medicine, University Hospital, Ludwig-Maximilians-University, 81377 Munich, Germany
2. Department of Surgery, Einthoven Laboratory for Experimental Vascular Medicine, Leiden University Medical Center, 2300 RC Leiden, The Netherlands
* Correspondence: elisabeth.deindl@med.uni-muenchen.de (E.D.); p.h.a.quax@lumc.nl (P.H.A.Q.); Tel.: +49-89-2180-76504 (E.D.); +31-71-526-1584 (P.H.A.Q.)

Received: 19 May 2020; Accepted: 22 May 2020; Published: 25 May 2020

This Special Issue enqueues a series of publications dealing with arteriogenesis, which is the growth of a natural bypass from pre-existing arteriolar connections, as defined by Wolfgang Schaper, Werner Risau and Ramon Munoz-Chapuli in the late nineties of the last century. In times of increasing numbers of patients with cardiovascular occlusive diseases not only in highly industrialized but in almost all countries of the world, it is of major importance to understand the molecular mechanisms of this tissue- and life-saving process, which was given to us by mother nature to compensate for the function of a stenosed coronary or peripheral artery non-invasively. Since our first investigations on collateral artery growth more than 20 years ago, a lot of progress has been made, which we try to give access to in this issue on arteriogenesis.

In the current special issue, entitled "Arteriogenesis – Molecular Regulation, Pathophysiology and Therapeutics II" in the *International Journal of Molecular Sciences*, Zeen Aref and Margreet de Vries, from the group around Paul Quax, give an overview of the currently available variations of murine hind limb models for the study of angiogenesis and arteriogenesis, and highlight their advantages and disadvantages [1]. Huan Zhang and Don Chalothron, from Jim Fabers´ group, describe the features of collateral vessels and supply insights into the unique phenotypes and features of collateral endothelial and smooth muscle cells [2].

The trigger for arteriogenesis is increased fluid shear stress, which is exerted on the endothelial cells of pre-existing collateral arteries by blood flow being redirected around stenosed vessels. For a long time, it was completely unknown how this increased mechanical stress results in local leukocyte recruitment promoting collateral artery growth. Co-workers of the group of Elisabeth Deindl describe the functional role of extracellular RNA in that process and highlight the role of this nucleic acid during ongoing arteriogenesis [3]. Moreover, the same group presents a simple flow cytometry-based method to identify and quantify tissue infiltrated leukocyte subpopulations [4]. Macrophages, which accumulate in the perivascular tissue of growing collateral arteries, are well described for their pro-arteriogenic feature. Co-workers of Kerstin and Christian Troidl delineate the relevance of alternatively and classically activated macrophages, and explain the function of IL10 in that context [5].

Arterial occlusion results in reduced perfusion, and hence ischemia, in distally located tissue. As a consequence of the thereto related hypoxia, angiogenesis is induced. In contrast to other ischemic conditions, where capillaries are required to supply tissue locally with oxygen and nutrients, capillaries in regions distal to occluded arteries are necessary for the removal of cell debris. Yvonn Heun and the group around Hanna Mannel show that the tyrosine phosphatase SHP-2 inhibits 26S proteasome and thereby activates hypoxia-induced HIF-1α (hypoxia inducible factor 1α). This mechanism, which was identified in wounds, seems to be generally applicable, and results in pro-angiogenic gene expression under hypoxic conditions in ischemic tissue [6].

The process of collateral artery growth is often severely compromised in patients with diabetes mellitus. Srinivasan Vedantham and Elisabeth Deindl investigated the role of insulin for arteriogenesis in diabetic mice. They were able to attribute to this peptide hormone a function in the expression of Egr-1 (early growth response-1), a transcription factor relevant for collateral outward remodeling [7]. Cathrine Gorick, John Chappell and Richard Price explain the technical possibilities of ultrasound together with microbubbles as a non-invasive and spatially targeted option to therapeutically stimulate revascularization and point to perspectives of such approaches [8].

Thomas-Schmitz-Rixen, Kerstin Troidl and co-workers have developed an exercise training protocol in mice allowing the investigation of the effect of this physical force on collateral artery growth in mice [9], and, together with co-workers of Winfried Banzer, they show the effect of resistance training with and without blood flow restriction on the expression of circulating micro RNAs, which are relevant for collateral artery growth, in healthy volunteers [10].

Last but not least, the interventional cardiologists and specialists in the field of arteriogenesis, Bigler Marius Reto and Christian Seiler, provide an overview of human coronary collateral circulation and introduce the different clinical therapeutic approaches for the promotion of arteriogenesis in patients. They explain the problematic nature of biochemical concepts involving, for example, G-CSF (granulocyte-colony stimulating factor) and GM-CSF (granulocyte-macrophage colony stimulating factor), review the feasibility of biophysical concepts such as physical exercise and ECP (external counterpulsation), and focus on the promising approach of permanent occlusion of the internal mammary arteries in promoting natural bypass growth in patients [11].

With all our investigations and efforts, we think that we have come much closer to the goal of all of us to understand the mechanisms of collateral artery growth, finally enabling clinicians to promote arteriogenesis effectively in patients with vascular occlusive diseases.

Conflicts of Interest: The authors declare no conflict of interest.

References

1. Aref, Z.; de Vries, M.R.; Quax, P.H.A. Variations in Surgical Procedures for Inducing Hind Limb Ischemia in Mice and the Impact of These Variations on Neovascularization Assessment. *Int. J. Mol. Sci.* **2019**, *20*, 3704. [CrossRef] [PubMed]
2. Zhang, H.; Chalothorn, D.; Faber, J.E. Collateral Vessels Have Unique Endothelial and Smooth Muscle Cell Phenotypes. *Int. J. Mol. Sci.* **2019**, *20*, 3608. [CrossRef] [PubMed]
3. Kluever, A.K.; Braumandl, A.; Fischer, S.; Preissner, K.T.; Deindl, E. The Extraordinary Role of Extracellular RNA in Arteriogenesis, the Growth of Collateral Arteries. *Int. J. Mol. Sci.* **2019**, *20*, 6177. [CrossRef] [PubMed]
4. Kumaraswami, K.; Salei, N.; Beck, S.; Rambichler, S.; Kluever, A.K.; Lasch, M.; Richter, L.; Schraml, B.U.; Deindl, E. A Simple and Effective Flow Cytometry-Based Method for Identification and Quantification of Tissue Infiltrated Leukocyte Subpopulations in a Mouse Model of Peripheral Arterial Disease. *Int. J. Mol. Sci.* **2020**, *21*, 3593. [CrossRef] [PubMed]
5. Gotze, A.M.; Schubert, C.; Jung, G.; Dorr, O.; Liebetrau, C.; Hamm, C.W.; Schmitz-Rixen, T.; Troidl, C.; Troidl, K. IL10 Alters Peri-Collateral Macrophage Polarization and Hind-Limb Reperfusion in Mice after Femoral Artery Ligation. *Int. J. Mol. Sci.* **2020**, *21*, 2821. [CrossRef] [PubMed]
6. Heun, Y.; Grundler Groterhorst, K.; Pogoda, K.; Kraemer, B.F.; Pfeifer, A.; Pohl, U.; Mannell, H. The Phosphatase SHP-2 Activates HIF-1alpha in Wounds In Vivo by Inhibition of 26S Proteasome Activity. *Int. J. Mol. Sci.* **2019**, *20*, 4404. [CrossRef] [PubMed]
7. Thulasingam, S.; Krishnasamy, S.; Raj, C.D.; Lasch, M.; Vedantham, S.; Deindl, E. Insulin Treatment Forces Arteriogenesis in Diabetes Mellitus by Upregulation of the Early Growth Response-1 (Egr-1) Pathway in Mice. *Int. J. Mol. Sci.* **2019**, *20*, 3320. [CrossRef] [PubMed]
8. Gorick, C.M.; Chappell, J.C.; Price, R.J. Applications of Ultrasound to Stimulate Therapeutic Revascularization. *Int. J. Mol. Sci.* **2019**, *20*, 3081. [CrossRef] [PubMed]

9. Bresler, A.; Vogel, J.; Niederer, D.; Gray, D.; Schmitz-Rixen, T.; Troidl, K. Development of an Exercise Training Protocol to Investigate Arteriogenesis in a Murine Model of Peripheral Artery Disease. *Int. J. Mol. Sci.* **2019**, *20*, 3956. [CrossRef] [PubMed]
10. Vogel, J.; Niederer, D.; Engeroff, T.; Vogt, L.; Troidl, C.; Schmitz-Rixen, T.; Banzer, W.; Troidl, K. Effects on the Profile of Circulating miRNAs after Single Bouts of Resistance Training with and without Blood Flow Restriction-A Three-Arm, Randomized Crossover Trial. *Int. J. Mol. Sci.* **2019**, *20*, 3249. [CrossRef] [PubMed]
11. Bigler, M.R.; Seiler, C. The Human Coronary Collateral Circulation, Its Extracardiac Anastomoses and Their Therapeutic Promotion. *Int. J. Mol. Sci.* **2019**, *20*, 3726. [CrossRef]

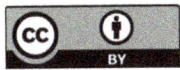

© 2020 by the authors. Licensee MDPI, Basel, Switzerland. This article is an open access article distributed under the terms and conditions of the Creative Commons Attribution (CC BY) license (http://creativecommons.org/licenses/by/4.0/).

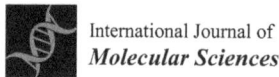

Review

Variations in Surgical Procedures for Inducing Hind Limb Ischemia in Mice and the Impact of These Variations on Neovascularization Assessment

Zeen Aref, Margreet R. de Vries and Paul H.A. Quax *

Department of Surgery, Einthoven Laboratory for Experimental Vascular Medicine, Leiden University Medical Center, 2300 RC Leiden, The Netherlands
* Correspondence: p.h.a.quax@lumc.nl; Tel.: +31-71-526-1584; Fax: + 31-71-526-6570

Received: 31 May 2019; Accepted: 25 July 2019; Published: 29 July 2019

Abstract: Mouse hind limb ischemia is the most common used preclinical model for peripheral arterial disease and critical limb ischemia. This model is used to investigate the mechanisms of neovascularization and to develop new therapeutic agents. The literature shows many variations in the model, including the method of occlusion, the number of occlusions, and the position at which the occlusions are made to induce hind limb ischemia. Furthermore, predefined end points and the histopathological and radiological analysis vary. These differences hamper the correlation of results between different studies. In this review, variations in surgical methods of inducing hind limb ischemia in mice are described, and the consequences of these variations on perfusion restoration and vascular remodeling are discussed. This study aims at providing the reader with a comprehensive overview of the methods so far described, and proposing uniformity in research of hind limb ischemia in a mouse model.

Keywords: arteriogenesis; angiogenesis; hind limb ischemia; animal model; mouse

1. Introduction

Peripheral arterial disease (PAD) is a major cause of morbidity and mortality [1]. PAD is caused by atherosclerotic plaque progression which leads to the occlusion of peripheral arteries and results in claudication intermittens, or in more severe cases, in critical limb ischemia. The prevalence of PAD increases with age to 20% in people over 70 years [1]. Furthermore, type II diabetes, obesity, and hypertension are known risk factors for atherosclerosis [2]. As increased life expectancy is leading to an increased number of elderly patients suffering from these comorbidities [2], the number of patients with PAD is expected to grow the coming years. Therefore, there is a need for developing new therapies to treat peripheral arterial disease. As a consequence, there is a need for representative models to study and validate these potential new therapies. Therapeutic neovascularization is an alternative therapeutic strategy aimed at improving blood flow to the lower extremities and promoting blood vessel growth. Neovascularization consists of the processes of arteriogenesis, angiogenesis, and vasculogenesis. These processes differ from each other. Arteriogenesis is initiated by shear stress and is the formation of collateral arteries from the pre-existing arteriolar network [3], and will mainly be found in the upper limb of the mice after ligation of the arteries in the limb. The molecular mechanism for arteriogenesis is based on shear stress regulated inflammatory responses, accompanied by the influx of inflammatory cells in the perivascular compartment around the collateral that are being formed.

Angiogenesis is the process of sprouting new capillaries from pre-existing microvasculature. Angiogenesis is mainly driven by ischemia and the upregulation of ischemia-induced transcription factors like HIF1a, and the genes that are responsive to these transcription factors, such as VEGFa and SDF1. In the mouse hind limb model, angiogenesis will mostly occur in the distal parts of the limbs, the gastrocnemius muscle, and the soleus muscle. Vasculogenesis describes the incorporation of circulating (progenitor) cells into the regenerating microvasculature [4], and will only be of relevance in the mouse hind limb ischemia model in cases of cell therapy related studies.

For the purpose of elucidating the cellular and molecular mechanisms underlying the process of neovascularization, and for developing and testing the new therapeutic approaches for neovascularization, a reliable and reproducible animal model is needed.

Animal models of hind limb ischemia have been developed in rabbits, pigs, rats, and mice. A mouse model is preferable over larger animal models because of practical circumstances, and over a rat model because of the wide range of transgenic mice that are available. These are not only mice lacking angiogenic factors like eNOS [5], but also mice deficient in various factors of inflammatory or immune pathways that can subsequently be related to the molecular mechanisms involved in angiogenesis and arteriogenesis [6–9]. Therefore, the mouse model of hind limb ischemia is the main model used in the preclinical studies. It has to be noted that the mouse model can be performed using different strains of mice, each having a specific pattern of blood flow recovery [10–14]. Applying to all local and governmental regulatory and ethical aspects regarding animal experimentation is, of course, essential.

In this model, limb ischemia is induced by ligation, electrocoagulation, or by applying an ameroid constrictor to occlude the femoral artery. The occlusion of the femoral artery results in arteriogenesis in the thigh and angiogenesis in the distal part of the limb to recover perfusion. Different positions of ligation trigger different pathways of neovascularization. Therefore, the position at which the ligation of the femoral artery should be performed in order to provide a proper model for investigating the perfusion recovery, arteriogenesis, and or angiogenesis remains a topic of research and debate [10]. This illustrates that variations in the model for inducing hind limb ischemia in mice may lead to differences in blood flow recovery and vascular repair or neovascularisation, and may also have consequences for the interpretation of the data obtained in relation to the underlying pathophysiological mechanisms. In the literature, the tourniquet-induced hindlimb ischemia-reperfusion method is also described to induce acute ischemia [15–17]. For the current review, this method is less relevant, since the induced ischemia is for such a short period that no effects on neovascularization are observed.

Moreover, as will be discussed below, it is essential to consider which mouse strain to use, because genetic background influences the outcome. Several studies have shown that different mouse strains display a high variability in the degree of neovascularization [13,14]. Many studies have shown fast recovery of limb perfusion in C57BL/6 after inducing hind limb ischemia in comparison to the slow recovering Balb/C mice. Furthermore, it is important to realize that immune-compromised mice such as nude mice or non-obese diabetic-severe combined immunodeficiency (NOD-SCID) mice that are frequently used for cell therapy studies [18] have an increased number of pre-existing collaterals and require a more fierce induction of ischemia, including the removal of arterial branches [18].

The aim of this paper is to review the techniques of inducing hind limb ischemia in a mouse model, providing a rationale with which to identify the optimal mouse model. To this end, we describe variations in anatomical nomenclature, variation in surgical methods, and histopathological and radiological techniques for the quantification of the end-points.

2. Mouse Model for Hind Limb Ischemia

The mouse model of hind limb ischemia was first described by Couffinhal et al. [19] based on the rabbit model for hind ischemia, as developed in the group of Wolfgang Schaper. They induced acute hind limb ischemia by ligating the proximal end of the femoral artery, and the distal portion of the saphenous artery, and subsequently excised the femoral artery and all side-branches. The recovery of the blood flow in the limbs was monitored for 5 weeks postoperatively by Laser Doppler Perfusion Imaging (LDPI). The blood flow was reduced postoperatively and the reduction maintained for 7 days; then, the flow was increased over the course of 14 days, reaching a plateau between days 21 and 28 [19]. Thereafter, many groups used the model and also developed new adapted approaches.

2.1. Vascular Anatomy of the Mouse

The mouse hind limb is perfused by the external iliac artery (EIA), which changes in the common femoral artery after it passes the inguinal ligament. The femoral artery gives rise to branches that further divide into collateral vessels that penetrate the muscles.

Kochi et al. described in detail the arterial anatomy of the mouse hind limb, the distribution of collaterals, and also three collateral arterial routes [20]. They indicated that there are collateral artery routes through the quadriceps femoris, the biceps femoris muscles, and medial thigh muscles [20]. The medial thigh muscles include the adductor muscles, and are perfused by the proximal caudal femoral artery, as named by Kochi et al.; however, the same artery is termed the deep femoral artery by Limbourg et al. [20,21]. It is the same artery which gives rise to collateral arteries that pervade the adductor muscle group and are the most evaluated muscle groups for arteriogenesis in the tissue after inducing hind limb ischemia.

Kochi et al. highlighted the confusion in the literature about the arterial anatomy due the embedding of the arteries in the musculature and the fact that some of the small arteries are only visualized after dilating and fixing the arteries and, if needed, dissecting the vein to better expose the artery. In order to compare the different approaches used to induce hind limb ischemia, it is important to name the structures identically, and it is more important to describe the procedure and, if possible, to add images of the ligation site to make comparisons possible between the studies and a correct interpretation of the results.

2.2. Technical Aspects of Inducing Mouse Limb Ischemia

For the induction of hind limb ischemia in mice, the blood flow in vessels supplying the limb needs to be interrupted by surgical intervention. The general steps of the procedure are described below, whereas the details on the variations in the procedure will be described in the following sections. After anesthetizing a mouse, it is positioned in dorsal decubitus with the hind limbs externally rotated. In one limb, ischemia was operatively induced by ligation or coagulation, with the other limb serving as an internal control. Ligation and coagulation are considered equal in inducing hind limb ischemia, even though coagulation may induce recoil of the femoral artery. For anesthesia two types are commonly used: inhalation, using isoflurane [22], and injectable, using different combinations. The most used combination is midazolam (5 mg·kg^{-1}) and medetomidine (0.5 mg·kg^{-1}) [10] or a combination of 100 mg/kg of ketamine (100 mg·kg^{-1}) and xylazine (10 mg·kg^{-1}) [23]. However, alpha-agonists induce early peripheral vasoconstriction and may disturb the results of the experiment [24]. Therefore, ketamine and alpha-agonist combinations are not suitable for studies of vascular smooth muscle cell rich vasculature [23]. For analgesics, fentanyl (0.05 mg·kg^{-1}) is most commonly used. For anesthesia reversal, atipamezole (1 mg·kg^{-1}) is used. After surgery, the skin can be closed with 6-0 (Ethilon) sutures.

2.3. Variants of Surgical Procedure

To induce hind limb ischemia, different surgical approaches have been used (Figure 1, Table 1), ranging from a single ligation of the femoral artery or iliac artery [11,25] to a complete excision of the femoral artery and its side-branches [19], sometimes even in combination with dissection of the vein and the nerve [26]. Also, there is a variation in the level of inducing the arterial occlusion ranging from proximal ligation of the iliac artery to distal ligation just proximal to the bifurcation of the saphenous artery and the popliteal artery.

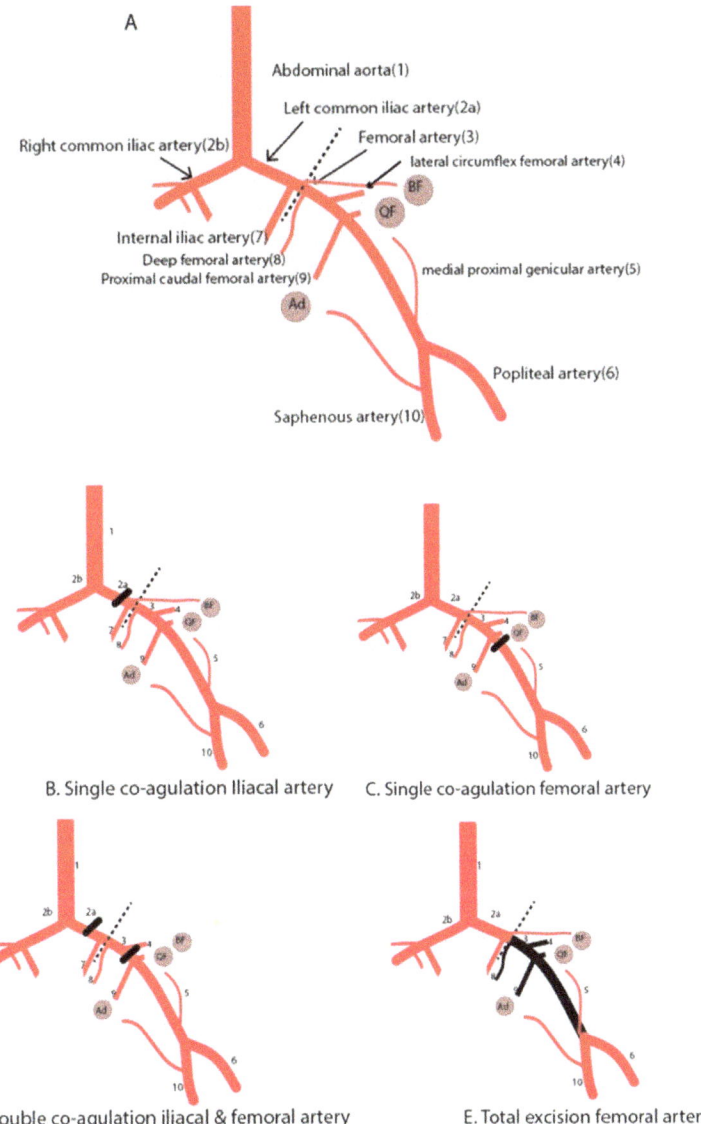

Figure 1. Schematic diagram illustrating the hind limb ischemia and different surgical methods to induce hind limb ischemia. (**A**) Hind limb vasculature. (**B**) Single electrocoagulation of the iliac artery. (**C**) Single electrocoagulation of the femoral artery. (**D**) Double electrocoagulation of the iliac and femoral artery. Alternatively, the electrocoagulation of the iliac artery can be replaced by a second electrocoagulation of the femoral artery just above the bifurcation of the saphenous and popliteal artery. (**E**) Total excision of the femoral artery. Round circles are muscle groups: (Ad) adductor muscle group. (QF) Quadriceps femoris. (BF) Biceps femoris. Dotted line is the inguinal ligament. Black beam is the occlusion site.

Table 1. Surgical methods used to induce hind limb ischemia, time course of blood reperfusion recovery, whether the method is suitable to assess arteriogenesis and angiogenesis, and if arteriogenesis takes place, where it will take place.

Surgical Method Used to Induce HLI	Time Course of Blood Reperfusion (Days)	Ischemia Rate	Suitable to Studying Arteriogenesis?	Which Collateral Group Can Be Studied?	Suitable to Studying Angiogenesis in Calf Muscle?
Electrocoagulation of common iliac artery	7–14 days	moderate	Yes	Medial thigh muscles (includes adductor muscles) Quadriceps femoris Biceps femoris	Yes
Electrocoagulation of the femoral artery, distal from origin of deep branch	7–14 days	mild	Yes	Adductor muscles Quadriceps femoris Biceps femoris	Yes
Electrocoagulation of the femoral artery, proximal from origin of deep branch	7–14 days	mild	Yes	Quadriceps femoris Biceps femoris	Yes
Total excision of the femoral artery	28 days	severe	No		Yes
Double electrocoagulation of iliac and femoral artery	28 days	moderate	Yes	Medial thigh muscles (includes adductor muscles) Quadriceps femoris Biceps femoris	Yes
Ameriod constrictors		mild	Unclear		No

2.3.1. Single Electrocoagulation or Ligation of Femoral Artery

This surgical method is the most used method to induce hind limb ischemia. Through an incision in the inguinal region, the femoral artery is exposed. Thereafter, the subcutaneous inguinal fat pad is pulled aside and the artery is dissected from the vein and the nerve. Then the femoral artery is ligated or coagulated. The anatomical level at which the occlusion of femoral artery is induced differs among studies. Limbourg et al. ligated the femoral artery distally to the origin of the deep branch [21], which leads to increase of blood flow and shear stress in the collaterals where remodeling occurs. The deep branch of the femoral artery gives rise to collaterals in the adductor muscles, and after ligation of femoral artery distally from it, remodeling will take place and collaterals will develop, as is the case in neovascularization in human PAD. In some studies, the electrocoagulation level is more proximal in the femoral artery. The most important consideration for the site of ligation is that collaterals need to form from proximal side branches of the femoral artery; thus, the ideal site of ligation should be distal of side branches of the artery.

Furthermore, ligation of the femoral artery also induces ischemia and triggers angiogenesis in the distal part of the limb, in the calf muscles, especially in the gastrocnemicus muscle.

2.3.2. Single Electrocoagulation of Iliac Artery

For the exposure of the iliac artery, two approaches are used; Westvik et al. performed a midline incision in the abdomen exposing the common iliac artery and vein and then ligated both, proximally from the origin of the internal iliac artery [26]. Hellingman et al. used the approach of making an incision in the inguinal region and retroperitoneally moving the peritoneum proximally with a cotton swab. Thereafter, the artery is prepared from the vein and the common iliac artery is electrocoagulated proximally from the origin of the internal iliac artery [10,18,27]. In this method arteriogenesis in the upper thigh muscles in all the three collateral compartments can be evaluated. Also, angiogenesis in the distal calf muscle can be evaluated. The recovery of blood perfusion in C57Bl6 mice analyzed by Laser Doppler Perfusion Imaging (LDPI) was complete in 7–14 days. This was the same as the blood reperfusion period in single electrocoagulation of the femoral artery [10].

2.3.3. Double Electrocoagulation of Both Femoral Artery and Iliac Artery

An incision in the inguinal region is made, and through the retroperitoneal approach, the peritoneum is moved proximally with a cotton swab. In this model, both the common iliac artery and femoral artery were electrocoagulated. The common iliac artery is ligated proximally of the internal iliac artery and the femoral artery is electro-coagulated proximal to the superficial epigastric artery [10]. Alternatively, a double electrocoagulation may be performed in the femoral artery, one just distally to the origin of the deep branch and the second one just above the bifurcation of the saphenous and popliteal artery. These double occlusion models are suitable for assessing both arteriogenesis and angiogenesis. The double electrocoagulation leads to severe ischemia and prolonged time course of blood flow recovery in C57Bl6 mice up to 21 days for reaching the plateau in flow recovery. This makes the method suitable for studying new therapeutic approaches, as it offers, due to a higher degree of tissue damage as well as ischemia, a therapeutic window in which improvements can be evaluated.

2.3.4. Total Excision of the Femoral Artery

Total excision of the femoral artery was the first described method by Couffinhal, Isner and colleagues [19]. An incision is made in the skin overlying the middle portion of the hind limb. The common femoral artery is exposed and dissected from the vein and nerve in the distal direction. All side branches of the artery were dissected free and coagulated. The distal ligation level was at the popliteal artery level, just distal from the bifurcation of the saphenous artery and the popliteal artery. After cutting the artery between the two ligatures proximal and distal, the whole artery was removed from the surrounding tissue. The advantage of this method is that a severe ischemia is induced in the calf muscle, and angiogenesis can be assessed. The disadvantage is that the collateral artery formation is impeded due to the disturbance of the pre-existing arterial bed and connections. Therefore, this method is not suitable for assessing arteriogenesis, but is very adequate for assessing angiogenesis in ischemic distal tissue.

2.3.5. Ameroid Constrictors

One of the shortcomings of all the aforementioned models is the fact that all are for acute induction of ischemia in the hind limb, whereas PAD patients mostly suffer from a gradual occlusion of the blood vessels in the legs. Yang et al. and Padgett et al. used ameroid constrictors to induce hind limb ischemia [6,28]. Ameroid constrictors are devices that occlude the artery over 1–3 days through gradually absorption of moisture from the surrounding tissues. By using this method, the blood flow fell to its lowest in 3 days instead of directly after surgery in the traditional hind limb ischemia model. The aim of this method was to develop a more subacute ischemia instead of an acute one. However, Yang et al. showed that this method leads to different responses in the thigh than the traditional ligation model. In the thigh, where the remodeling of collaterals occurs, was a lack of upregulation of shear stress responsive genes and inflammatory genes, which are essential for the process of arteriogenesis, despite the formation of collaterals. There are also technical challenges, namely that commercially-available ameroid constrictors are variable in depth and shape. Furthermore, the severity of the induced ischemia is influenced by the vessel size which depends on age, and age differences of only a few weeks can lead to vessel size differences.

This model has potential. However, for studying the effects of flow recovery, it is hampered by the fact that gradual occlusion leads to a gradual induction of collateral formation to compensate for the occlusions. Consequently, distal ischemia, and thus angiogenesis, is hardly observed. Although this model has to potential to better mimic the situation in patients with chronic ischemia, more research is needed to optimize the method.

3. Analysis of Blood Flow Perfusion and Neovascularization/End-Points

Different approaches are used to visualize the blood flow recovery and evaluate the arteriogenic effects and the angiogenic effects.

3.1. Laser Doppler Perfusion Imaging

The essential readout of the model is the time course and extent of the blood flow recovery in the ischemic limb. The blood reperfusion in the ischemic limb and control limb is mainly analyzed by Laser Doppler Perfusion Imaging (LDPI). LDPI is based on the principle whereby the Doppler effect caused by the interaction between the laser light and red blood cells is depicted on a color scale. The blood perfusion values are measured per pixel and the region of interest can be indicated on the images by manually drawing these regions of interest. The mean of perfusion in this region is calculated. The ratio of blood flow in the ischemic to the control limb is the general method to express the blood flow reperfusion.

Laser Doppler Perfusion Imaging is a non-invasive method and is reproducible and repeatable under the same experimental conditions at different time points. The perfusion signal is influenced by various experimental conditions including the presence of hair, the type of anesthesia that mice are subjected to and body temperature [23]; it is also associated with movement. Therefore, standardization of the analysis conditions including the environmental temperature is essential. Keeping the animals at physiological temperatures ~37 °C during the Laser Doppler measurements is strongly recommended using e.g., a body temperature control pad or a 37 °C double glass water bowl.

For measuring the recovery of the blood flow, different regions of interest can be used. These regions vary from whole limb with or without the inguinal region, or the footpad. A critical point in whole limb analysis is that increased angiogenesis due to wound healing at the site of the incision should be taken into account. The footpad is the most reliable region, since it is hairless, and shaving is not required. Shaving can irritate the skin, and therefore, influences the flow signal. The hair absorbs laser light and prevents it from interacting with red blood cells. Other methods for removing the hair such as the use of hair removal creams can be considered, but usually require that the mouse be under anesthesia for a longer period, and can irritate the skin too.

The LPDI analysis is generally performed at predetermined time points; before the surgery, directly after the surgery, after 3 and 7 days, and thereafter weekly over a period of 2 or 4 weeks.

3.2. Immunohistochemical Analysis

Next to evaluating the blood flow restoration, usually a histological analysis is performed to study arteriogenic and angiogenic responses in the tissue. Immunohistochemical analysis can be used to detect neovessels, as well as inflammatory cells that infiltrate the tissue. In addition, histological analysis can also be used for analysis of skeletal muscle remodeling, damage, and necrosis.

Arteriogenesis is studied in the proximal part of the limb, in the adductor muscle group. The collateral formation is determined by immunohistochemical staining using antibodies against alpha-Smooth Muscle Actin (a-SMA) to demonstrate the arterial nature of the newly formed vessels in the adductor muscle [7].

For assessing angiogenic capillary density in the distal part of the limb, the ischemic calf muscle, is most commonly used. The angiogenic capillaries are detected by using immunohistochemical techniques to identify endothelial cells (e.g., CD31 or von Willebrand factor) [29,30].

3.3. Other Methods for Assessment of Collateral Formation and Limb Perfusion

For assessments of vascular remodeling, both the evaluation of the anatomic dimensions and the functionality of the newly formed vessels are of interest. Methods for evaluations will be discussed in the following section and are summarized in Table 2.

Table 2. Methods of assessment of collateral formation and limb perfusion.

Techniques	Results Obtained	Advantages	Disadvantages
Micro-CT	- Anatomical visualization of vasculature circulation - Extent of vasculature formation	- Non-invasive - Reproducible - Repeatable - 3D reconstruction	- Challenging to discriminate arteries from veins - Ionizing radiation
Ex vivo Micro-CT of polymer casted vasculature	- Extent of vasculature formation - Quantification of changes in the microvasculature	- Only arteries - 3D reconstruction	- Invasive - Repeated measurement not possible
X-ray microangiography	- Gross anatomical view of the circulation	- Overview of the vascular anatomy	- Invasive - Technically challenging - Only 2D projection images
Post-mortem X-ray microangiography	- Gross anatomical view of the circulation	- Overview of the vascular anatomy	- Repeated measurement not possible
MRA	- Detecting arterial blood flow - Determine collateral formation - Follow collateral arterial formation	- Repeated measurements possible - 3D reconstructions	- Invasive (vascular access for injecting contrast) - Long scan times
MRI TOF	- Visualizing flow within vessels - Quantitative evaluation of arterial blood flow - Determine collateral formation	- Non-invasive - Repeated measurements possible - 3D reconstructions	- Long scan times
SPECT	-Analyzing perfusion recovery	-Non-invasive -Accurate	-Special facility is needed

The traditionally-used X-ray microangiography after administration of an iodinated contrast agent can provide a gross anatomical view of the circulation visualizing the vessels in the range of 25 to 50 μm in diameter. This method is invasive and provides only 2-D projection images. Furthermore, the need for anesthesia and vascular access makes this technique technically challenging.

A different method is to inject the aorta with polyacrylamide-bismuth contrast inducing vasodilation followed by post-mortem angiographic images to study the collateral vessel growth [31]. Although technically less demanding, the obvious disadvantage of this method is that it is acquired post-mortem, and therefore, repeated measurements are not possible.

For the anatomical visualization of the arterial circulation, high-resolution micro-computed tomography (Micro-CT) is the best method, which is reproducible, and the 2D images can be reconstructed as 3D images [32]. Also, for the quantification of the extent of arteriogenesis, micro-CT can be used by analyzing the obtained images for the number, volume and length of the newly-formed collateral arteries [33]. Using Micro-CT in combination with the administration of intra-arterial contrast medium makes it possible to visualize vessels of 8 μm in diameter [34]. The challenge of this technique is discriminating arteries from veins after administration of the contrast agent. Also, underfilling the arteries with the contrast agent, or conversely, overfilling leading to extravasation of the contrast agent, are possible problems impairing comparisons between different measurements.

Another method is casting the vasculature with a silicone radiopaque casting agent (Microfill) and post-mortem imaging using Micro-CT to quantify changes in the microvasculature [35].

For the functional assessment of blood flow recovery and tissue perfusion, magnetic resonance imaging (MRI) is a promising technique to detect arterial blood flow and to follow the collateral arterial formation after occlusion of the femoral artery in the hind limb ischemia model. There are two MR imaging techniques, namely contrast-enhanced MRA with a gadolinium-based contrast agent and the time-of-flight (TOF) sequence technique. TOF is an MRI technique to visualize flow within vessels, and is based on flow-related increase of spins entering into a single image slice; as a result of being unsaturated, these spins of the blood give more signal than the stationary spins of the surrounding tissue [36,37]. Wagner et al. showed that the use of MRI angiograms is an effective technique for determining the collateral formation, and whether the collateral arteries in the quadriceps muscles are better developed than those in the adductor muscle group [38]. In another study, Wagner et al.

showed that TOF MRI imaging without using a contrast agent is effective in mice, and can be used for quantitative evaluations of arterial blood flow. The advantage of this method is that it does not require a contrast agent, and therefore, no vascular access for injection of contrast is needed; furthermore, repetitive analyses on one animal is feasible, without considering the residue of the used contrast agent [37]. Using a non-invasive MRI technique to follow the development of collateral arteries is a promising technique, now even more so as the images can be combined using a reconstruction technique of maximum intensity projection (MIP) to acquire a 3D image of the vessels, similarly to conventional angiography.

Hendrikx et al. showed that single photon emission computed tomography (SPECT) perfusion imaging using radioisotope-based tracers can be used to analyze perfusion recovery and muscular damage in the mouse hind limb model [39]. This nuclear perfusion imaging and myocyte damage imaging are non-invasive and have high resolution. The results of the study demonstrated that LDPI analysis underestimates the revascularization processes in the hind limb ischemia model. When interpreting the results of LDPI, researchers should take into account that the main blood flow recovery occurs in the first 7 days. The disadvantage of this method is that it needs special facilities to work with the radioisotope-based tracers.

Microsphere injection and contrast enhanced ultrasounds are two further techniques currently in early experimental phases of research.

3.4. Methods to Further Differentiate the Results of HLI and Neovascularisation

3.4.1. Matrigel Plug Assay

Studies using the mouse hind limb ischemia model are often directed at the discovery of factors that improve or impair blood flow recovery. As mentioned, the blood flow recovery is dependent on the processes of arteriogenesis, angiogenesis, or both. A method to further differentiate whether the blood recovery is due arteriogenesis or angiogenesis is performing an in vivo Matrigel plug assay.

The in vivo Matrigel plug assay is an assay solely intended to assess angiogenesis; it is performed by injecting Matrigel into the subcutaneous space on the dorsal side of the mice on both the left and right flank [7]. Post-implantation, after 7 to 14 days, the mice are sacrificed and the Matrigel plugs are excised and processed for immunohistological analysis. Paraffin sections could be stained with a general staining such as Hematoxylin, Eosin or Hematoxylin, Phloxine and Saffron, and anti-CD31. The CD31 staining affirms the endothelial nature of the infiltrating capillary structures. The extent of the angiogenesis is determined by assessing the vascular ingrowth in the Matrigel plug. The vascular ingrowth is scored by measuring the depth of ingrowth and the length of the capillary structures, and provides information on the angiogenic potential of the condition or compound being studied.

3.4.2. Pre-existing Collateral Density

The dominant mechanism responsible for the restoration of the blood flow after arterial occlusion is the remodeling of the pre-existing collateral arterioles into mature functioning collateral arteries.

There are pre-existing interarterial collateral connections in the peripheral circulation. The amount of these pre-existing arterioles varies between different strains, and different factors can influence the pre-existing vascular bed. Pre-existing collateral density can be determined in pial circulation of the pia mater [40]. The pre-existing collateral density in the cerebral pial circulation gives an indication of collateral density in skeletal muscle [8].

To determine the pial circulation in mice, after anesthesia, the thoracic aorta is cannulated retrograde, and the circulation is maximally dilated by infusion of sodium-nitroprusside and papaverine in PBS at approximately 100 mmHg prior to vascular casting. After craniotomy, Microfil is infused under a stereomicroscope. The dorsal cerebral circulation is then fixed by the topical application of 4% paraformaldehyde (PFA) to prevent any degradation in vessel dimensions after Microfil injection. The brains are fixed overnight in 4% PFA, and subsequently incubated for several days to improve the contrast of the visualization of the vasculature. The number of pre-existing collaterals in the semi-hemispheres of the pia mater is subsequently quantified, and can be used as a general degree for pre-existing arterioles in the particular strain of mice [14,41].

4. Discussion

The mouse hind limb ischemia model is the most used model for basic research and for pre-clinical studies investigating therapeutic neovascularization. It is considered a proper model, as it is reproducible, and strongly mimics the specific features of human peripheral arterial disease.

To perform this model, occlusions at different anatomical levels of the iliac and femoral artery are used, as well as different technical approaches. Based on the knowledge that arteriogenesis can only occur after increasing shear stress in the pre-existing arterioles proximal to the occlusion, the correct level of ligation of the femoral artery is distal to the origin of the collateral branches. However, in methods in which the femoral artery is ligated proximal to the origin of the collateral branches, arteriogenesis is also observed. Kochi et al. demonstrated that the number of collaterals is higher than previously thought. This may explain the unexpected arteriogenesis after ligation of the femoral artery at the proximal end. Kochi et al. also demonstrated the presence of collateral arteries in other muscle groups in the upper thigh besides the adductor muscle group. Furthermore, recent MRI research demonstrated that the collateral arteries in the quadriceps muscles are better developed than those in the adductor muscle group. This suggests that the analysis of the other muscle groups may yield valuable information on arteriogenesis, and should be included in experimental studies.

The hind limb ischemia mouse model has limitations. One of the major limitations is the acute nature of the ischemia induced in this model, while the PAD in patients is a chronic process, and critical limb ischemia arises slowly as a result of a gradual build-up of atherosclerosis. Yang et al. [28] and Padgett et al. [6] used ameroid constrictors to progressively induce hind limb ischemia and mimic the gradual occlusion that occurs in patients. However, this method is not yet representative of the cellular response in the thigh after occlusion in PAD patients; therefore, further optimization of the method is needed.

Another limitation related to the hind limb ischemia model is that the procedure is predominately performed in young and healthy mice, which do not reflect patients with PAD. PAD patients are old and have co-morbidities like diabetes mellitus, hypercholesterolaemia, and hypertension. Westvik et al. showed that old mice show a slower perfusion recovery after inducing hind limb ischemia compared to young mice [26]. Young wild-type mice do not show the comorbidities of PAD patients. It is well known that these comorbidities accelerate the development of atherosclerosis and affect vascular remodeling [12]. The extent to which these comorbidities affect vascular remodeling varies. Van Weel et al. investigated arteriogenesis using a hind limb ischemia model in different mouse types and showed that hypercholesterolaemia is more than hyperglycemia or hyperinsulinemia associated with impaired arteriogenesis [12]. Hypercholesterolaemia leads to impaired arteriogenesis due elevated blood cholesterol levels which affect monocyte chemotaxis, whereby monocyte influx is reduced [42]. These data suggest that the changed lipid metabolism in diabetes patients may affect the arteriogenesis more than a disturbed glucose metabolism. Moreover, diabetes mellitus causes endothelial dysfunction which is multifactorial and results in reduced angiogenesis [43].

Hypertension activates angiotensin, which is associated with endothelial dysfunction due increased oxidative stress. However, Angiotensin activation can initiate and stimulate arteriogenesis due to inflammation regulation. Hypertension can also stimulate arteriogenesis through the increase of shear stress and activation of the renin-angiotensin system [42].

The mouse hind limb ischemia model and PAD patients frequently show similar neovascularization patterns with arteriogenic responses that are close to the occlusions to form collaterals arteries and an angiogenic response in the distal ischemic tissue, as was illustrated by comparing the angiogenic response and VEGF expression in the muscle biopsies of CLI patients and mice after induction of HLI [31,44,45]. However, there may also be differences in neovascularization patterns observed. In the mouse HLI model, neovascularization occurs in a standard, homogenous fashion, due to the fairly standard way of blocking the blood flow, i.e., by occluding the major arteries in the upper limb in an acute way. This may be a crucial difference with the situation in PAD patients, where occlusion usually occurs gradually, but most importantly, it may occur at various locations in the vascular tree. It is obvious that an occlusion of one of the major arteries above the knee may have different consequences on endogenous collateral formation and neovascularization than an occlusion below the knee. Therefore, the neovascularization required to restore the blood flow in PAD patients with critical limb ischemia will be quite heterogeneous in nature, whereas the mouse models usually focus on a more standardized neovascularization induction. Unfortunately, mimicking the human situation is still complex, and really predictive (larger) animal models are not available yet, making the mouse model the most used model at present.

Furthermore, to choose an appropriate model, it is essential to consider which mouse strain to use, because the genetic background influences the outcomes. Several studies have shown high variability between mouse strains in restoring the limb perfusion after the induction of ischemia, and variability in ability of neovascularization [13,14]. Different strains show different blood recovery patterns after surgically-induced hind limb ischemia. Many studies have exhibited fast recovery of limb perfusion in C57BL/6 after inducing hind limb ischemia in comparison to the slow recovery of Balb/C mice. It has been suggested that the difference in vascular remodeling is due to a specific gene locus in chromosome 7 of the mouse [46,47]. Also, a wide variation in the extent of the native pre-existing collaterals is observed in different mouse strains, whereby C57BL/6 and BALB/c demonstrate the largest difference [40]. Due to their slow recovery, Balb/c mice are often used for hind limb ischemia studies, based on the assumption that this slow response better mimics the situation in patients with PAD. Recently Nossent et al. showed that especially in Balb/c mice, a stronger upregulation of pro-angiogenic and pro-arteriogenic genes is observed when compared to C57Bl6 mice, despite the poorer blood perfusion recovery in Balb/c [7]. This suggests Balb/c mice lack a thus far unknown factor that is crucial for vascular remodeling, rather than that this model better mimics the situation in patients with peripheral arterial disease.

Schmidt et al. recently demonstrated more muscle injury within 6 h after inducing ischemia in Balb/c mice compared to C57BL/6 mice [48]. The muscle injury may contribute to the ability of the vascular bed to recover after ischemia, and to regenerate. This suggests that understanding of etiology of the ischemic muscle and its contribution to the restoration of blood flow is needed, and that more research on this topic is required.

The techniques for the assessment of the results of the hind limb ischemia model are diverse. However, LDPI remains the essential readout method because of feasibility and reproducibility. The other techniques can serve as additional techniques since they mostly lack the capability to perform robust and fast analysis of the blood flow in larger series of mice.

5. Conclusions

The mouse hind limb ischemia model is performed in many variants. No single method for inducing hind limb ischemia that is appropriate for all research questions. The researchers should recognize the variants to be able to choose the most suitable model for their experiments, and they should describe the method and the used anatomical landmarks in order to make comparisons possible among studies.

Author Contributions: Z.A., M.R.d.V., and P.Q. all contributed to conceptualizing, writing and editing the manuscript.

Funding: This research forms part of the Project P1.03 PENT of the research program of the Biomedical Materials institute, co-funded by the Dutch Ministry of Economic Affairs, Agriculture and Innovation.

Conflicts of Interest: The authors declare no conflict of interest.

References

1. Norgren, L.; Hiatt, W.R.; Dormandy, J.A.; Nehler, M.R.; Harris, K.A.; Fowkes, F.G. Inter-Society Consensus for the Management of Peripheral Arterial Disease (TASC II). *J. Vasc. Surg.* **2007**, *45*, 5–67. [CrossRef] [PubMed]
2. Van Oostrom, M.C.; van Oostrom, O.; Quax, P.H.; Verhaar, M.C.; Hoefer, I.E. Insights into mechanisms behind arteriogenesis: What does the future hold? *J. Leukoc. Biol.* **2008**, *84*, 1379–1391. [CrossRef] [PubMed]
3. Heil, M.; Eitenmuller, I.; Schmitz-Rixen, T.; Schaper, W. Arteriogenesis versus angiogenesis: Similarities and differences. *J. Cell. Mol. Med.* **2006**, *10*, 45–55. [CrossRef] [PubMed]
4. Annex, B.H. Therapeutic angiogenesis for critical limb ischaemia. *Nat. Rev. Cardiol.* **2013**, *10*, 387–396. [CrossRef]
5. Murohara, T.; Asahara, T.; Silver, M.; Bauters, C.; Masuda, H.; Kalka, C.; Kearney, M.; Chen, D.; Symes, J.F.; Fishman, M.C.; et al. Nitric oxide synthase modulates angiogenesis in response to tissue ischemia. *J. Clin. Investig.* **1998**, *101*, 2567–2578. [CrossRef]
6. Padgett, M.E.; McCord, T.J.; McClung, J.M.; Kontos, C.D. Methods for Acute and Subacute Murine Hindlimb Ischemia. *J. Vis. Exp. JoVE* **2016**. [CrossRef]
7. Nossent, A.Y.; Bastiaansen, A.J.; Peters, E.A.; de Vries, M.R.; Aref, Z.; Welten, S.M.; de Jager, S.C.; van der Pouw Kraan, T.C.; Quax, P.H. CCR7-CCL19/CCL21 Axis is Essential for Effective Arteriogenesis in a Murine Model of Hindlimb Ischemia. *J. Am. Heart Assoc.* **2017**, *6*. [CrossRef]
8. Wang, S.; Zhang, H.; Dai, X.; Sealock, R.; Faber, J.E. Genetic architecture underlying variation in extent and remodeling of the collateral circulation. *Circ. Res.* **2010**, *107*, 558–568. [CrossRef]
9. Bastiaansen, A.J.; Karper, J.C.; Wezel, A.; de Boer, H.C.; Welten, S.M.; de Jong, R.C.; Peters, E.A.; de Vries, M.R.; van Oeveren-Rietdijk, A.M.; van Zonneveld, A.J.; et al. TLR4 accessory molecule RP105 (CD180) regulates monocyte-driven arteriogenesis in a murine hind limb ischemia model. *PLoS ONE* **2014**, *9*, e99882. [CrossRef]
10. Hellingman, A.A.; Bastiaansen, A.J.; de Vries, M.R.; Seghers, L.; Lijkwan, M.A.; Lowik, C.W.; Hamming, J.F.; Quax, P.H. Variations in surgical procedures for hind limb ischaemia mouse models result in differences in collateral formation. *Eur. J. Vasc. Endovasc. Surg* **2010**, *40*, 796–803. [CrossRef]
11. Van Weel, V.; Toes, R.E.; Seghers, L.; Deckers, M.M.; de Vries, M.R.; Eilers, P.H.; Sipkens, J.; Schepers, A.; Eefting, D.; van Hinsbergh, V.W.; et al. Natural killer cells and CD4+ T-cells modulate collateral artery development. *Arterioscler. Thromb. Vasc. Biol.* **2007**, *27*, 2310–2318. [CrossRef]
12. Van Weel, V.; de Vries, M.; Voshol, P.J.; Verloop, R.E.; Eilers, P.H.; van Hinsbergh, V.W.; van Bockel, J.H.; Quax, P.H. Hypercholesterolemia reduces collateral artery growth more dominantly than hyperglycemia or insulin resistance in mice. *Arterioscler. Thromb. Vasc. Biol.* **2006**, *26*, 1383–1390. [CrossRef]
13. Helisch, A.; Wagner, S.; Khan, N.; Drinane, M.; Wolfram, S.; Heil, M.; Ziegelhoeffer, T.; Brandt, U.; Pearlman, J.D.; Swartz, H.M.; et al. Impact of mouse strain differences in innate hindlimb collateral vasculature. *Arterioscler. Thromb. Vasc. Biol.* **2006**, *26*, 520–526. [CrossRef]
14. Chalothorn, D.; Faber, J.E. Strain-dependent variation in collateral circulatory function in mouse hindlimb. *Physiol. Genom.* **2010**, *42*, 469–479. [CrossRef]
15. Bonheur, J.A.; Albadawi, H.; Patton, G.M.; Watkins, M.T. A noninvasive murine model of hind limb ischemia-reperfusion injury. *J. Surg. Res.* **2004**, *116*, 55–63. [CrossRef]
16. Tran, T.P.; Tu, H.; Pipinos, I.I.; Muelleman, R.L.; Albadawi, H.; Li, Y.L. Tourniquet-induced acute ischemia-reperfusion injury in mouse skeletal muscles: Involvement of superoxide. *Eur. J. Pharmacol.* **2011**, *650*, 328–334. [CrossRef]
17. Drysch, M.; Wallner, C.; Schmidt, S.V.; Reinkemeier, F.; Wagner, J.M.; Lehnhardt, M.; Behr, B. An optimized low-pressure tourniquet murine hind limb ischemia reperfusion model: Inducing acute ischemia reperfusion injury in C57BL/6 wild type mice. *PLoS ONE* **2019**, *14*, e0210961. [CrossRef]
18. Hellingman, A.A.; Zwaginga, J.J.; van Beem, R.T.; Hamming, J.F.; Fibbe, W.E.; Quax, P.H.; Geutskens, S.B. T-cell-pre-stimulated monocytes promote neovascularisation in a murine hind limb ischaemia model. *Eur. J. Vasc. Endovasc. Surg* **2011**, *41*, 418–428. [CrossRef]
19. Couffinhal, T.; Silver, M.; Zheng, L.P.; Kearney, M.; Witzenbichler, B.; Isner, J.M. Mouse model of angiogenesis. *Am. J. Pathol.* **1998**, *152*, 1667–1679.
20. Kochi, T.; Imai, Y.; Takeda, A.; Watanabe, Y.; Mori, S.; Tachi, M.; Kodama, T. Characterization of the arterial anatomy of the murine hindlimb: Functional role in the design and understanding of ischemia models. *PLoS ONE* **2013**, *8*, e84047. [CrossRef]

21. Limbourg, A.; Korff, T.; Napp, L.C.; Schaper, W.; Drexler, H.; Limbourg, F.P. Evaluation of postnatal arteriogenesis and angiogenesis in a mouse model of hind-limb ischemia. *Nat. Protoc.* **2009**, *4*, 1737–1746. [CrossRef]
22. Niiyama, H.; Huang, N.F.; Rollins, M.D.; Cooke, J.P. Murine model of hindlimb ischemia. *J. Vis. Exp: JoVE* **2009**. [CrossRef]
23. Greco, A.; Ragucci, M.; Liuzzi, R.; Gargiulo, S.; Gramanzini, M.; Coda, A.R.; Albanese, S.; Mancini, M.; Salvatore, M.; Brunetti, A. Repeatability, reproducibility and standardisation of a laser Doppler imaging technique for the evaluation of normal mouse hindlimb perfusion. *Sensors* **2012**, *13*, 500–515. [CrossRef]
24. Medgett, I.C.; Ruffolo, R.R., Jr. Alpha adrenoceptor-mediated vasoconstriction in rat hindlimb: Innervated alpha-2 adrenoceptors in the saphenous arterial bed. *J. Pharmacol. Exp. Ther.* **1988**, *246*, 249–254.
25. Stabile, E.; Burnett, M.S.; Watkins, C.; Kinnaird, T.; Bachis, A.; la Sala, A.; Miller, J.M.; Shou, M.; Epstein, S.E.; Fuchs, S. Impaired arteriogenic response to acute hindlimb ischemia in CD4-knockout mice. *Circulation* **2003**, *108*, 205–210. [CrossRef]
26. Westvik, T.S.; Fitzgerald, T.N.; Muto, A.; Maloney, S.P.; Pimiento, J.M.; Fancher, T.T.; Magri, D.; Westvik, H.H.; Nishibe, T.; Velazquez, O.C.; et al. Limb ischemia after iliac ligation in aged mice stimulates angiogenesis without arteriogenesis. *J. Vasc. Surg.* **2009**, *49*, 464–473. [CrossRef]
27. Hellingman, A.A.; van der Vlugt, L.E.; Lijkwan, M.A.; Bastiaansen, A.J.; Sparwasser, T.; Smits, H.H.; Hamming, J.F.; Quax, P.H. A limited role for regulatory T cells in post-ischemic neovascularization. *J. Cell Mol. Med.* **2012**, *16*, 328–336. [CrossRef]
28. Yang, Y.; Tang, G.; Yan, J.; Park, B.; Hoffman, A.; Tie, G.; Wang, R.; Messina, L.M. Cellular and molecular mechanism regulating blood flow recovery in acute versus gradual femoral artery occlusion are distinct in the mouse. *J. Vasc. Surg.* **2008**, *48*, 1546–1558. [CrossRef]
29. Simons, K.H.; Aref, Z.; Peters, H.A.B.; Welten, S.P.; Nossent, A.Y.; Jukema, J.W.; Hamming, J.F.; Arens, R.; de Vries, M.R.; Quax, P.H.A. The role of CD27-CD70-mediated T cell co-stimulation in vasculogenesis, arteriogenesis and angiogenesis. *Int. J. Cardiol.* **2018**, *260*, 184–190. [CrossRef]
30. Pusztaszeri, M.P.; Seelentag, W.; Bosman, F.T. Immunohistochemical expression of endothelial markers CD31, CD34, von Willebrand factor, and Fli-1 in normal human tissues. *J. Histochem. Cytochem. J. Histochem. Soc.* **2006**, *54*, 385–395. [CrossRef]
31. Van Weel, V.; Deckers, M.M.; Grimbergen, J.M.; van Leuven, K.J.; Lardenoye, J.H.; Schlingemann, R.O.; van Nieuw Amerongen, G.P.; van Bockel, J.H.; van Hinsbergh, V.W.; Quax, P.H. Vascular endothelial growth factor overexpression in ischemic skeletal muscle enhances myoglobin expression in vivo. *Circ. Res.* **2004**, *95*, 58–66. [CrossRef]
32. Nebuloni, L.; Kuhn, G.A.; Vogel, J.; Muller, R. A novel in vivo vascular imaging approach for hierarchical quantification of vasculature using contrast enhanced micro-computed tomography. *PLoS ONE* **2014**, *9*, e86562. [CrossRef]
33. Simons, M. Chapter 14. Assessment of arteriogenesis. *Methods Enzymol.* **2008**, *445*, 331–342. [CrossRef]
34. Simons, M.; Alitalo, K.; Annex, B.H.; Augustin, H.G.; Beam, C.; Berk, B.C.; Byzova, T.; Carmeliet, P.; Chilian, W.; Cooke, J.P.; et al. State-of-the-Art Methods for Evaluation of Angiogenesis and Tissue Vascularization: A Scientific Statement from the American Heart Association. *Circ. Res.* **2015**, *116*, e99–e132. [CrossRef]
35. Liu, X.; Terry, T.; Pan, S.; Yang, Z.; Willerson, J.T.; Dixon, R.A.; Liu, Q. Osmotic drug delivery to ischemic hindlimbs and perfusion of vasculature with microfil for micro-computed tomography imaging. *J. Vis. Exp. JoVE* **2013**. [CrossRef]
36. Wehrli, F.W.; Shimakawa, A.; Gullberg, G.T.; MacFall, J.R. Time-of-flight MR flow imaging: selective saturation recovery with gradient refocusing. *Radiology* **1986**, *160*, 781–785. [CrossRef]
37. Wagner, S.; Helisch, A.; Bachmann, G.; Schaper, W. Time-of-flight quantitative measurements of blood flow in mouse hindlimbs. *J. Magn. Reson. Imaging JMRI* **2004**, *19*, 468–474. [CrossRef]
38. Wagner, S.; Helisch, A.; Ziegelhoeffer, T.; Bachmann, G.; Schaper, W. Magnetic resonance angiography of collateral vessels in a murine femoral artery ligation model. *NMR Biomed.* **2004**, *17*, 21–27. [CrossRef]
39. Hendrikx, G.; Vries, M.H.; Bauwens, M.; De Saint-Hubert, M.; Wagenaar, A.; Guillaume, J.; Boonen, L.; Post, M.J.; Mottaghy, F.M. Comparison of LDPI to SPECT perfusion imaging using (99m)Tc-sestamibi and (99m)Tc-pyrophosphate in a murine ischemic hind limb model of neovascularization. *EJNMMI Res.* **2016**, *6*, 44. [CrossRef]

40. Zhang, H.; Prabhakar, P.; Sealock, R.; Faber, J.E. Wide genetic variation in the native pial collateral circulation is a major determinant of variation in severity of stroke. *J. Cereb. Blood Flow Metab. J. Int. Soc. Cereb. Blood Flow Metab.* **2010**, *30*, 923–934. [CrossRef]
41. Bastiaansen, A.J.; Ewing, M.M.; de Boer, H.C.; Tineke, C.P.K.; de Vries, M.R.; Peters, E.A.; Welten, S.M.; Arens, R.; Moore, S.M.; Faber, J.E.; et al. Lysine acetyltransferase PCAF is a key regulator of arteriogenesis. *Arterioscler. Thromb. Vasc. Biol/* **2013**, *33*, 1902–1910. [CrossRef]
42. De Groot, D.; Pasterkamp, G.; Hoefer, I.E. Cardiovascular risk factors and collateral artery formation. *Eur. J. Clin. Investig.* **2009**, *39*, 1036–1047. [CrossRef]
43. Kolluru, G.K.; Bir, S.C.; Kevil, C.G. Endothelial dysfunction and diabetes: effects on angiogenesis, vascular remodeling, and wound healing. *Int. J. Vasc. Med.* **2012**, *2012*, 918267. [CrossRef]
44. Van Weel, V.; Seghers, L.; de Vries, M.R.; Kuiper, E.J.; Schlingemann, R.O.; Bajema, I.M.; Lindeman, J.H.; Delis-van Diemen, P.M.; van Hinsbergh, V.W.; van Bockel, J.H.; et al. Expression of vascular endothelial growth factor, stromal cell-derived factor-1, and CXCR4 in human limb muscle with acute and chronic ischemia. *Arterioscler. Thromb. Vasc. Biol.* **2007**, *27*, 1426–1432. [CrossRef]
45. Van Weel, V.; van Tongeren, R.B.; van Hinsbergh, V.W.; van Bockel, J.H.; Quax, P.H. Vascular growth in ischemic limbs: a review of mechanisms and possible therapeutic stimulation. *Ann. Vasc. Surg.* **2008**, *22*, 582–597. [CrossRef]
46. Sealock, R.; Zhang, H.; Lucitti, J.L.; Moore, S.M.; Faber, J.E. Congenic fine-mapping identifies a major causal locus for variation in the native collateral circulation and ischemic injury in brain and lower extremity. *Circ. Res.* **2014**, *114*, 660–671. [CrossRef]
47. Dokun, A.O.; Keum, S.; Hazarika, S.; Li, Y.; Lamonte, G.M.; Wheeler, F.; Marchuk, D.A.; Annex, B.H. A quantitative trait locus (LSq-1) on mouse chromosome 7 is linked to the absence of tissue loss after surgical hindlimb ischemia. *Circulation* **2008**, *117*, 1207–1215. [CrossRef]
48. Schmidt, C.A.; Amorese, A.J.; Ryan, T.E.; Goldberg, E.J.; Tarpey, M.D.; Green, T.D.; Karnekar, R.R.; Yamaguchi, D.J.; Spangenburg, E.E.; McClung, J.M. Strain-Dependent Variation in Acute Ischemic Muscle Injury. *Am. J. Pathol.* **2018**, *188*, 1246–1262. [CrossRef]

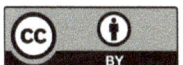

© 2019 by the authors. Licensee MDPI, Basel, Switzerland. This article is an open access article distributed under the terms and conditions of the Creative Commons Attribution (CC BY) license (http://creativecommons.org/licenses/by/4.0/).

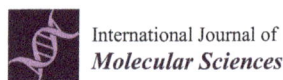

Article

Collateral Vessels Have Unique Endothelial and Smooth Muscle Cell Phenotypes

Hua Zhang, Dan Chalothorn and James E Faber *

Department of Cell Biology and Physiology, Curriculum in Neuroscience, McAllister Heart Institute, University of North Carolina, Chapel Hill, NC 27599-7545, USA
* Correspondence: jefaber@med.unc.edu; Tel.: +919-966-0327; Fax: +919-966-6927

Received: 29 May 2019; Accepted: 19 July 2019; Published: 24 July 2019

Abstract: Collaterals are unique blood vessels present in the microcirculation of most tissues that, by cross-connecting a small fraction of the outer branches of adjacent arterial trees, provide alternate routes of perfusion. However, collaterals are especially susceptible to rarefaction caused by aging, other vascular risk factors, and mouse models of Alzheimer's disease—a vulnerability attributed to the disturbed hemodynamic environment in the watershed regions where they reside. We examined the hypothesis that endothelial and smooth muscle cells (ECs and SMCs, respectively) of collaterals have specializations, distinct from those of similarly-sized nearby distal-most arterioles (DMAs) that maintain collateral integrity despite their continuous exposure to low and oscillatory/disturbed shear stress, high wall stress, and low blood oxygen. Examination of mouse brain revealed the following: Unlike the pro-inflammatory cobble-stoned morphology of ECs exposed to low/oscillatory shear stress elsewhere in the vasculature, collateral ECs are aligned with the vessel axis. Primary cilia, which sense shear stress, are present, unexpectedly, on ECs of collaterals and DMAs but are less abundant on collaterals. Unlike DMAs, collaterals are continuously invested with SMCs, have increased expression of *Pycard*, *Ki67*, *Pdgfb*, *Angpt2*, *Dll4*, *Ephrinb2*, and eNOS, and maintain expression of *Klf2/4*. Collaterals lack tortuosity when first formed during development, but tortuosity becomes evident within days after birth, progresses through middle age, and then declines—results consistent with the concept that collateral wall cells have a higher turnover rate than DMAs that favors proliferative senescence and collateral rarefaction. In conclusion, endothelial and SMCs of collaterals have morphologic and functional differences from those of nearby similarly sized arterioles. Future studies are required to determine if they represent specializations that counterbalance the disturbed hemodynamic, pro-inflammatory, and pro-proliferative environment in which collaterals reside and thus mitigate their risk factor-induced rarefaction.

Keywords: collateral circulation; cerebral collaterals; endothelial cells; ischemic stroke; primary cilia

1. Introduction

Obstructive disease, i.e., stroke and atherosclerosis of the coronary and peripheral arteries, is the leading cause of morbidity and mortality. Collateral circulation, which is composed of anastomotic vessels called collaterals, is the most important system capable of mitigating the effects of obstructive disease [1–5]. However, the number and diameter of collaterals in tissues vary greatly among individuals for reasons that are only beginning to be understood [1]. Moreover, little is known about the basic biology of collaterals, in part because of their small diameter and low density in tissues, difficulty in distinguishing them from other vessels, and lack of methodologies allowing study of their endothelial cells (ECs) and smooth muscle cells (SMCs) in cell culture. It is known, however, that collaterals are unique with regard to their: mechanism of formation during development (collaterogenesis) and its high sensitivity to genetic background-dependent variation, anatomic location in the circulation, hemodynamic forces acting on their ECs and SMCs, hallmark tortuosity, high susceptibility to risk factor-induced rarefaction, robust shear stress-dependent outward remodeling, and protective function in ischemic disease [1–5].

In mice, collaterals form late during gestation by the sprouting of ephrin-B2$^+$ ECs off of a small number of distal arterioles that subsequently undergo a tip cell-led proliferation, migration, and lumenization process to establish anastomoses between adjacent arterial trees [6–8]. This process varies greatly due to naturally-occurring polymorphisms in certain genes in the collaterogenesis pathway, resulting in wide differences in collateral extent and thus collateral-dependent blood flow and tissue injury in experimental models of occlusive arterial disease [9–11]. Collateral blood flow also varies widely in humans suffering stroke [3,4], coronary, and peripheral artery diseases [12,13], with recent evidence supporting involvement of the same key variant gene identified in the mouse [14]. Since collaterals interconnect adjacent arterial trees, there is little or no pressure drop across them in the absence of obstructive disease. Thus, blood flow within collaterals is near zero, oscillating slowly toward one or the other tree that they anastomose [6,15]. Endothelial cells and SMCs that compose the collateral wall are therefore continuously exposed to low and disturbed shear stress, high circumferential wall stress, and low blood oxygen content. Accompanying this adverse hemodynamic environment, which favors vascular inflammation and endothelial dysfunction elsewhere in the circulation, collaterals in mice undergo a progressive decline in number and a loss of diameter with aging, presence of vascular risk factors, and in models of Alzheimer's disease [16–21]. Supportive evidence, based on measurement of collateral-dependent flow induced by acute ischemic stroke, has been reported in humans with aging and presence of vascular risk factors [22–24]. This so call "collateral rarefaction" has been linked in mice to chronic low-level inflammation, endothelial dysfunction, and increased proliferation of collateral ECs and SMCs [16–20,25]. Collaterals are also capable of undergoing robust anatomic outward remodeling in steno-occlusive disease, compared to similarly sized arterioles [2,5,9,10]. Additionally, different from arterioles in the trees that they interconnect, collaterals lack myogenic responsiveness and have less SMC tone at baseline [26,27].

Despite these important unique features of collaterals, no studies have examined cellular and molecular aspects of their endothelial and smooth muscle cells to determine whether they differ from those of similarly sized arterioles. For example, blood flow in arteries and arterioles of healthy tissues, and thus fluid shear stress experienced by their ECs, is laminar, orthograde, and high velocity, with the exception of the inner curvature of the aortic arch and sites immediately downstream of arterial bifurcations where flow varies from high-velocity and orthograde to low-velocity with transient flow reversals in a fraction of the fluid laminae during each cardiac cycle (i.e., "disturbed" flow) [28–31]. Endothelial cells at these sites of disturbed shear stress are cobblestone in shape, as opposed to elsewhere where they are elongated and aligned with the vessel axis. They also evidence higher levels of proliferation, apoptosis, permeability, lipid uptake, oxidative stress, and markers of inflammation and aging, i.e., displaying the well-known pro-atherogenic EC phenotype specific to these sites. Flow and shear stress in collaterals in the absence of obstruction share similarly disturbed conditions [6,15]. Yet this is the normal environment in which collateral ECs and SMCs reside.

The purpose of this study was to examine the hypothesis that collateral ECs and SMCs express unique morphological and functional phenotypes that serve as adaptations or specializations to maintain the integrity of the collateral wall and balance against collateral rarefaction favored by the low and disturbed shear stress, high wall stress, and low blood oxygen levels—the latter caused by low flow-induced hemoglobin unloading to tissue. Such differences, if present, could offer insights into how collaterals are able to persist in healthy individuals but also why they are so susceptible to rarefaction with aging and other vascular risk factors. In addition, knowledge concerning the molecular features of collateral wall cells is fundamental to better understand how collaterals form during development, remodel in obstructive disease, and undergo risk factor-induced rarefaction, and to investigate possible treatments to augment or intervene with these processes.

2. Results

2.1. Collateral Endothelial Cells Are Aligned with the Vessel Axis Despite their Chronic Exposure to Low and Oscillatory Shear Stress

As a first-test of the hypothesis that collateral wall cells have unique phenotypes, we assessed the orientation of collateral ECs using scanning electron microscopy (SEM) and staining of the junctional protein zona occludens-1 (ZO-1). Despite the unique low and disturbed shear stress present in collaterals, ECs of collaterals were aligned with the vessel axis to the same extent, i.e., ~4 degrees off the longitudinal axis, which was present in nearby distal-most arterioles (DMAs) and in the descending thoracic aorta where blood flow is high-velocity and laminar (Figures 1 and 2). The area, perimeter, length, and width of collateral ECs were also comparable to ECs lining DMAs (Figure S1).

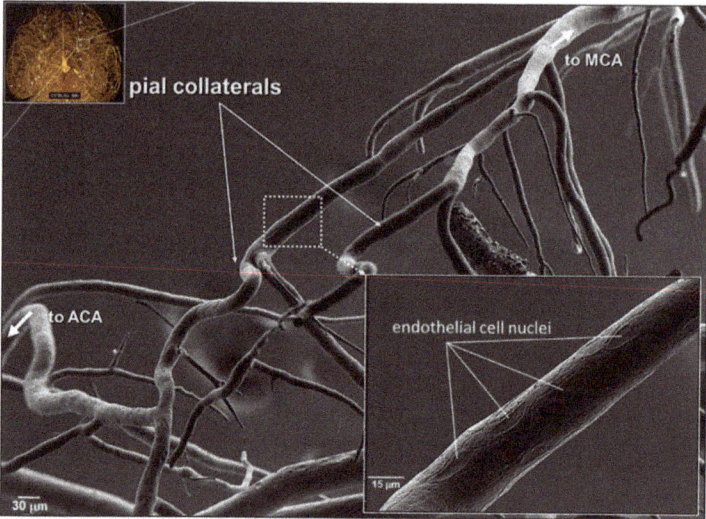

Figure 1. Pial collateral endothelial cells are aligned with the vessel axis. Scanning electron micrograph (SEM) of a corrosion cast of Batson's #17-filled cerebral pial arterial vessels and 2 collaterals, fixed after maximal dilation, which overlie the watershed zone between the anterior (ACA) and middle (MCA) cerebral artery trees. Upper inset, Microfil® cast of arterial vessels and collaterals (stars) in optically cleared brain. SEMs were obtained from six mice (see also Figure S1). Penetrating arterioles are evident branching from collaterals and pial arterioles.

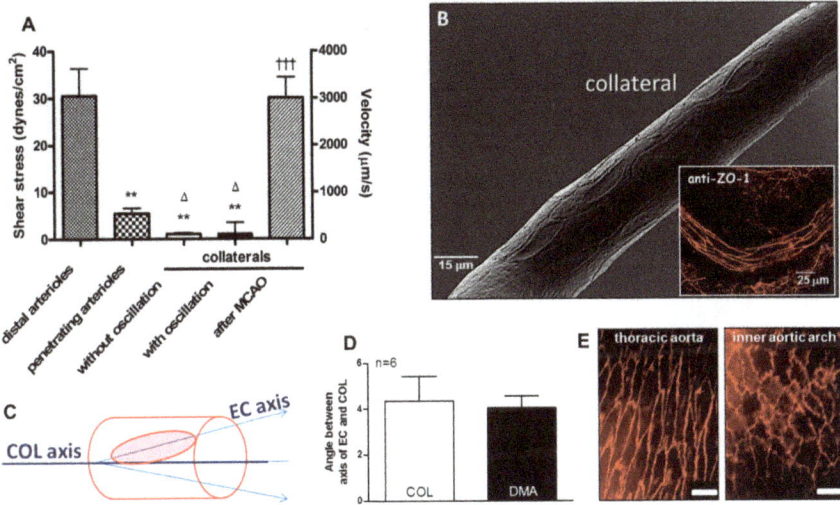

Figure 2. Collateral endothelial cells are aligned with the vessel axis despite having low and oscillatory flow/shear stress in the absence of arterial obstruction. (**A**) Data were obtained in anesthetized mice via cranial window and previously published in reference [6]; unlike distal-most arterioles (DMAs) with diameters comparable to collaterals (COLs) and penetrating arterioles, COLs examined over 30 s intervals have either no flow or slowly oscillating, low velocity, to-and-fro flow with ~zero net-direction. After ligation of the MCA trunk (MCAO), flow to its territory reaches that evident in DMAs within 10–30 s. (**B–E**) Collateral endothelial cells (ECs) have the same "anti-inflammatory" alignment (~4 degrees from horizontal) as ECs of DMAs and the descending thoracic aorta, despite having low/disturbed shear stress at baseline. This is in contrast to the "pro-inflammatory" non-alignment present in the inner curvature of the aortic arch. In this and subsequent figures, data are means ± SE for "n" number of mice. Data in D determined from SEM images, $n = 6$ mice. Panel E magnification bar is 25 µm. Panel A 2-sided t-tests for shear stress followed by Bonferroni correction for ** $p < 0.01$ vs distal arterioles; Δ $p < 0.05$ vs penetrating arterioles; 2-sided t-test for ttt $p < 0.001$ vs before MCAO. ZO-1, zona occludens-1 immunohistochemistry.

2.2. Endothelial Cells of Collaterals and Distal-Most Arterioles Have Primary Cilia; Collaterals Have Fewer

While examining EC orientation using SEM we noticed the presence of casts of channels penetrating into a fraction of the ECs lining collaterals (Figure 3). Based on studies in other cell types including bovine aorta and human umbilical vein ECs [32–34], these are invaginations of the plasmalemma that abut the ciliary membrane to form the ciliary pocket, which houses the proximal end of luminal primary cilia (PrC) that were removed by shearing forces ("depilated/de-ciliated") during infusion of Batson's #17. The Batson's-filled ciliary pockets (i.e., PrC) were commonly located near the nucleus, in accordance with the base of the cilium being associated with the basal body [34–40]. Distal arterioles also have cilia (Figure S1). One, two, or rarely three cilia were present in ECs that expressed them (Figure 3, Figure S2). More than one cilium per EC has not been found in previous studies, to our knowledge; however, previous reports have only examined large conduit vessels. The above method, which serendipitously identified PrC, is indirect since ciliary pockets were what were detected. We therefore confirmed their presence using immunofluorescence (Figure 4). Eighteen percent of collateral ECs expressed PrC, as compared to 28% of DMAs; thus ECs lining collaterals had 34% fewer cilia. We have not found other reports that ECs within vessels of the microcirculation express primary cilia.

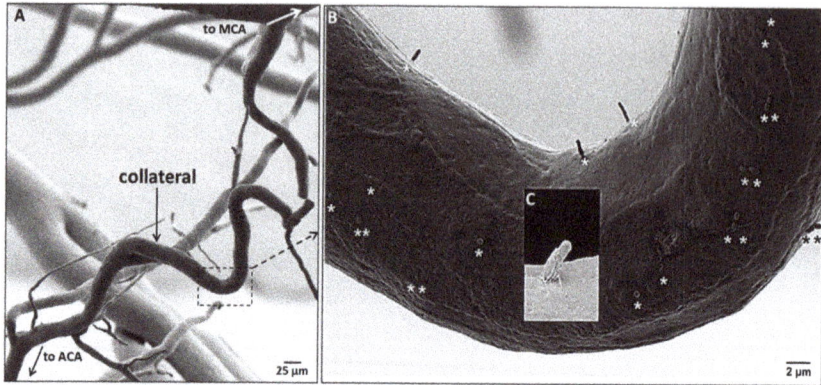

Figure 3. Collateral endothelial cells have primary cilia. (**A**) SEM of a corrosion cast of pial arterial vessels and a collateral, fixed at maximal dilation. (**B**) Stars identify casts of plasmalemmmal invaginations that contain the proximal end of the primary cilia (PrC) filled with Batson's #17 after removal of the PrC by shearing during infusion of the casting agent; each EC has 0–3 PrC. (**C**) Higher magnification SEM of a ~2 µm long PrC invagination.

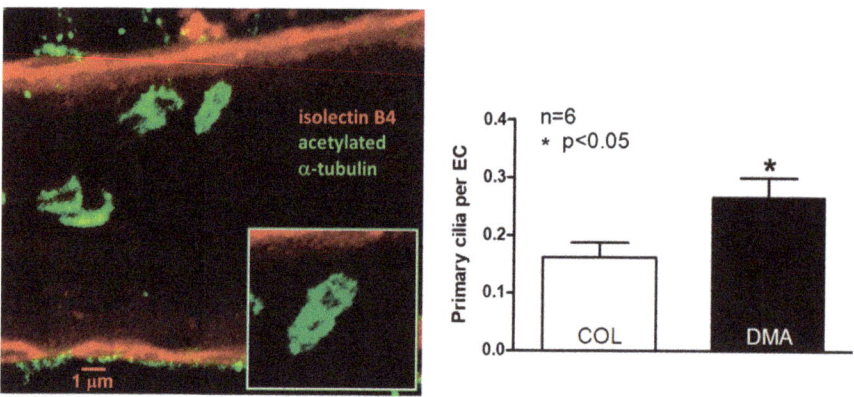

Figure 4. Collateral endothelial cells have fewer primary cilia than distal-most arterioles (DMA). Immunofluorescent-stained collaterals (COL) with focal plane set within the lumen above the far-wall, showing primary cilia. Figure S2 shows cilia on DMAs. Inset, higher magnification. Right panel, $n = 6$ mice, 2-sided t-test.

2.3. Collaterals Are Invested with a Continuous Layer of Smooth Muscle Cells, unlike Distal-Most Arterioles Whose Smooth Muscle Cells Are Discontinuous

Smooth muscle cells (SMCs) become sparse and discontinuous on distal arterioles in many tissue types [41–43]. Unlike arterioles that have orthograde flow, collateral blood flow converges from opposite directions, resulting in an average flow of near or at zero in the center-most segment of the collateral in the absence of occlusion (Figure 2A). The kinetic energy of flow is therefore converted to potential energy, which increases the circumferential wall stress of collaterals. Accordingly, we reasoned that SMC investment of collaterals might be greater than that present on DMAs to balance this increased wall stress. Figure 5 supports this hypothesis.

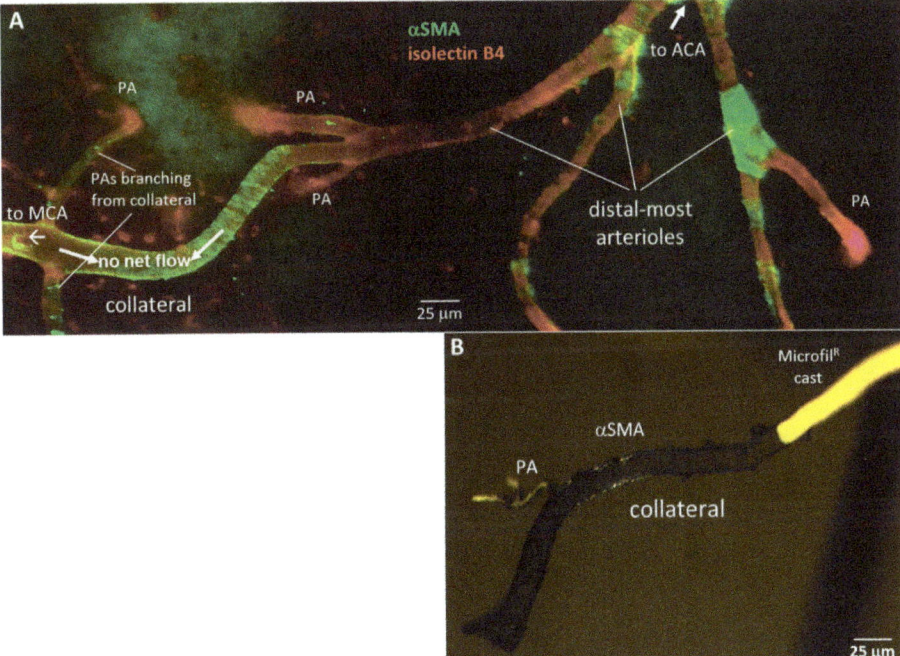

Figure 5. Collaterals are invested with a continuous layer of smooth muscle cells (SMCs), unlike distal-most arterioles (DMAs) that lack or have discontinuous SMCs. (**A**), Immuno-fluorescent staining of SMCs (αSM-actin) and ECs (IB4-lectin). Representative image of pial collaterals, DMAs and penetrating arterioles (PA). (**B**), Brightfield image of αSMA-stained collateral and PA filled with yellow Microfil®, then freed from surrounding pial membrane.

2.4. Gene Expression Differs for Collaterals Versus Distal-Most Arterioles

Given the disturbed hemodynamic, pro-oxidative stress (i.e., low blood oxygen content) environment in which collateral mural cells reside, plus the high susceptibility of collaterals to undergo rarefaction with aging, vascular risk factor presence, and eNOS/NO deficiency [16–21,25] compared to nearby DMAs [17], we postulated that expression of genes involved with inflammation, cell proliferation, aging, and angiogenesis differ for collaterals and DMAs. To test this hypothesis, we measured transcript levels of 22 such genes (Figure 6), as well as eNOS immunofluorescence (Figure 7). Collaterals had increased expression of *Pycard*, *Ki67*, *Pdgfb*, *Angpt2*, *Dll4*, *Ephrinb2*, and eNOS, whereas 16 other genes were not significantly different. Of note, expression of the EC shear stress-sensitive transcription factors Klf2 and Klf4, which promote anti-proliferative, -inflammatory, and -angiogenic processes, upregulate eNOS, and are sharply downregulated at vascular sites of low and disturbed shear stress [35–37,44,45], were, in contrast, not downregulated in collaterals compared to DMAs with laminar high-velocity flow.

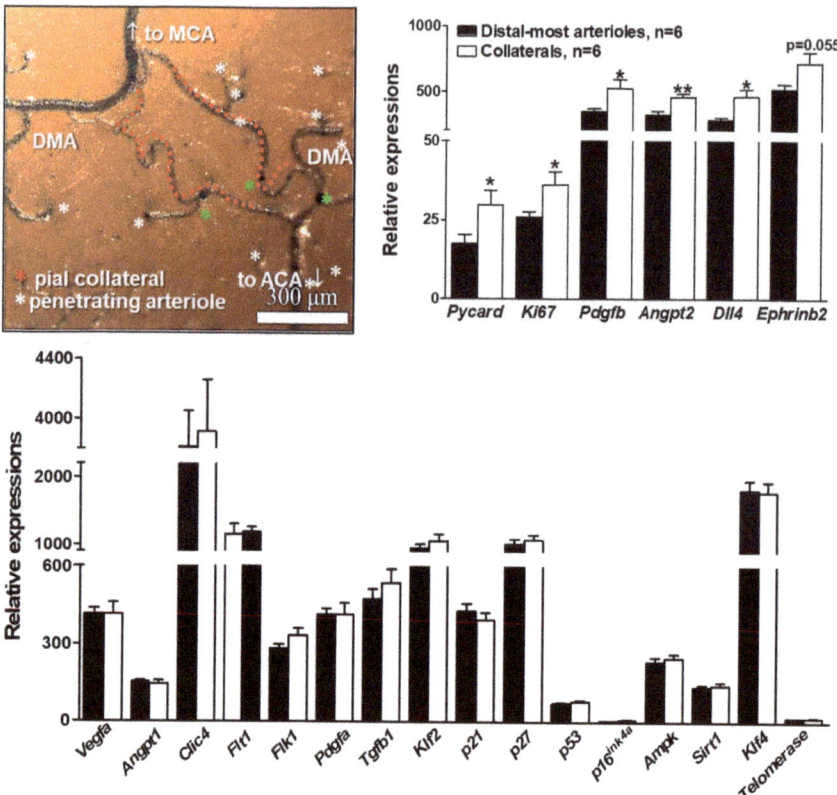

Figure 6. Gene expression differs for collaterals versus distal-most arterioles. Upper left panel, pial arterial vasculature perfusion-fixed at maximal dilation then filled with PU4ii polyurethane. Stars identify penetrating arterioles, including three that bifurcate and descend into the cortex immediately below the arteriole or collateral (green stars). Ten collaterals and 10 nearby similarly-sized distal-most arterioles DMAs were dissected from each of 36 mice and pooled into six samples for extraction of RNA. Transcript abundance was determined by Nanostring n-Counter® for 22 genes, each normalized to one of six housekeeping genes (*Gapdh, βactin, Tubb5, Hprt1, Ppia, Tbp*) selected for comparable level of expression [46]. * $p < 0.05$, ** $p < 0.01$ by 2-sided t-test for collaterals versus DMAs.

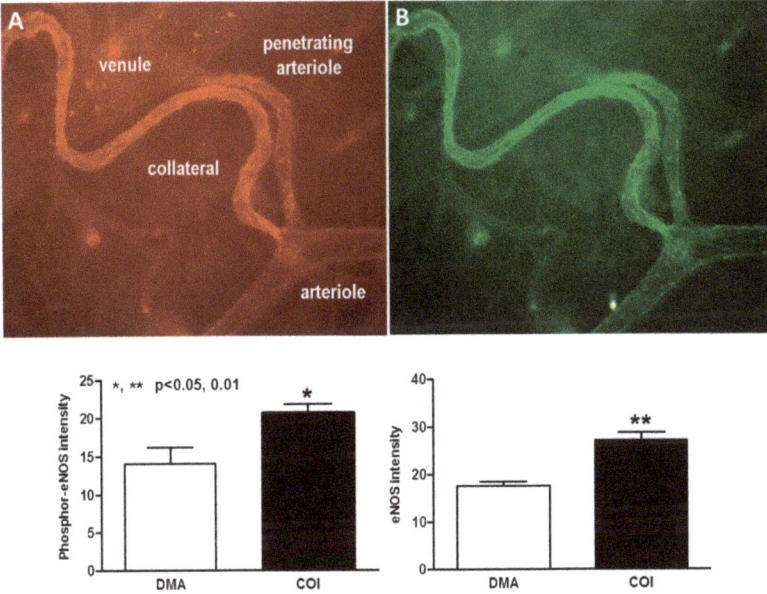

Figure 7. Collaterals express increased levels of phospho- and total eNOS compared to arterioles. Top panels, immunohistochemistry for phospho- (**A**, red) and total (**B**, green) eNOS, n = 4 mice, 1-sided t-tests, 163x magnification. * $p < 0.05$, ** $p < 0.01$.

2.5. Changes in Tortuosity over a Collateral's "Lifetime" Suggests Accelerated Proliferative Senescence of their Mural Cells

We previously reported that aging, hypertension, and other vascular risk factors cause a loss of collateral number and a smaller diameter in those that remain [17–19,25]. Aging-induced rarefaction becomes evident in late middle-age in mice (16 months of age), is not seen in DMAs, is accelerated in onset by the presence of other vascular risk factors, and is associated with increased cellular markers of oxidative stress, inflammation, proliferation, and aging, as well as increased vessel tortuosity [17–19,25]. Tortuosity is a hallmark of collaterals. We postulated that it arises from a persistently increased rate of proliferation of collateral wall cells (confirmed in [18]) that is driven by the disturbed hemodynamic conditions present in collaterals. The above studies did not examine tortuosity at time points earlier than 3 months of age. To determine whether collaterals begin to acquire tortuosity from formation onward, we examined mice on embryonic day E15.5 (collaterals form between E15.5 and E18.5 [6,7]) and on post-natal day-1 and day-21. Tortuosity was absent at E15.5 but became evident by P1 and was significant by P21 (Figure 8). When viewed in context with our previous data for tortuosity at later ages (Figure 9; human year-equivalents for the latter five bars are approximately 13, 19, 49, 69, 84 years [47]), these findings support the hypothesis that collateral rarefaction, which becomes evident in late middle-age in mice [17], is caused by proliferative senescence of collateral ECs and SMCs due to a lifetime elevation in proliferation in excess of apoptosis that is caused by the disturbed hemodynamic conditions in which collaterals reside.

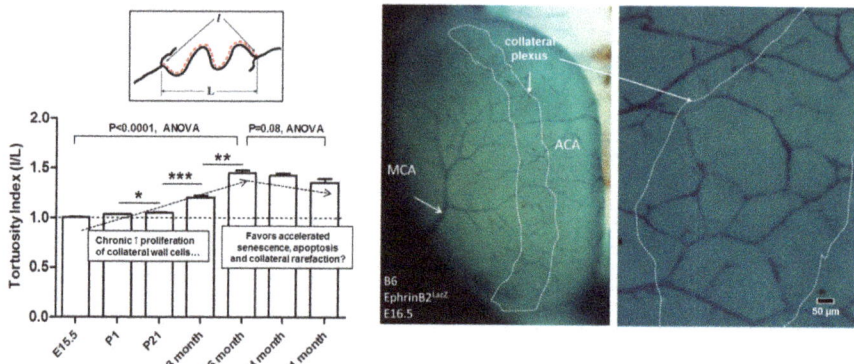

Figure 8. Tortuosity increases progressively with time after formation of collaterals. Images at right, ephrin-B2^{LacZ} reporter mouse (construction of mutant described in [6]) showing embryonic collaterals. Bar graph, tortuosity index = l/L (axial length of collateral ÷ scalar length connecting collateral endpoints). E, embryonic day, P, post-natal day. Data for last four bars from Faber et al. [17] who also showed that collateral diameter and number begin to decline at or after 16 months of age. Number of mice (C57BL/6, B6) for bars 1–7: 8,9,8,9,10,7,8. For each mouse tortuosity, was determined for all MCA–ACA collaterals and averaged. ANOVA followed by 1-sided Bonferroni t-tests, *, **, ***, $p < 0.05$, 0.01, 0.001, respectively.

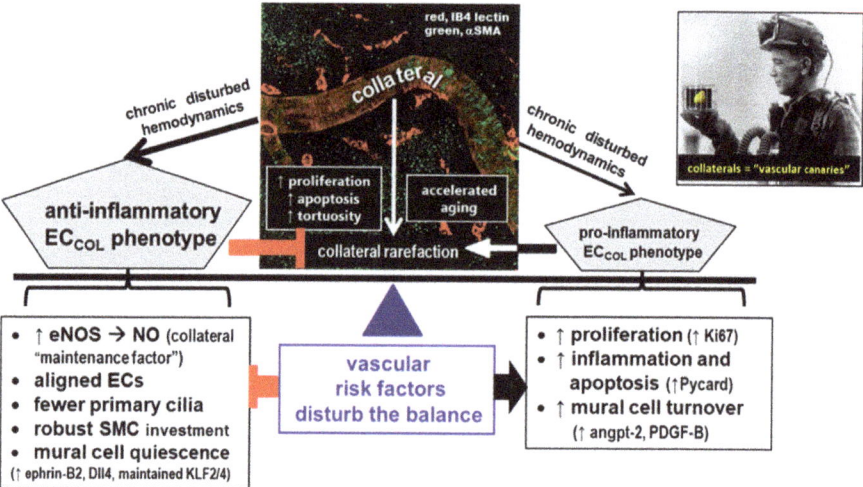

Figure 9. Persistence/maintenance versus rarefaction/pruning of collaterals "hangs in the balance". Proposed model whereby collateral (COL) mural cells reside in an environment of low/disturbed shear stress, high circumferential wall stress, and low blood oxygen content. This favors a pro-inflammatory, pro-proliferative, pro-apoptotic, and accelerated aging EC phenotype, leading to loss of collateral number and diameter (rarefaction). Compared to distal arterioles, collaterals have specializations and differential gene expression (left box) that provide adaptations that mitigate against factors that promote collateral rarefaction (right box). Vascular risk factors, e.g., aging, hypertension, EC dysfunction, and oxidative stress, disturb the balance. Collaterals are more sensitive than other vessels to these environmental risk factors, like "canaries in a mine-shaft".

3. Discussion

The present study identified a number of distinct features of collateral ECs and SMCs that may underlie or contribute to the unique characteristics of collaterals outlined in the Introduction. We found that despite the low and oscillatory shear stress present in collaterals at baseline in the absence of obstruction, their ECs are aligned with the vessel axis to the same degree present in distal-most arterioles and the descending aorta—vessels with high-velocity orthograde laminar flow. Endothelial cells of both collaterals and arterioles have primary cilia, and collaterals possess fewer of them. Smooth muscle cells of collaterals are continuous, unlike those of DMAs. Collaterals have higher levels of expression of genes associated with both pro- and anti-inflammatory and pro- and anti-proliferation pathways, compared to DMAs. A bias towards a higher rate of cell proliferation in collateral mural cells [18] is supported by the observation that collaterals begin to acquire tortuosity shortly after their formation in the embryo that increases through middle age (16 months, 49 human year-equivalents [47]). The above findings provide insights into structural and molecular specializations that may underlie the unique features and functions of collateral vessels.

Convergence of blood flow in collaterals at baseline imposes low and "disturbed" flow/shear stress forces on their mural cells, i.e., either absence of flow or very low flow that oscillates to-and-fro (~1–10 times per minute) and averages zero [6,15]. This results in increased wall stress according to the Bernoulli relationship. When present elsewhere in the arterial circulation, e.g., at bifurcations, the inner arch of the aorta or downstream of plaques, low and disturbed shear stress favors a non-aligned cobblestoned EC morphology that is associated with increased oxidative stress, inflammation, markers of aging, and low eNOS/NO activity (i.e., endothelial dysfunction) [28–31,44,45]. Surprisingly, however, we found that collateral ECs have the same alignment (and cell dimensions) as ECs in DMAs and the descending aorta. We did not investigate how this anti-inflammatory structural phenotype is specified. It is possible that one or more of the other unique features that we identified are involved (see below). On the other hand, the data in Figure 2 for flow and shear stress were obtained in anesthetized animals. During awake behaviors, collaterals may have periods of sustained flow in one or the other direction induced by changes in regional metabolic activity in the territory supplied by the arterial trees that they cross-connect. It is not known if collaterals contribute in this way to physiological metabolic regulation of blood flow and oxygen delivery, i.e., neurovascular coupling in brain and functional hyperemia elsewhere. However, such periods of sustained unidirectional flow could promote the EC orientation we observed. Irrespective of underlying cause, we speculate that the aligned phenotype of collateral ECs is part (or a marker) of a group of protective mechanisms that favor maintenance of collaterals and mitigate their rarefaction (Figure 9).

To our knowledge, this is the first report showing that ECs lining collaterals and arterioles have primary cilia. They are much more abundant than reported previously for conduit vessels from healthy individuals (i.e., absent or present on less than 1% of ECs [32,34]): 18% of collateral ECs have PrC compared to 28% for DMAs. Primary cilia on ECs were described in 1984 by Haust in aorta of rabbits and humans with atherosclerosis [48]. Subsequent reports described ciliated ECs in capillaries of the pineal gland of a 20 week-old human fetus [49], developing heart and aortic valve leaflets [33,50,51], and references therein], surrounding atheromas [52], ectopically in the common carotid artery of $ApoE^{-/-}$ mice, and in healthy individuals at bifurcations of conduit arteries and the inner curvature of the aortic arch; by contrast cilia are absent or nearly so in regions of arteries where shear stress is laminar [33,40,50]. Most other cell types express PrC during development, under certain conditions of cell culture [53], and in adults [35–37]. Depending on cell type, PrC participate in specification of embryo asymmetry, centriole disposition, proliferation/cell cycle regulation, autophagy, flow-sensing mechanotransduction, chemoception, and compartmentalization and trafficking of signaling proteins among the cilioplasm, cytoplasm, and nucleoplasm (e.g., for Gli and PDGFRα) [35–37]. When present, cilia are most abundant in non-proliferating cells, with the proximal end anchored in an invagination of the plasmalemma (ciliary pocket) in ECs and other but not all cell types [33,34,36]. Primary cilia are complexed with the mother centriole of the basal body that links to the microtubule-organizing center

(MTOC) [32,35–37,54]. Disassembly/resorption of the cilium during S-phase and centriole liberation are essential for cell division [36,37,54]. Since PrC are linked to the cytoskeleton via the MTOC, flow-induced ciliary bending in ECs [55] is capable of being transmitted throughout the cell, including to cell–cell and cell–matrix junctions [33,37]. Primary cilia transduce fluid shear stress in renal tubular epithelial cells and ECs through a pathway that that is exceptionally sensitive to shear stress and involves polycystin-1 and polycystin-2, which are encoded by *Pkd1* and *Pkd2* [35–37]. Polycystin-1 has mechanosensitive properties while polycystin-2 is a TRP calcium channel. Both proteins are required to sense shear stress and in turn release nitric oxide [33,37]. Defects in PrC are associated with many abnormalities. For example, mutations of *PKD1* and *PKD2* are causal for autosomal dominant polycystic kidney disease, with kidney ECs and tubular cells of patients evidencing deficient calcium and NO responses and increased proliferation [33,35–37].

Primary cilia are absent in human umbilical vein ECs maintained under laminar shear stress and proliferative quiescence in cell culture. In human umbilical veins less than one percent of ECs have cilia that protrude into the lumen, while in a larger fraction the cilia are located intracellularly [34,55]. Embryonic aorta and ECs cultured from it have a single cilium that projects into the lumen [38–40]. Endothelial cilia are present in regions of high shear stress during embryonic development, along with expression of the shear stress-sensitive transcription factor, KLF2, which transactivates *eNOS* and other anti-inflammatory and anti-proliferative genes [44,45]. In regions with low or disturbed shear stress PrC are disassembled/absent and expression of *Klf2* and *eNOS* are abolished and reduced, respectively [33,56]. Expression of *Klf2* is also inhibited in non-ciliated ECs isolated from embryonic arteries, and chemical removal of PrC from ECs in culture has a similar effect, i.e., abolishing *Klf2* expression [57]. Interestingly, in ECs of adult $ApoE^{-/-}$ mice, which have endothelial dysfunction but do not develop plaques, cilia are expressed ectopically in the common carotid artery despite the presence of laminar flow, compared to wildtype mice that are devoid of cilia [33]. Cilia were lost when high shear stress was induced via implantation of a flow-restricting cast around the vessel. Casting of common carotids in wildtype mice induced ciliogenesis only in regions of low and disturbed shear stress. These findings suggest that expression of PrC on ECs in vivo in adults is limited to regions of low/disturbed shear stress but can occur ectopically in arteries with laminar flow in the presence of endothelial dysfunction caused by hyperlipidemia [33] and possibly other vascular risk factors. Of note, in highly ciliated, disturbed-flow areas such as the inner curvature of the aortic arch or downstream of plaques, approximately 25% of ECs have a single cilium while the rest are devoid [33], a percentage similar to what we observed in arterioles and collaterals.

Our findings that PrC are also present on arterioles and collaterals in healthy young adult mice highlight the need for studies examining cilia function in these vessel types. This includes determining whether our observation of fewer cilia on collateral ECs than arterioles has functional significance. Endothelial cells are coupled mechanically, electrically, and diffusionally to adjacent ECs and SMCs [58], thus only a fraction of ECs may need to express cilia for transduction of mechano-sensitive or other signals. High shear stress causes disassembly of cilia in cultured ECs, while oscillatory flow reversal induces their expression [33]. We speculate that cilia on arteriole and collateral ECs may reflect the lower flow/shear stress in arterioles and very low and disturbed flow in collaterals and that fewer PrC on collateral ECs may serve to reduce their sensitivity to the prevailing disturbed shear stress environment. In other words, fewer cilia on collateral ECs may be part of a repertoire of adaptations that balance against or oppose—through maintained or increased expression of KLF2/4, eNOS, and other anti-inflammatory/anti-proliferative factors—the low-grade inflammatory, oxidative, proliferative, and apoptotic signals promoted by the disturbed hemodynamic environment present in collaterals (Figure 9). Egorova et al. [36] proposed something similar, i.e., that since presence of PrC on ECs is associated with KLF2 expression, endothelial cilia may signal a brake on EC activation in regions of low and disturbed flow. A protective role for cilia in these regions [36,37] is supported by the recent report that removal of endothelial cilia using conditional deletion of *Ift88* increased atherosclerosis and inflammatory gene expression, and decreased eNOS activity in $Apoe^{-/-}$ mice fed a high-fat diet [59], and that the endothelium becomes sensitized in athero-prone regions to undergo osteogenic differentiation in Tg737 (orpk/orpk) cilium-defective mice [60]. It is also possible that if PrC are protective, fewer of them in collaterals could contribute to the high susceptibility of these vessels to rarefaction from aging and other vascular risk factors. However, fewer cilia on collaterals might simply reflect a secondary or bystander effect, being a consequence, for example, of a higher inherent proliferation rate of collateral ECs as evidenced by the progressive increase in collateral tortuosity (discussed below), since presence of PrC and their association with the basal body is believed to favor removal of cells from the cell cycle [35–37]. Future studies will be required to determine if our finding of multiple cilia on ECs reflects ECs that have undergone proliferative senescence and associated failed cytokinesis and nuclear polyploidy [39].

It has recently been shown that ECs in the developing mouse retina rely on PrC to stabilize vessel connections during remodeling of the vascular plexus in regions with low to intermediate shear stress [61]. Endothelial cilia sense flow in zebrafish embryos, participate in recruitment of mural cells to arterial fated vessels, and are required for normal vascular morphogenesis [62,63]. The number and diameter of collaterals declines beginning in middle age [17]. This age-induced rarefaction is strongly accelerated by genetic or pharmacologically induced eNOS/NO deficiency or the presence of vascular risk factors [16,19]. Increased shear stress induces collateral outward remodeling following acute or slowly developing arterial obstruction [1,2,5]. $Pkd1^{+/-}$ mice and patients with autosomal dominant polycystic kidney disease have endothelial eNOS/NO dysfunction [64]. It will be important to examine in future studies whether collateral PrC participate in one or more of the above functions using EC-specific knockdown of polycystin-1, since: 1) deficiency in it leads to altered ciliary function, 2) polycystin-1 together with polycystin-2 participate in flow-sensing by PrC, 3) mutant forms of either protein cause polycystic kidney disease [35–37], 4) there is evidence that VHL, independent of its role in the degradation of Hif1α, together with GSK3β are required for structural maintenance of the cilium [65], and 5) the protein Rabep2, which is required for collaterogenesis [11], is a novel substrate of GSK3β [66], localizes at the cilium–basal body complex, and knockdown of it leads to defective ciliogenesis [67]. Other approaches to interfere with cilia presence and function, e.g., with knockdown of other ciliary proteins such as Pkd2 and Ift88, also will need to be examined.

In contrast to distal arterioles, which have sparse and discontinuous SMCs in various tissues including retina (we were unable to identify studies in brain) [41–43], SMCs were continuous on collaterals. We speculate this may be an adaptive increase in wall thickness to balance the increase in circumferential wall stress caused by the Bernoulli-specified conversion of kinetic energy of flow to increased potential energy (transmural pressure) as a consequence of flow-convergence in collaterals. It would be interesting to examine whether the composition and amount of extracellular matrix, which could assist SMCs in balancing the increased wall stress in collaterals, differs in collaterals versus arterioles. Of note, despite their increased SMC coverage, collaterals have less rather than more tone compared to similarly-sized arterioles, and lack myogenic responsiveness—additional unique features of collateral vessels [26,27].

The disturbed hemodynamic, pro-oxidative environment in which collateral mural cells reside led us to examine whether expression of genes involved in inflammation, cell proliferation, aging, and angiogenesis differ for collaterals versus distal arterioles. Collaterals displayed increased mRNA levels for the pro-inflammatory, pro-apoptosis inflammasome gene, Pycard, the pro-proliferative genes, Ki67, Pdgfb, and Angpt2, the anti-proliferative gene, Dll4, and the differentiated arterial-type EC marker gene, Ephrinb2. However, expression of cell cycle inhibitor genes, p21, p27, and p53, were not different, nor were other genes associated with proliferation, cell cycle arrest, and aging ($p16^{Ink4a}$, Ampk, Sirt1, telomerase). Neither were there differences in expression of other genes associated with EC and/or SMC proliferation (Vegfa, Flk1, Clic4, Pdgfa, Flt1) and that are required (in the case of the first three genes [7,8]) for formation of collaterals during development or involved with specifying EC and SMC differentiation and quiescence (Tgfb, Angpt1). Increased expression by collaterals of the above pro-proliferation genes is consistent with our tortuosity measurements, which suggest that collateral mural cells have a higher proliferation rate, compared to other arterial vessels: collateral tortuosity was evident by the first day after birth, continued to increase through middle age, and then declined. The latter occurred at the same time that collaterals experience a decline in number and diameter with advanced aging [17]. These findings support the hypothesis that age-associated collateral rarefaction is caused by proliferative senescence and subsequent apoptosis of collateral ECs and SMCs due to a lifetime elevation in proliferation rate caused by the disturbed hemodynamic and low blood oxygen content environment in which collaterals reside (Figure 9).

Collaterals also displayed increased activity of eNOS, which previous studies have shown opposes rarefaction of collaterals caused by aging and other vascular risk factors [16,18,19]. eNOS-derived NO inhibits oxidative stress, inflammation, proliferation, leukocyte adhesion, platelet aggregation, and cellular aging and promotes SMC relaxation [58,68]. Since shear stress is a proximate stimulus for eNOS-derived NO, increased eNOS/NO in collaterals with their low and disturbed shear stress environment may lessen the effect of factors promoting collateral rarefaction (Figure 9). Likewise, maintained expression of the EC shear stress-sensitive transcription factors, *Klf2* and *Klf4*, in collaterals despite their low and oscillatory flow, which inhibits expression of these factors elsewhere in the arterial vasculature with disturbed flow [44], may act as additional "balancing" factors or collateral specializations, along with increased eNOS, aligned ECs, fewer cilia, robust SMC coverage, and increased ephrin-B2 and Dll4. Expression of KLF2 and KLF4, which negatively regulate proliferation, inflammation, and angiogenesis, upregulate eNOS, and are sharply downregulated at sites of low and disturbed shear stress, were not different in collaterals versus DMAs. Interestingly, PrC promote *Klf2*, *Klf4*, and *eNOS* expression [35–37,44,69,70].

A limitation of the above studies is that RNA was obtained from dissected vessels, which are composed of ECs, SMCs, and, although less so, pericytes, fibroblasts, and resident myeloid cells. Studies are needed that employ separation of cell types and examination of a wider array of genes and their respective protein levels. However, the difficulty in manually dissecting collaterals and distal arterioles in the required numbers, the effect of cell dissociation techniques on baseline levels of RNA and protein, the absence of cell culture models of "collateral" ECs and SMCs, and the as of yet lack of any collateral-specific marker gene, preclude the use of these approaches. Of note, however, expression of several of the genes examined are specific or enriched for ECs, e.g., *Flk1*, *Angpt1*, *Angpt2*, *Ephrinb2*, *DLL4*, *eNOS*, *Clic4*, *Klf2*, and *Klf4*. However, analysis of gene transcription does not always reflect changes in protein level or function; thus the investigation of oxidative stress, inflammatory, proliferation, or senescence markers at the protein level may better reflect differences in cellular characteristics.

4. Materials and Methods

Three to 4 month-old male C57BL/6 (B6) wildtype (lab colony, Jackson Laboratories breeders, Bar Harbor, ME, USA) or genetically modified mice were studied. Scanning electron microscopy was performed on the cerebral arterial vasculature that was filled with Batson's #17. Angiography and morphometry were performed after filling with yellow Microfil® [18]. Prior to infusion of the casting agents, and also for immunohistochemistry, the vasculature was cleared of blood and perfusion-fixed after maximal dilation with 10^{-4} M nitroprusside. Filling was confined to the pre-capillary vessels by adjusting the viscosity and input pressure of the casting material. All pial collaterals between the anterior cerebral artery (ACA) and middle (MCA) trees of both hemispheres were identified; tortuosity (axial length of the collateral ÷ scalar length connecting the collateral's endpoints [17]) and lumen diameter, EC orientation, and other morphometrics were obtained at midpoint for each collateral and an average value obtained for each animal unless indicated otherwise in the figure legends. Permanent MCA occlusion was by electro-cautery occlusion of the M1-MCA just distal to the lenticulostriate branches [18]. Right femoral artery (FA) occlusion was achieved by ligating the superficial FA immediately proximal and distal to the superior epigastric artery, which was also ligated [18]. Hindlimb perfusion was measured by laser Doppler perfusion imaging of the plantar foot and the adductor thigh regions. Values reported are means ± SE, with significance at $p < 0.05$; n-sizes (number of animals studied) and statistical tests are given in the figure legends.

All applicable international, national, and/or institutional guidelines for the care and use of animals were followed, including the National Institutes of Health Guide for the Care and Use of Laboratory Animals (UNC IACUC #18-123.0-A, 1 April 2019). This article does not contain any studies with human participants performed by any of the authors.

4.1. Angiography and Morphometry

As previously described in detail [20] animals were anesthetized deeply with ketamine and xylazine and heparinized. The distal thoracic aorta was cannulated, right atrium perforated, and the mouse was perfused with PBS containing freshly prepared sodium nitroprusside (10^{-4} M, for maximal dilation) and Evans blue dye (for light staining of brain and the endothelial surface) at ~100 mmHg. One ml of yellow Microfil (Flowtech Inc, Carver, MA, USA) was infused at a viscosity adjusted to fill the entire pial arterial and collateral circulations with sufficient pressure (~100 mmHg) and duration to cause limited capillary transit and venous filling to assure complete filling of all precapillary vessels and collaterals. After the Microfil had set for 20 min, brains were kept in 4% PFA and collaterals were imaged the next day using a Leica fluorescent stereomicroscope. All collaterals between the anterior cerebral artery (ACA) and middle cerebral artery (MCA) trees of both hemispheres were counted and divided by 2 to give the average number per hemisphere. Images were subsequently analyzed (ImageJ, NIH, Bethesday, MD, USA): Collateral lumen diameter was determined at midpoint at 50X for all ACA-MCA collaterals and averaged for each mouse.

4.2. Permanent Middle Cerebral Artery Occlusion (pMCAO)

As previously described [20], mice were anesthetized with ketamine and xylazine (100 and 10 mg/kg, ip, respectively) and rectal temperature was maintained at 37 ± 0.5 °C. The temporalis muscle between the eye and ear on one side was retracted after a 4 mm incision. After a 2 mm craniotomy (18000-17 drill, FST, Foster City, CA, USA), the dura was incised with a 27 gauge needle tip and reflected to reveal the main trunk of the MCA which was cauterized (18010-00, FST, modified) distal to the lenticulostriate branches. The incision was closed with suture and Vetbond (3M, Minneapolis, MN, USA), intramuscular cefazolin 50 mg/kg and buprenorphine were administered, and the animal was monitored in a warmed cage during recovery from anesthesia to maintain the above rectal temperature. Mice were euthanized 4 days after pMCAO. Pial collateral morphometry was then performed as described above.

4.3. Laser Doppler Perfusion Imaging and Hindlimb Ischemia Model

Femoral artery ligation (FAL) was performed and hindlimb perfusion was measured using a laser Doppler perfusion imager (Model LDI2-IR, Moor Instruments, Wilmington, DE, USA, ~2 mm penetration and high resolution) as described previously [71]. Briefly, the anterior thigh and adductor regions were depilated followed by 24 h to recover from any erythema. Mice were then anesthetized with 1.25% isoflurane/O_2, rectal temperature was maintained at 37 ± 0.5 °C. A 3 mm incision was made overlying the femoral vessels 5 mm proximal to the knee. The femoral artery was gently isolated and ligated twice with 7-0 suture immediately distal to the lateral caudal femoral artery and 1 mm further distally, followed by transection between the ligatures. The superficial epigastric artery was also ligated. The skin was closed using 5-0 silk. Mice were placed in a heated chamber to block ambient light, and rectal temperature was maintained at 37 ± 0.5 °C. Less than 5 min after ligation, the plantar and adductor regions of both legs were laser-scanned. Average perfusion within the region of interest, drawn to outline the plantar surface of the paws, was calculated using Moor LDI Image Processing V5.0 software and reported as the ratio of ligated to the non-ligated hindlimb, where the region of interest was defined according to anatomic landmarks as described previously [71].

4.4. Quantitative NanoString Expression Analysis

As described previously [46], mice placed under deep anesthesia (ketamine and xylazine, 100 and 10 mg/kg, ip, respectively) were perfused with 1 ml RNAlater®(Sigma-Aldrich Corp, St. Louis, MO, USA) premixed with 10% Evans blue dye through the thoracic aorta. The brain was then removed and immersed in RNAlater®. Approximately 10 pial collaterals and 10 nearby similarly sized distal-most arterioles per mouse (total 36 mice) were micro-dissected and pooled in RNAlater®as 6 samples. Samples were homogenized (TH, Omni International, Marietta, GA, USA) in Trizol Reagent (Invitrogen, Carlsbad, CA, USA). Total RNA was purified using the RNeasy Micro Kit according to the manufacturer (Qiagen, Valencia, CA, USA). RNA concentration and quality were determined by NanoDrop 1000 (Thermo Scientific, Wilmington, DE, USA) and Bioanalyzer 2100 (Agilent, Foster City, CA, USA), respectively. Measurement of transcript number was conducted for 22 selected genes by the genomics facility at UNC using NanoString custom-synthesized probes (NanoString, Seattle, WA, USA). Transcript number for each gene was normalized to one of the following 6 housekeeping genes selected to be in range of the target gene under analysis: *Gapdh*, *βactin*, *Tubb5*, *Hprt1*, *Ppia* and *Tbp*.

4.5. Immunohistochemistry

Mice under deep anesthesia (ketamine and xylazine, 100 and 10 mg/kg, ip, respectively) were perfused with nitroprusside (10^{-4} M) in PBS at ~100 mmHg with a reservoir for 3 minutes for maximal dilation and then with 2% PFA for 15 min for fixation. Brains were blocked with 10% goat serum in 0.3% PBS-triton 1 hr at room temperature. Then the cortex area were incubated with 1:50 anti-eNOS rabbit IgG (sc-654, Santa Cruz Biotechnology, Santa Cruz, CA, USA); 1:100 anti-phospho eNOS rabbit IgG (ab75639, Abcam, Cambridge, MA, USA), 1:100 anti-acetylated-tubulin (T7451, Sigma), 1:100 anti-ZO1 (ab96587, Abcam), 1;400 anti-aSMA (Abcam, 32575, clone E184), overnight, 4 °C in a shaker, followed by incubation of 1:200 goat anti rabbit-fluorescent conjugated with Alexa fluor®568 (A10042, ThermoFisher Scientific, Grand Island, NY, USA) or Alexa fluor®488 (A21208). Images of eNOS and phorpho-eNOS for pial collaterals and DMAs were taken using a Leica fluorescent stereomicroscope (Richmond, IL, USA), and the signal strength was measured using ImageJ (Bethesda, MD, USA). Endothelial cells were probed with Isolectin-GS-IB4-Alexa568 (I121415, ThermoFisher Scientific). Primary cilia (probed with anti-acetylated-tubulin antibody) in the lumen of pial collaterals were observed with a Zeiss 710 confocal microscope (Thornwood, NT, USA), with z stack scanning from the top of cortex down to a depth of ~30 um. Endothelial junctions (probed with ZO-1) were visualized with a Zeiss 710 confocal microscope.

4.6. Collateral Primary Cilia and Endothelial Orientation Assessed by Scanning Electron Microscopy

Mice were perfused with maximal vessel dilation as described above. Brain arterial vasculature was then casted using a Batson's No 17 Plastic Replica and Corrosion Kit (Polysciences, Inc, Warrington, PA, USA). Briefly, 1 ml of Batson's 17 was infused through the thoracic aorta. After fully curing, the brain tissue was removed using maceration solution, and the cerebral vasculature including the pial collateral regions were carefully persevered for emission scanning electron microscopy. The vasculature was observed under a Zeiss Supra 25 Field emission scanning electron microscope. Images of pial collateral and DMAs were saved for analysis of primary cilia and endothelial cell morphology. To measure the orientation of collateral endothelial cells, we use Photoshop to draw a line coordinate with the collateral axis and a second line coordinate with the endothelial cell axis (see Figure 2, panel C), and the angle formed was measured.

4.7. Statistics

Experiments were performed in accordance with the University of North Carolina's Institutional Animal Care and Use Committee, the NIH Guide for the Care and Use of Laboratory Animals, the ARRIVE guidelines, and the following suggested STAIR criteria [72]: investigators were blinded during data analysis where possible; no data points were identified as outliers by statistical test and none were excluded; all results were fully disclosed including negative results; the review, discussion and citation of the literature was unbiased; pMCAO was used to permanently recruit blood flow across pial collaterals. Values are mean ± SEM. Statistical analysis ($p < 0.05$ = significant) is described in the figure legends.

5. Conclusions

In conclusion, collaterals are unique among blood vessel types with regard to their formation, structure, function, prevailing shear stress, and susceptibility to variation in their extent caused primarily by differences in genetic background but also by environmental factors such as aging and risk factors. The present study provides our first look into how differences in collateral endothelial and smooth muscle cells may accommodate and contribute to these unique features. Moreover, the model/hypothesis shown in Figure 9, if correct, may begin to provide answers to two perplexing questions: Why do collaterals undergo rarefaction with aging and other vascular risk factors? They are chronically exposed to adverse hemodynamic conditions. How do they resist more extensive pruning away? Their mural cells have specializations or adaptations in structure and expression of factors that mitigate the effects of these conditions.

Supplementary Materials: Supplementary materials can be found at http://www.mdpi.com/1422-0067/20/15/3608/s1.

Author Contributions: H.Z. performed angiography, morphometry, in vivo experiments, immunostaining, expression analysis, animal husbandry, and statistical analysis; D.C. performed SEM and determined collateral tortuosity in perinatal mice; J.E.F. designed the experiments, data analysis, and figures and wrote the manuscript.

Funding: National Institutes of Health, National Institute of Neurological Diseases and Stroke (grant NS083633), and National Heart Lung and Blood Institute (grant HL111070).

Acknowledgments: We thank Kirk McNaughton for histological tissue sectioning and Katy Liu for assistance in preparation of the SEM samples.

Conflicts of Interest: The authors declare no conflict of interest.

Abbreviations

ACA	anterior cerebral artery
B6	C57BL/6 mouse strain
COL	collateral
DMA	distal-most arteriole
EC	endothelial cell
eNOS	endothelial nitric oxide synthase
Flt 1	VEGF receptor 1
Flk1	VEGF receptor 2
MCA	middle cerebral artery
NO	nitric oxide
PA	penetrating arteriole
Pkd1	gene that encodes polycystin-1
PrC	primary cilia
SMC	smooth muscle cell
VECAD	vascular endothelial cell adhesion protein, selectively expressed by ECs
WT	wildtype littermate controls

References

1. Faber, J.E.; Chilian, W.M.; Deindl, E.; van Royen, N.; Simons, M. A brief etymology of the collateral circulation. *Atheroscler. Thromb. Vasc. Biol.* **2014**, *34*, 1854–1859. [CrossRef] [PubMed]

2. Nishijima, Y.; Akamatsu, Y.; Weinstein, P.R.; Liu, J. Collaterals: Implications in cerebral ischemic diseases and therapeutic interventions. *Brain Res.* **2015**, *1623*, 18–29. [CrossRef] [PubMed]
3. Bang, O.Y.; Goyal, M.; Liebeskind, D.S. Collateral circulation in ischemic stroke: Assessment tools and therapeutic strategies. *Stroke* **2015**, *46*, 3302–3309. [CrossRef]
4. Ginsberg, M.D. The cerebral collateral circulation: Relevance to pathophysiology and treatment of stroke. *Neuropharmacology* **2018**, *134*, 280–292. [CrossRef] [PubMed]
5. Schaper, W. Collateral circulation: Past and present. *Basic Res. Cardiol.* **2009**, *104*, 5–21. [CrossRef] [PubMed]
6. Chalothorn, D.; Faber, J.E. Formation and maturation or the murine native cerebral collateral circulation. *J. Mol. Cell. Cardiol.* **2010**, *49*, 251–259. [CrossRef] [PubMed]
7. Lucitti, J.L.; Mackey, J.K.; Morrison, J.C.; Haigh, J.J.; Adams, R.H.; Faber, J.E. Formation of the collateral circulation is regulated by vascular endothelial growth factor-A and A disintegrin and metalloprotease family members 10 and 17. *Circ. Res.* **2012**, *111*, 1539–1550. [CrossRef] [PubMed]
8. Lucitti, J.L.; Tarte, N.J.; Faber, J.E. Chloride intracellular channel 4 is required for maturation of the cerebral collateral circulation. *Am. J. Physiol. Heart Circ. Physiol.* **2015**, *309*, H1141–H1150. [CrossRef] [PubMed]
9. Zhang, H.; Prabhakar, P.; Sealock, R.; Faber, J.E. Wide genetic variation in the native pial collateral circulation is a major determinant of variation in severity of stroke. *J. Cereb. Blood Flow Metab.* **2010**, *30*, 923–934. [CrossRef]
10. Chalothorn, D.; Faber, J.E. Strain-dependent variation in native collateral function in mouse hindlimb. *Physiol. Genom.* **2010**, *42*, 469–479. [CrossRef]
11. Lucitti, J.L.; Sealock, R.; Buckley, B.K.; Zhang, H.; Xiao, L.; Dudley, A.C.; Faber, J.E. Variants of Rab GTPase-effector binding protein-2 cause variation in the collateral circulation and severity of stroke. *Stroke* **2016**, *47*, 3022–3031. [CrossRef] [PubMed]
12. Seiler, C.; Stoller, M.; Pitt, B.; Meier, P. The human coronary collateral circulation: Development and clinical importance. *Eur. Heart J.* **2013**, *34*, 2674–2682. [CrossRef] [PubMed]
13. Traupe, T.; Ortmann, J.; Stoller, M.; Baumgartner, I.; de Marchi, S.F.; Seiler, C. Direct quantitative assessment of the peripheral artery collateral circulation in patients undergoing angiography. *Circulation* **2013**, *128*, 737–744. [CrossRef] [PubMed]
14. Rost, N.S.; Giese, A.K.; Worrall, B.B.; Williams, S.; Malik, R.; Cloonan, L.; Furie, K.L.; Lindgren, A.; Frid, P.; Wasselius, J.; et al. RABEP2 (Rab GTPase-effector binding protein-2) is associated with ischemic stroke phenotypes: a translational replication study. *Eur. Stroke J.* **2018**, *3*, 42–43.
15. Toriumi, H.; Tatarishvili, J.; Tomita, M.; Tomita, Y.; Unekawa, M.; Suzuki, N. Dually supplied T-junctions in arteriolo-arteriolar anastomosis in mice: Key to local hemodynamic homeostasis in normal and ischemic states? *Stroke* **2009**, *40*, 3378–3383. [CrossRef] [PubMed]
16. Dai, X.; Faber, J.E. eNOS deficiency causes collateral vessel rarefaction and impairs activation of a cell cycle gene network during arteriogenesis. *Circ. Res.* **2010**, *106*, 1870–1881. [CrossRef] [PubMed]
17. Faber, J.E.; Zhang, H.; Lassance-Soares, R.M.; Prabhakar, P.; Najafi, A.H.; Burnett, M.S.; Epstein, S.E. Aging causes collateral rarefaction and increased severity of ischemic injury in multiple tissues. *Arterioscler. Thromb. Vasc. Biol.* **2011**, *31*, 1748–1756. [CrossRef] [PubMed]
18. Moore, S.M.; Zhang, H.; Maeda, N.; Doerschuk, C.; Faber, J.E. Cardiovascular risk factors cause premature rarefaction of the collateral circulation and greater ischemic tissue injury. *Angiogenesis* **2015**, *18*, 265–281. [CrossRef]
19. Rzechorzek, W.; Zhang, H.; Buckley, B.K.; Hua, H.; Pomp, D.; Faber, J.E. Exercise training prevents rarefaction of pial collaterals and increased severity of stroke with aging. *J. Cereb. Blood Flow Metab.* **2017**, *37*, 3544–3555. [CrossRef]
20. Zhang, H.; Jin, B.; Faber, J.E. Mouse models of Alzheimer's disease cause loss of pial collaterals and increased severity of ischemic stroke. *Angiogenesis* **2018**, *22*, 263–279. [CrossRef]
21. Hecht, N.; He, J.; Kremenetskaia, I.; Nieminen, M.; Vajkoczy, P.; Woitzik, J. Cerebral hemodynamic reserve and vascular remodeling in C57/BL6 mice are influenced by age. *Stroke* **2012**, *43*, 3052–3062. [CrossRef] [PubMed]
22. Menon, B.K.; Smith, E.E.; Coutts, S.B.; Welsh, D.G.; Faber, J.E.; Damani, Z.; Goyal, M.; Hill, M.D.; Demchuk, A.M.; Hee Cho, K.H.; et al. Leptomeningeal collaterals are associated with modifiable metabolic risk factors. *Ann. Neurol.* **2013**, *74*, 241–248. [CrossRef] [PubMed]

23. Malik, N.; Hou, Q.; Vagal, A.; Patrie, J.; Xin, W.; Michel, P.; Eskandari, A.; Jovin, T.; Wintermark, M. Demographic and clinical predictors of leptomeningeal collaterals in stroke patients. *J. Stroke Cerebrovasc. Dis.* **2014**, *23*, 2018–2022. [CrossRef] [PubMed]
24. Arsava, E.M.; Vural, A.; Akpinar, E.; Gocmen, R.; Akcalar, S.; Oguz, K.K.; Topcuoglu, M.A. The detrimental effect of aging on leptomeningeal collaterals in ischemic stroke. *J. Stroke Cerebrovasc. Dis.* **2014**, *23*, 421–426. [CrossRef] [PubMed]
25. Wang, J.; Peng, X.; Lassance-Soares, R.M.; Najafi, A.H.; Alderman, L.O.; Sood, S.; Xue, Z.; Chan, R.; Faber, J.E.; Epstein, S.E.; et al. Aging-induced collateral dysfunction: Impaired responsiveness of collaterals and susceptibility to apoptosis via dysfunctional eNOS signaling. *J. Cardiovasc. Transl. Res.* **2011**, *4*, 779–789. [CrossRef] [PubMed]
26. Chan, S.L.; Sweet, J.G.; Bishop, N.; Cipolla, M.J. Pial collateral reactivity during hypertension and aging: Understanding the function of collaterals for stroke therapy. *Stroke* **2016**, *47*, 1618–1625. [CrossRef] [PubMed]
27. Beard, D.J.; Murtha, L.A.; McLeod, D.D.; Spratt, N.J. Intracranial pressure and collateral blood flow. *Stroke* **2016**, *47*, 1695–1700. [CrossRef] [PubMed]
28. Davies, P.F.; Civelek, M.; Fang, Y.; Fleming, I. The atherosusceptible endothelium: Endothelial phenotypes in complex haemodynamic shear stress regions in vivo. *Cardiovasc. Res.* **2013**, *99*, 315–327. [CrossRef]
29. Abe, J.; Berk, B.C. Novel mechanisms of endothelial mechanotransduction. *Arterioscler. Thromb. Vasc. Biol.* **2014**, *34*, 2378–2386. [CrossRef]
30. Zhou, J.; Li, Y.S.; Chien, S. Shear stress-initiated signaling and its regulation of endothelial function. *Arterioscler. Thromb. Vasc. Biol.* **2014**, *34*, 2191–2198. [CrossRef]
31. Zakkar, M.; Angelini, G.D.; Emanueli, C. Regulation of vascular endothelium inflammatory signaling by shear stress. *Curr. Vasc. Pharmacol.* **2016**, *14*, 181–186. [CrossRef]
32. Briffeuil, P.; Thibaut-Vercruyssen, R.; Ronveaux-Dupal, M.F. Ciliation of bovine aortic endothelial cells in culture. *Atherosclerosis* **1994**, *106*, 75–81. [CrossRef]
33. Van der Heiden, K.; Hierck, B.P.; Krams, R.; de Crom, R.; Cheng, C.; Baiker, M.; Pourquie, J.; Alkemade, F.E.; DeRuiter, M.C.; Gittenberger-de Groot, A.C.; et al. Endothelial primary cilia in areas of disturbed flow are at the base of atherosclerosis. *Atherosclerosis* **2008**, *196*, 542–550. [CrossRef] [PubMed]
34. Geerts, W.J.; Vocking, K.; Schoonen, N.; Haarbosch, L.; van Donselaar, E.G.; Regan-Klapisz, E.; Post, J.A. Cobblestone HUVECs: A human model system for studying primary ciliogenesis. *J. Struct. Biol.* **2011**, *176*, 350–359. [CrossRef]
35. Satir, P. Cilia: Before and after. *Cilia* **2017**, *6*. [CrossRef]
36. Egorova, A.D.; van der Heiden, K.; Poelmann, R.E.; Hierck, B.P. Primary cilia as biomechanical sensors in regulating endothelial function. *Differentiation* **2012**, *83*, S56–S61. [CrossRef]
37. Pala, R.; Jamal, M.; Alshammari, Q.; Nauli, S.M. The roles of primary cilia in cardiovascular diseases. *Cells* **2018**, *7*, 233. [CrossRef] [PubMed]
38. Nauli, S.M.; Kawanabe, Y.; Kaminski, J.J.; Pearce, W.J.; Ingber, D.E.; Zhou, J. Endothelial cilia are fluid shear sensors that regulate calcium signaling and nitric oxide production through polycystin-1. *Circulation* **2008**, *117*, 1161–1171. [CrossRef] [PubMed]
39. AbouAlaiwi, W.A.; Ratnam, S.; Booth, R.L.; Shah, J.V.; Nauli, S.M. Endothelial cells from humans and mice with polycystic kidney disease are characterized by polyploidy and chromosome segregation defects through survivin down-regulation. *Hum. Mol. Genet.* **2011**, *20*, 354–367. [CrossRef]
40. Abdul-Majeed, S.; Moloney, B.C.; Nauli, S.M. Mechanisms regulating cilia growth and cilia function in endothelial cells. *Cell. Mol. Life Sci.* **2012**, *69*, 165–173. [CrossRef]
41. Price, R.J.; Owens, G.K.; Skalak, T.C. Immunohistochemical identification of arteriolar development using markers of smooth muscle differentiation. Evidence that capillary arterialization proceeds from terminal arterioles. *Circ. Res.* **1994**, *75*, 520–527. [CrossRef] [PubMed]
42. Murfee, W.L.; Skalak, T.C.; Peirce, S.M. Differential arterial/venous expression of NG2 proteoglycan in perivascular cells along microvessels: Identifying a venule-specific phenotype. *Microcirculation* **2005**, *12*, 151–160. [CrossRef] [PubMed]
43. Reagan, A.M.; Gu, X.; Paudel, S.; Ashpole, N.M.; Zalles, M.; Sonntag, W.E.; Ungvari, Z.; Csiszar, A.; Otalora, L.; Freeman, W.M.; et al. Age-related focal loss of contractile vascular smooth muscle cells in retinal arterioles is accelerated by caveolin-1 deficiency. *Neurobiol. Aging.* **2018**, *71*. [CrossRef] [PubMed]

44. Niu, N.; Xu, S.; Xu, Y.; Little, P.J.; Jin, Z.G. Targeting mechanosensitive transcription factors in atherosclerosis. *Trends Pharmacol. Sci.* **2019**, *40*, 253–266. [CrossRef] [PubMed]
45. Baeyens, N.; Bandyopadhyay, C.; Coon, B.G.; Yun, S.; Schwartz, M.A. Endothelial fluid shear stress sensing in vascular health and disease. *J Clin. Invest.* **2016**, *126*, 821–828. [CrossRef] [PubMed]
46. Wang, S.; Zhang, H.; Wiltshire, T.; Sealock, R.; Faber, J.E. Genetic dissection of the *Canq1* locus governing variation in extent of the collateral circulation. *PLOS One* **2012**, *7*, e31910. [CrossRef] [PubMed]
47. Flurkey, K.; Currer, J.M.; Harrison, D.E. *The Mouse in Biomedical Research*, 2nd ed.; Elsevier: Amsterdam, The Netherlands, 2007; pp. 637–672.
48. Haust, M.D. Endothelial cilia in human aortic atherosclerotic lesions. *Virchows Arch. A* **1987**, *410*, 317–326. [CrossRef]
49. Yamamoto, K.; Fujimoto, S. Endothelial cilium in the capillaries of the human fetal pineal gland. *Microscopy* **1980**, *29*, 256–258.
50. Toomer, K.A.; Fulmer, D.; Guo, L.; Drohan, A.; Peterson, N.; Swanson, P.; Brooks, B.; Mukherjee, R.; Body, S.; Lipschutz, J.H.; et al. A role for primary cilia in aortic valve development and disease. *Dev. Dyn.* **2017**, *246*, 625–634. [CrossRef]
51. Blom, J.N.; Feng, Q. Cardiac repair by epicardial EMT: Current targets and a potential role for the primary cilium. *Pharmacol. Ther.* **2018**, *186*, 114–129. [CrossRef]
52. Bystrevskaya, V.B.; Lichkun, V.V.; Antonov, A.S.; Perov, N.A. An ultrastructural study of centriolar complexes in adult and embryonic human aortic endothelial cells. *Tissue Cell* **1988**, *20*, 493–503. [CrossRef]
53. Lim, Y.C.; McGlashan, S.R.; Cooling, M.T.; Long, D.S. Culture and detection of primary cilia in endothelial cell models. *Cilia* **2015**, *4*, 11. [CrossRef] [PubMed]
54. Pan, J.; Snell, W. The primary cilium: Keeper of the key to cell division. *Cell* **2007**, *129*, 1255–1257. [CrossRef] [PubMed]
55. Boselli, F.; Goetz, J.G.; Charvin, G.; Vermot, J. A quantitative approach to study endothelial cilia bending stiffness during blood flow mechanodetection in vivo. *Methods Cell Biol.* **2015**, *127*, 161–173. [PubMed]
56. Wang, N.; Miao, H.; Li, Y.S.; Zhang, P.; Haga, J.H.; Hu, Y.; Young, A.; Yuan, S.; Nguyen, P.; Wu, C.C.; et al. Shear stress regulation of Krüppellike factor 2 expression is flow pattern-specific. *Biochem. Biophys. Res. Commun.* **2006**, *341*, 1244–1251. [CrossRef] [PubMed]
57. Hierck, B.P.; Van der Heiden, K.; Alkemade, F.E.; Van de Pas, S.; Van Thienen, J.V.; Groenendijk, B.C.; Bax, W.H.; Van der Laarse, A.; Deruiter, M.C.; Horrevoets, A.J.; et al. Primary cilia sensitize endothelial cells for fluid shear stress. *Dev. Dyn.* **2008**, *237*, 725–735. [CrossRef] [PubMed]
58. Hu, X.; De Silva, T.M.; Chen, J.; Faraci, F.M. Cerebral vascular disease and neurovascular injury in ischemic stroke. *Circ. Res.* **2017**, *120*, 449–471. [CrossRef] [PubMed]
59. Dinsmore, C.; Reiter, J.F. Endothelial primary cilia inhibit atherosclerosis. *EMBO Rep.* **2016**, *17*, 156–166. [CrossRef]
60. Sánchez-Duffhues, G.; de Vinuesa, A.G.; Lindeman, J.H.; Mulder-Stapel, A.; DeRuiter, M.C.; Van Munsteren, C.; Goumans, M.J.; Hierck, B.P.; Ten Dijke, P. SLUG is expressed in endothelial cells lacking primary cilia to promote cellular calcification. *Arterioscler. Thromb. Vasc. Biol.* **2015**, *35*, 616–627. [CrossRef]
61. Vion ACAlt, S.; Klaus-Bergmann, A.; Szymborska, A.; Zheng, T.; Perovic, T.; Hammoutene, A.; Oliveira, M.B.; Bartels-Klein, E.; Hollfinger, I.; Rautou, P.E.; et al. Primary cilia sensitize endothelial cells to BMP and prevent excessive vascular regression. *J. Cell. Biol.* **2018**, *217*, 1651–1665. [CrossRef]
62. Chen, X.; Gays, D.; Milia, C.; Santoro, M.M. Cilia control vascular mural cell recruitment in vertebrates. *Cell Rep.* **2017**, *18*, 1033–1047. [CrossRef] [PubMed]
63. Goetz, J.G.; Steed, E.; Ferreira, R.R.; Roth, S.; Ramspacher, C.; Boselli, F.; Charvin, G.; Liebling, M.; Wyart, C.; Schwab, Y.; et al. Endothelial cilia mediate low flow sensing during zebrafish vascular development. *Cell Rep.* **2014**, *6*, 799–808. [CrossRef] [PubMed]
64. Devuyst, O. Variable renal disease progression in autosomal dominant polycystic kidney disease: A role for nitric oxide? *J. Nephrol.* **2003**, *16*, 449–452. [PubMed]
65. Thoma, C.R.; Frew, I.J.; Krek, W. The VHL tumor suppressor: Riding tandem with GSK3beta in primary cilium maintenance. *Cell Cycle* **2007**, *6*, 1809–1813. [CrossRef] [PubMed]

66. Logie, L.; Van Aalten, L.; Knebel, A.; Force, T.; Hastie, C.J.; MacLauchlan, H.; Campbell, D.G.; Gourlay, R.; Prescott, A.; Davidson, J.; et al. Rab-GTPase binding effector protein 2 (RABEP2) is a primed substrate for glycogen synthase kinase-3 (GSK3). *Sci. Rep.* **2017**, *7*, 17682. [CrossRef] [PubMed]
67. Airik, R.; Schueler, M.; Airik, M.; Cho, J.; Ulanowicz, K.A.; Porath, J.D.; Hurd, T.W.; Bekker-Jensen, S.; Schrøder, J.M.; Andersen, J.S.; et al. SDCCAG8 interacts with RAB effector proteins RABEP2 and ERC1 and is required for hedgehog signaling. *PLOS One* **2016**, *11*, e0156081. [CrossRef] [PubMed]
68. Katusic, Z.S.; Austin, S.A. Neurovascular protective function of endothelial nitric oxide—Recent advances. *Circ. J.* **2016**, *80*, 1499–1503. [CrossRef] [PubMed]
69. Zhong, F.; Lee, K.; He, J.C. Role of Krüppel-like factor-2 in kidney disease. *Nephrology* **2018**, *23*, 53–56. [CrossRef] [PubMed]
70. Cheng, Z.; Zou, X.; Jin, Y.; Gao, S.; Lv, J.; Li, B.; Cui, R. The role of KLF4 in Alzheimer's disease. *Front. Cell. Neurosci.* **2018**, *12*, 325. [CrossRef] [PubMed]
71. Sealock, R.; Zhang, H.; Lucitti, J.L.; Moore, S.M.; Faber, J.E. Congenic fine-mapping identifies a major causal locus for variation in the native collateral circulation and ischemic injury in brain and lower extremity. *Circ. Res.* **2014**, *114*, 660–671. [CrossRef]
72. RIGOR. Improving the Quality of NINDS-Supported Preclinical and Clinical Research through Rigorous Study Design and Transparent Reporting. 2012. Available online: http://www.ninds.nih.gov/funding/transparency_in_reporting_guidance.pdf (accessed on 1 May 2019).

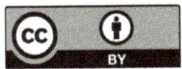

© 2019 by the authors. Licensee MDPI, Basel, Switzerland. This article is an open access article distributed under the terms and conditions of the Creative Commons Attribution (CC BY) license (http://creativecommons.org/licenses/by/4.0/).

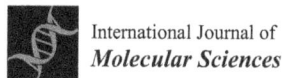

Review

The Extraordinary Role of Extracellular RNA in Arteriogenesis, the Growth of Collateral Arteries

Anna-Kristina Kluever [1], Anna Braumandl [1], Silvia Fischer [2], Klaus T. Preissner [2] and Elisabeth Deindl [1,*]

[1] Walter-Brendel-Center of Experimental Medicine, University Hospital, Ludwig-Maximilians-University, 81377 Munich, Germany; A.Kluever@campus.lmu.de (A.-K.K.); Anna.Braumandl@med.uni-muenchen.de (A.B.)
[2] Institute of Biochemistry, Medical School, Justus-Liebig-University, 35392 Giessen, Germany; Silvia.Fischer@biochemie.med.uni-giessen.de (S.F.); klaus.t.preissner@biochemie.med.uni-giessen.de (K.T.P.)
* Correspondence: elisabeth.deindl@med.uni-muenchen.de; Tel.: +49-89-2180-76504

Received: 18 November 2019; Accepted: 6 December 2019; Published: 7 December 2019

Abstract: Arteriogenesis is an intricate process in which increased shear stress in pre-existing arteriolar collaterals induces blood vessel expansion, mediated via endothelial cell activation, leukocyte recruitment and subsequent endothelial and smooth muscle cell proliferation. Extracellular RNA (eRNA), released from stressed cells or damaged tissue under pathological conditions, has recently been discovered to be liberated from endothelial cells in response to increased shear stress and to promote collateral growth. Until now, eRNA has been shown to enhance coagulation and inflammation by inducing cytokine release, leukocyte recruitment, and endothelial permeability, the latter being mediated by vascular endothelial growth factor (VEGF) signaling. In the context of arteriogenesis, however, eRNA has emerged as a transmitter of shear stress into endothelial activation, mediating the sterile inflammatory process essential for collateral remodeling, whereby the stimulatory effects of eRNA on the VEGF signaling axis seem to be pivotal. In addition, eRNA might influence subsequent steps of the arteriogenesis cascade as well. This article provides a comprehensive overview of the beneficial effects of eRNA during arteriogenesis, laying the foundation for further exploration of the connection between the damaging and non-damaging effects of eRNA in the context of cardiovascular occlusive diseases and of sterile inflammation.

Keywords: arteriogenesis; VEGF; extracellular RNA; shear stress; endothelial activation; mast cell degranulation; macrophages; sterile inflammation; collateral artery growth; TACE

---

1. Introduction

Cardiovascular diseases such as ischemic heart disease, stroke or peripheral arterial occlusive disease are a major public health burden, accounting for approximately 30% of deaths worldwide in 2017 [1]. These diseases are commonly treated with percutaneous coronary interventions involving stents or with coronary bypass surgery. Interestingly enough, the body has a natural non-invasive way of forming a bypass around an occluded vessel called arteriogenesis. During arteriogenesis, blood flow is redirected through preexisting collateral arterioles upon occlusion of a supplying artery [2]. The main stimulus to initiate arteriogenesis in the pre-existing arteriolar vessels is increased fluid shear stress, which subsequently leads to endothelial cell activation, leukocyte extravasation and vessel wall (endothelial and smooth muscle cell) proliferation, substantially increasing the luminal diameter and restoring perfusion [2]. Whilst many of the steps leading to leukocyte extravasation and vessel growth have been uncovered, the crucial missing link of how intravascular shear stress is translated into local endothelial activation and vascular cell growth remained unknown.

Extracellular RNA (eRNA) released upon increased fluid shear stress during arteriogenesis in vivo has recently been suggested to be this missing link by initiating the cascade of arteriogenesis through vascular endothelial growth factor (VEGF)/VEGF receptor 2 (VEGFR2) signaling [3]. eRNA is released from cells upon cellular stress or damage and is mainly composed of rRNA [3,4]. Other forms of extracellular RNA such as microRNA have also been suggested to have a regulatory effect on collateral remodeling during arteriogenesis through modulation of intracellular signaling pathways; however, whether this effect is positive or negative seems to depend on the specific microRNA [5–8]. In terms of cardiovascular disease, eRNA released upon cellular damage has proven to have adverse effects in, e.g., ischemia/reperfusion injury, transplantation or atherosclerosis by mediating vascular edema, thrombus formation and inflammation [9–14]. This review aims to further elucidate the beneficial role of eRNA during the various stages of arteriogenesis.

2. The Role of eRNA in Arteriogenesis

2.1. eRNA Acts as a Translator of Shear Stress during Arteriogenesis through an Endothelial Mechanosensory Complex

The initiating stimulus for collateral remodeling in arteriogenesis is increased arteriolar fluid shear stress as a result of the occlusion of the main supplying artery [15]. In sharp contrast to other forms of vessel growth such as vasculogenesis or angiogenesis, vessel remodeling in arteriogenesis is stimulated by mechanical forces rather than by conditional factors such as hypoxia or ischemia [15,16]. Various mechanisms for shear stress sensing in endothelial cells have been described such as mechano-sensitive ion channels or the entire cytoskeleton transmitting changes in membrane tension (tensegrity architecture) [17]. However, it has recently been suggested that shear stress is in fact translated into endothelial cell activation through a mechanosensory complex, which was previously found to be located on endothelial cells in murine aortas predominantly at sites of non-laminar blood flow [18]. This complex comprises platelet endothelial cell adhesion molecule 1 (PECAM-1), vascular endothelial cell cadherin (VE-cadherin) and VEGFR2, whereby PECAM-1 acts as a mechano-sensor and together with VE-cadherin mediates VEGFR2 activation and subsequent intracellular signaling (Figure 1) [18]. VE-cadherin is an essential component of the endothelial adherens junction, mediating interactions with cytoskeletal anchoring molecules, and has been demonstrated to promote endothelial cell survival by enhancing VEGF-A signaling via VEGFR2 and subsequent phosphatidylinositol-3-OH-kinase activation as well as by activating protein kinase B (Akt) [19,20]. PECAM-1, also an adhesion molecule, has been shown to be involved in collateral remodeling in arteriogenesis as deficiency of PECAM-1 led to an attenuated increase in collateral luminal diameter and leukocyte recruitment to the perivascular space in a murine model of peripheral arteriogenesis [21]. Interestingly, in mice deficient in PECAM-1, the diameter of preexisting collaterals was larger than in wildtype mice; however, the number of preexisting collateral arterioles was comparable in both groups [21]. The signaling pathways activated by this mechanosensory complex that could also be highly relevant in arteriogenesis include (1) VEGFR2 activation, crucial for endothelial proliferation and von Willebrand factor (vWF) release, (2) nuclear factor κB (NFκB) activation, important for enhancing cytokine release and adhesion molecule expression, and (3) phosphatidylinositol-3-OH-kinase and protein kinase B (Akt) activation, essential for promoting endothelial cell survival [18].

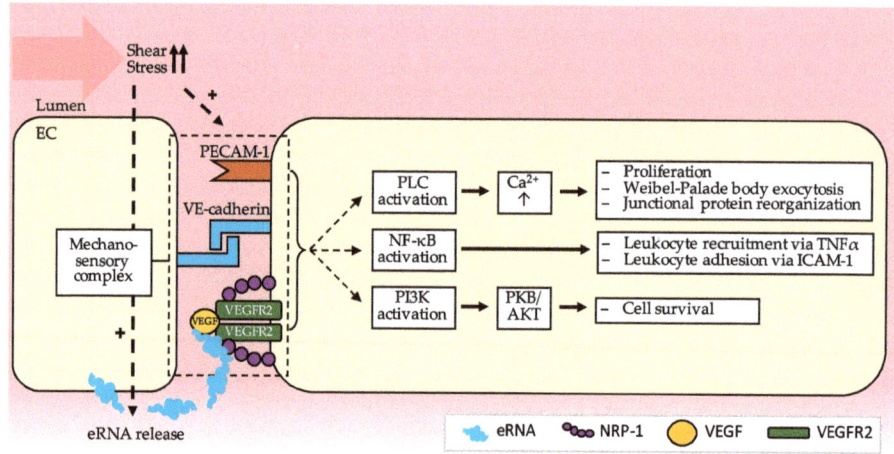

Figure 1. Proposed signaling mechanism downstream of the mechano-sensory complex composed of PECAM-1 (Platelet endothelial cell adhesion molecule (1), VE-cadherin (Vascular endothelial cadherin) and VEGFR2 (Vascular endothelial growth factor receptor (2) which could be relevant in arteriogenesis. eRNA released from EC (endothelial cells) upon shear stress enhances binding of VEGF to VEGFR2 and NRP-1 (Neuropilin-1) thus inducing the signaling mechanisms leading to endothelial cell activation and proliferation as well as leukocyte recruitment and adhesion. The intracellular compartment (EC) is depicted in yellow, the extracellular vessel lumen in red. Arrows indicate the various steps of the signaling pathways. [NF-κB (nuclear factor 'kappa-light-chain-enhancer' of activated B-cells); PI3K (Phosphoinositide 3-kinases); PLC (Phospholipase C); PKB/AKT (Protein kinase B)].

2.1.1. eRNA Initiates Arteriogenesis by Locally Enhancing VEGF/VEGFR2 Signaling

VEGF is a glycoprotein produced by a variety of cell types including leukocytes such as neutrophils or monocytes [22–25] and is critically involved in enhancing endothelial cell proliferation, permeability, and angiogenesis [26–28]. The role of VEGF in arteriogenesis remained uncertain for a long time; however, it has now been established that its downstream signaling events are crucial for this process [3,25]. While it has been demonstrated that the expression of the isoform VEGF-A is not increased in collateral vessels during the process of arteriogenesis and that administration of additional VEGF does not significantly improve collateral vessel development [16,29], antibodies blocking either VEGF or the cognate receptor (VEGFR2) have been shown to interfere greatly with vessel remodeling [25,30,31]. This indicates that VEGFR2 signaling is relevant in arteriogenesis but that endogenous VEGF levels are sufficient for this process [25]. Under physiological conditions, the activation of VEGFR2 induces its dimerization and subsequent tyrosine kinase auto-phosphorylation and endocytosis, thus activating phospholipase C (PLC) and raising intracellular calcium levels [32]. These intracellular signaling events ultimately lead to endothelial activation including the release of Weibel–Palade bodies. Hereby, the co-receptor neuropilin-1 (NRP-1) plays an essential role in linking VEGF and its receptor and in enhancing subsequent intracellular signaling (Figure 2) [32]. In vitro and in vivo studies have demonstrated that NRP-1 is also relevant in arteriogenesis [33,34], whereby its cytoplasmic domain mediates both the co-endocytosis of NRP-1 and VEGFR2 as well as its interaction with synectin [32–34]. These results indicate that the VEGF/VEGFR2 system plays a part in arteriogenesis; nevertheless, they do not explain how VEGFR2 is locally activated in collaterals upon increased shear stress. This is where eRNA comes into play.

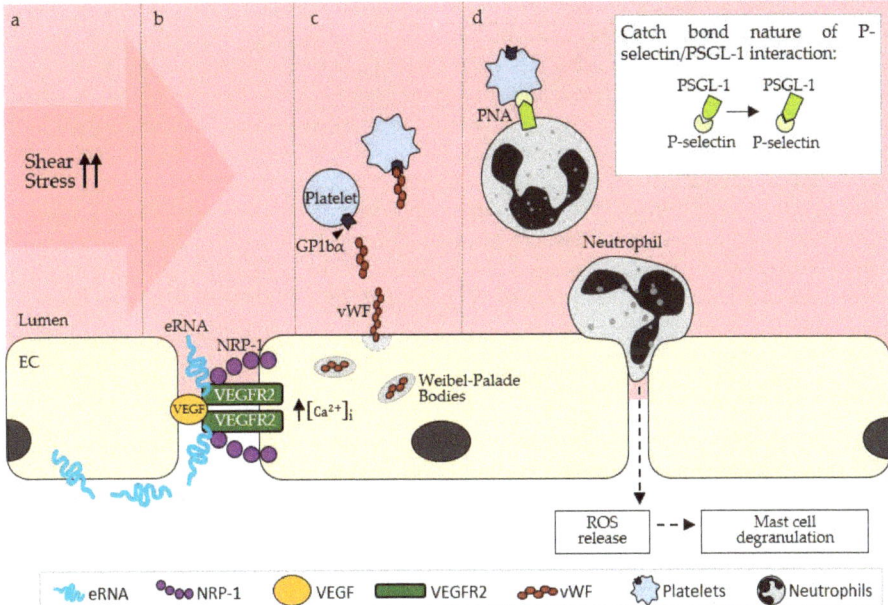

Figure 2. (a) Shear stress-induced activation of endothelial cells (EC) leads to the release of eRNA (extracellular RNA) on their abluminal side. (b) eRNA enhances the binding of VEGF (vascular endothelial growth factor) to NRP-1 (neuropilin (1) thus promoting VEGFR2 (VEGF Receptor (2) intracellular signaling. (c) VEGFR2 mediated raise of intracellular Ca^{2+} leads to the exocytosis of Weibel–Palade bodies and vWF (von Willebrand factor) release, which activates platelets via their GP1bα (Glycoprotein 1bα) receptor. (d) Upon activation, platelets express P-selectin, which subsequently binds its ligand PSGL-1 (P-selectin glycoprotein ligand-1) on neutrophils, inducing the formation of PNAs (platelet-neutrophil aggregates). The bond between P-selectin and PSGL-1 induces a deformational change, which promotes binding in these molecules (catch bond nature). PNA formation enhances neutrophil extravasation followed by ROS (reactive oxygen species) release which promotes mast cell degranulation. The intracellular compartment (EC) is depicted in yellow, the extracellular vessel lumen in red. Arrows indicate the subsequent steps during arteriogenesis.

VEGFR2 activation and signaling have been demonstrated to be involved in mediating the pro-inflammatory and permeability-enhancing effects of eRNA on endothelial cells. Binding studies of eRNA to different VEGF isoforms ($VEGF_{165}$ and $VEGF_{121}$) confirmed that eRNA directly interacts with VEGF, most likely via its heparin binding domain [12]. Whilst eRNA does not alter the expression of either VEGF [12] or of VEGFR2 in vitro [35], it has been shown to enhance the binding of VEGF to NRP-1 in vitro [35]. The formation of this complex of eRNA with VEGF, NRP-1 and VEGFR2 thus promotes PLC-dependent intracellular signaling mechanisms. Since eRNA is released from endothelial cells upon shear stress in vitro [3], it was proposed that eRNA could also play a role in the early steps of arteriogenesis by activating the VEGF/VEGFR2 signaling pathway and thereby inducing endothelial activation. Accordingly, in a murine model of peripheral arteriogenesis, eRNA—mostly rRNA—was found to be released from endothelial cells of developing collaterals, which were exposed to increased shear stress, on their abluminal side [3]. The levels of VEGF bound to the glycocalyx of endothelial cells might be sufficient for initial local signaling induced by eRNA; however, as collateral remodeling progresses, leukocytes might take over the role of supplying VEGF [24,25]. Crucially, this shear stress-induced release of eRNA during arteriogenesis is not related to cellular injury, as no lactate dehydrogenase was released into cell supernatants in vitro [3]. In contrast, eRNA, which is involved in other pathological situations such as stroke, was liberated mostly as a result of tissue damage [9,12]. eRNA seems to play a stimulatory part in arteriogenesis as treatment of mice with RNA-degrading RNase1 led to a smaller increase in luminal diameter of the growing collateral vessels compared to saline-treated control mice and also impaired perfusion recovery in vivo [3,36]. In contrast, administration of DNase or inactive RNase1 did not alter perfusion recovery [3], supporting the notion that the observed effects of RNase1 resulted from the hydrolysis of eRNA rather than from other functions of the endonuclease. In accordance with this, the administration of an RNase inhibitor improved perfusion recovery as well [3], which is highly relevant since eRNA is rapidly degraded in the circulation by RNases under physiological conditions [37]. Therefore, eRNA released upon increased fluid shear stress seems to play a pivotal role in the early processes of arteriogenesis by mediating endothelial cell activation through an enhanced VEGF/NRP-1/VEGFR2 interaction and subsequent intracellular signaling.

2.1.2. Contribution of eRNA in the Promotion of Collateral Remodeling through Stimulation of Endothelial NFκB Signaling

The extravasation of leukocytes, particularly of monocytes, is critical in arteriogenesis, since the cytokines and growth factors released by these cells are essential stimulators of endothelial and smooth muscle cell proliferation [38,39]. eRNA has previously been established as a strong promoter of leukocyte adhesion and extravasation, especially of monocytes, as demonstrated in a murine cremaster model and a murine model of atherosclerosis [11,14]. This pro-inflammatory effect was also confirmed in the process of arteriogenesis [3], where RNase1 treatment reduced the extravasation of neutrophils and monocytes in vivo [3]. In this case, no change in blood levels of leukocytes was observed [3], indicating that eRNA affects local cell interactions but not the systemic cell count. Physiologically and in arteriogenesis, leukocyte transmigration is facilitated by the interaction between endothelial adhesion molecules such as intercellular adhesion molecule 1 (ICAM-1) and leukocyte ligands such as macrophage-1 antigen (Mac-1) [40,41]. The expression of ICAM-1 has independently been shown to be upregulated on the one hand by fluid shear stress in vitro and in vivo [42,43] and on the other hand by eRNA in vitro [14,44]. In an in vivo model of peripheral arteriogenesis, the effects of eRNA on endothelial cell signaling were also demonstrated to be relevant for subsequent leukocyte adhesion, as inhibition of eRNA through RNase administration reduced the perivascular macrophage count to a similar degree as seen in ICAM-1 deficient mice [3].

Two possible ways through which eRNA might affect the expression of ICAM-1 are through stimulation of the NFκB or of the VEGFR2 signaling pathways. VEGF has been shown to induce the upregulation of ICAM-1 in a transgenic mouse model of psoriasis [45], whereby its effects on ICAM-1 expression were demonstrated to be the result of an enhanced VEGF/NRP-1 interaction in a retinal mouse model [46]. Since eRNA enhances the formation of an activated VEGF/NRP-1/VEGFR2 complex during arteriogenesis, it might promote the expression of adhesion molecules on endothelial cells through this avenue of signaling. Nevertheless, eRNA has also been shown to promote the activity of NFκB, which also enhances ICAM-1 expression [47], by inducing the phosphorylation of the cytoplasmic inhibitor of κB (IκB) in vitro [14]. The role of NFκB signaling in arteriogenesis has not yet been studied in detail; however, this pathway was found to be continuously activated in situations of disturbed blood flow such as in atherosclerosis [18]. Furthermore, an increase in the nuclear translocation of NFκB and hence an increase in the expression of its target genes was observed in a rat mesenteric model of collateral growth [48]. Moreover, NFκB is also able to induce the expression of VEGF [49], suggesting that there might be an interplay between these two avenues of signaling in mediating the effects of eRNA on endothelial activation during arteriogenesis.

2.2. eRNA Is Relevant for Mast Cell Degranulation during Arteriogenesis by Stimulating vWF Release and PNA Formation

2.2.1. eRNA Mediates vWF Release from Endothelial Weibel–Palade Bodies by Promoting VEGF/VEGFR2 Signaling

Through its stimulatory effect on VEGF/VEGFR2 signaling, eRNA mediates endothelial activation and the release of vWF from Weibel–Palade bodies, which is essential for subsequent platelet activation and platelet-neutrophil aggregate (PNA) formation in arteriogenesis (Figure 2). Endothelial cell activation as seen in arteriogenesis is characterized to a large extent by a loss of vascular barrier function, luminal expression of adhesion molecules for leukocytes and release of cytokines and pro-coagulatory molecules [50]. eRNA has been associated with all of these events, since it mediates hyper-permeability and vascular edema formation under conditions of ischemia/reperfusion injury or transplantation by disrupting endothelial tight junctions and since it promotes thrombus formation by activating the contact phase system of intrinsic coagulation [4,10,12,13]. In the inflammatory setting of arteriogenesis where eRNA plays such a prominent role, this raises the question of how thrombus formation is inhibited, which will be discussed at a later stage of this review. In addition to these pro-inflammatory and pro-coagulatory effects, eRNA also stimulates the exocytosis of endothelial cell storage granules, designated as Weibel–Palade bodies, which contain vWF, P-Selectin and other cytokines [51–53], as indicated by increased vWF release from endothelial cells upon eRNA exposure in vitro [35]. The exocytosis of Weibel–Palade bodies can also be induced by various other stimuli including thrombin, VEGF and reactive oxygen species (ROS) [54–56]. Weibel–Palade body exocytosis by eRNA was inhibited by an antibody against VEGF [35], suggesting that eRNA stimulates vWF release from endothelial cells via VEGF/VEGFR2 signaling as described above [12]. In the context of arteriogenesis, the ability of eRNA to induce endothelial activation and vWF release via VEGFR2 activation was confirmed, since RNase1 treatment in a murine model of peripheral arteriogenesis decreased luminal vWF levels to a similar extent as seen with vWF deficiency or VEGFR2 inhibition [3].

2.2.2. eRNA-Mediated vWF Release Is Pivotal for PNA Formation

vWF is an adhesive and prothrombotic glycoprotein, constitutively produced by endothelial cells and released from endothelial Weibel–Palade bodies upon cell stimulation. It forms large and ultralarge multimers and plays a key role in the tethering and adhesion of platelets to the injured vessel wall, particularly under fluid shear stress conditions [57,58]. In arteriogenesis, the release of vWF and its interaction with platelets have been demonstrated as pivotal, triggering the activation of platelets and the formation of PNAs (Figure 2) [59,60]. PNAs in turn have been implicated in the recruitment and priming of neutrophils during inflammatory processes and were shown to be relevant for the release of reactive oxygen species (ROS) [61], both of which are relevant in arteriogenesis [60,62]. Following neutrophil extravasation and ROS release, perivascular mast cells are activated and the subsequent extravasation of leukocytes and their release of cytokines and growth factors are increased. In this way, the proliferation of endothelial cells and smooth muscle cells is stimulated, collateral vessels are able to expand, and perfusion can be sufficiently restored. PNAs are also crucial for the formation of neutrophil extracellular traps (NETs), comprising the entire decondensated chromatin of neutrophils, whose formation has also been induced following stimulation of neutrophils with extracellular nucleic acids [63]. In the context of arteriogenesis, though, the formation of NETs has not yet been described. However, since the application of DNase had no effect on perfusion recovery in vivo [3], one can assume that even if NETs are formed during arteriogenesis, they would not have a negative effect on vessel remodeling.

While free platelets do not usually interact with vWF, they are able to transiently bind to vWF via their receptor glycoprotein Ibα (GPIbα) under high fluid shear stress, resulting in platelet activation and adhesion [64]. GPIbα also binds to other pro-coagulatory factors such as thrombin or factors XI and FXII as well as to adhesion molecules such as P-selectin or Mac-1 on immune cells, thereby facilitating cell-cell contacts [65]. Interestingly, the vWF-GPIbα interaction appears to be optimal at high fluid shear stress, a condition which is predominantly found in arterioles [64–66], which is also where vessel remodeling takes places during arteriogenesis. This seems to be due to the fact that shear stress induces conformational changes in the vWF multimers [64], which then facilitate their interactions with platelets. These interactions are also vital in the high shear stress setting of arteriogenesis, where both platelet deficiency and GPIbα deficiency resulted in reduced perfusion recovery in vivo [59]. Once platelets are activated through vWF/GPIbα binding, they express P-selectin on their surface, which is subsequently able to bind to the corresponding P-selectin glycoprotein ligand-1 (PSGL-1) on neutrophils [67,68], enabling the formation of PNAs [60]. The expression of P-selectin has been demonstrated to be increased by shear stress as well [67], and additionally, it was suggested that the resulting adhesive bonds between P-selectin and PSGL-1 are stronger under high fluid shear stress owing to the catch bond nature of selectins [40]. P-selectin and PSGL-1 seem to mediate the interactions of platelets with neutrophils at higher rates of shear stress in vitro, while integrin-mediated interactions seem to be more relevant at lower levels of fluid shear stress [69]. The formation of PNAs was also observed in vivo in the high fluid shear stress setting of arteriogenesis, whereby this binding of platelets to neutrophils was abolished in GPIbα knock-out mice [59], underlining the relevance of vWF release and binding to GPIbα for PNA formation in arteriogenesis.

This important step during collateral remodeling might also be influenced indirectly by eRNA, marking another point where eRNA could play a role during arteriogenesis. In a murine model of arteriogenesis, RNase1 treatment decreased the formation of PNAs to a similar extent as was seen in mice which were either deficient in vWF or treated with a VEGFR2 inhibitor [3], suggesting that VEGF/VEGFR2-dependent eRNA-mediated effects on vWF release also ultimately affect PNA formation. Critically, the administration of RNase1 did not change the blood levels of platelets or neutrophils [3], indicating that eRNA-mediated effects are not systemic but localized to collaterals and do not involve enhanced release of effector cells from the bone marrow. In addition, activated platelets are able to trigger the expression of P-selectin on endothelial cells, thus enabling leukocyte rolling along the activated vessel wall [70]. Such transient interactions of platelets with endothelial cells were also observed in arteriogenesis [59]. In summary, the release of vWF from endothelial Weibel–Palade bodies is a critical step in arteriogenesis as vWF subsequently leads to the activation of platelets and the formation of PNAs, and these processes depend on eRNA, which enhances VEGF/VEGFR2 signaling and endothelial activation.

2.2.3. The Possible Role of ADAMTS13 in the Suppression of Thrombus Formation in Arteriogenesis

The activation of platelets together with the secretion of highly reactive multimeric vWF from endothelial cells under inflammatory conditions during the process of arteriogenesis would provide an ideal setting for thrombus formation. Yet, such an outcome has never been observed, and it remains to be studied in which way local thrombus formation is inhibited during arteriogenesis. Following activation of endothelial cells and the initial release of vWF in a multimeric form to promote platelet adhesion under flow, the readily coagulable nature of these large vWF multimers needs to be weakened at a later phase to prevent the formation of microthrombi [71]. vWF can be cleaved via limited proteolysis by the circulating plasma metalloprotease ADAMTS13 (a disintegrin and metalloprotease with a thrombospondin type 1 motif, member 13) [57]. The deficiency of this protease has been associated with a thrombotic pathology known as thrombotic thrombocytopenic purpura [72]. The interaction between vWF and ADAMTS13 was revealed to be increased under high shear stress in vitro and was maintained even after shear stress was eliminated [58,73]. This effect has been attributed to unfolding of the vWF molecule from a globular to an elongated form upon exposure to shear stress and subsequent exposition of scissile bonds for cleavage by ADAMTS13 [57]. Cleavage of vWF by ADAMTS13 could therefore be a potential mechanism through which thrombus formation could be inhibited in arteriogenesis. In fact, platelet adhesion and aggregation reactions were increased in the arterioles of ADAMTS13-deficient mice compared to wild-type mice; however, this situation could be reversed by the administration of recombinant ADAMTS13 [74]. Furthermore, in a murine model of stroke, ADAMTS13 deficiency was associated with impaired angiogenesis and brain capillary perfusion [75]. The pro-angiogenic properties of ADAMTS13 have been proposed to be due to the phosphorylation of VEGFR2 and upregulation of VEGF, both in vivo and in vitro [75,76], which was also reflected by the fact that an in vitro siRNA-induced knockdown of ADAMTS13 reduced VEGF levels in the cell lysate as well as endothelial proliferation [77]. ADAMTS13 therefore seems to influence VEGF signaling, and since the effect of eRNA on this signaling pathway has proven to be pivotal in arteriogenesis, there might be a link between eRNA and ADAMTS13 in arteriogenesis as well. Yet, the exact role of ADAMTS13 during this process still needs to be assessed.

2.2.4. eRNA is Relevant for Mast Cell Degranulation Following PNA Formation

Following PNA formation, the extravasation of neutrophils is mediated through urokinase-type plasminogen activator (uPA) [60], which, in contrast to tissue plasminogen activator, has been shown to be vital for the transmigration of leukocytes during arteriogenesis in vivo [62]. The subsequent release of NADPH oxidase 2 (Nox2)-derived ROS from neutrophils is crucial for inducing mast cell degranulation [60], whereby neutrophils in PNAs were shown to produce more ROS than non-complexed neutrophils [61]. Both the surface expression of uPA as well as ROS formation via Nox2 were reduced in P-selectin-deficient and PSGL-1-deficient cells in vitro [60], underlining the importance of PNAs in triggering the steps leading to mast cell degranulation in arteriogenesis. Perivascular mast cells in turn have been established as key players during collateral remodeling and have been suggested to act in three ways: (1) by releasing cytokines, which promote the recruitment of growth factor producing leukocytes, (2) by themselves supplying growth factors for the growing collateral, and (3) by activating matrix metalloproteases (MMPs), responsible for extracellular matrix remodeling (Figure 3) [60]. Mast cell degranulation in arteriogenesis has also been shown to be promoted following eRNA stimulation of endothelial VEGF/VEGFR2 signaling, as RNase1 administration impaired mast cell degranulation in an in vivo model of arteriogenesis to a comparable degree as VEGFR2 inhibition and vWF deficiency did without affecting the perivascular mast cell count [3].

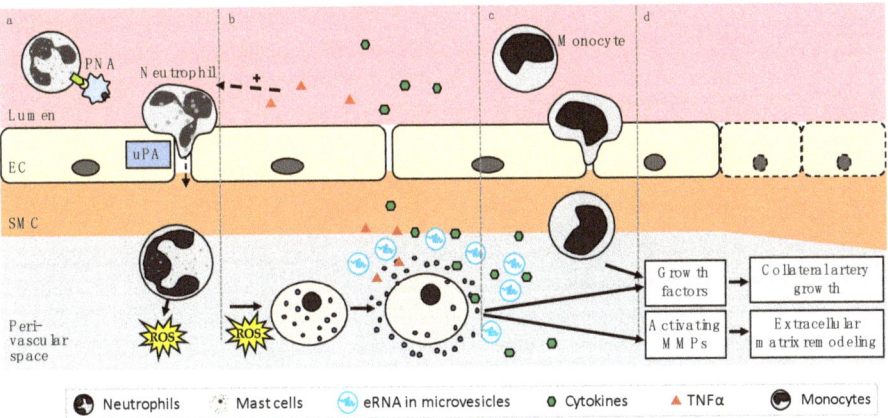

Figure 3. (a) PNA (platelet neutrophil aggregate) formation leads to uPA (Urokinase-type plasminogen activator) mediated neutrophil extravasation and subsequent ROS (reactive oxygen species) release. (b) ROS, released from neutrophils, initiates mast cell degranulation and consecutive release of cytokines, growth factors and eRNA in microvesicles. (c) eRNA and cytokine (especially MCP-1) mediated recruitment and extravasation of monocytes enhances local inflammatory processes leading to (d) collateral artery growth (arteriogenesis) and extracellular matrix remodeling. The extracellular vessel lumen is depicted in red, EC in yellow, SMC in orange, and the perivascular space in gray. Arrows indicate the subsequent steps during arteriogenesis. [EC: endothelial cells; SMC: smooth muscle cells].

2.3. eRNA Released from Mast Cells Provides a Second Stimulatory Boost for Collateral Remodeling

As previously described, eRNA released by endothelial cells upon cellular stress such as fluid shear stress has been attributed an essential role as the translator of shear stress into endothelial activation during the initial stages of collateral remodeling. However, eRNA is rapidly degraded by circulating RNases and could thus only unfold its actions over a short period of time [37]. Arteriogenesis, on the contrary, is a chronic process. Mast cells, whose degranulation is stimulated by the downstream effects of endothelial cell-derived eRNA, also release eRNA in the form of microvesicles concomitantly with degranulation [44]. This release of eRNA has been shown to promote local inflammatory processes and leukocyte extravasation [44]. Microvesicles (MV) are a type of extracellular vesicles that have been described to be released from a variety of cell types including endothelial cells, leukocytes, platelets and mast cells [78–81], often upon cell stress [82], to be involved in cell communication and inflammation including during angiogenesis [82,83], and to be selectively enriched with different types of RNA [84]. Microvesicles/microparticles are generated via budding from the cell membrane and can reach a diameter of up to 1000 nm, whereas exosomes, another type of extracellular vesicle, are released via exocytosis and are generally smaller than 100 nm [82]. In the context of arteriogenesis, this additional release of eRNA in microvesicles might act as a booster of the initial effects mediated by endothelial cell-derived eRNA. What remains to be determined is the exact mechanism through which mast cell-derived eRNA unfolds its effects. However, it is plausible that it also stimulates VEGF/VEGFR2 signaling in endothelial cells. This is supported by the fact that various leukocytes including neutrophils and monocytes, whose extravasation is critical in arteriogenesis, secrete VEGF and have been demonstrated to do so in arteriogenesis [22–25]. In addition, treatment of endothelial cells with MVs derived from mast cells potentiated the release of vWF from endothelial cells just as endothelial cell-derived eRNA did [44]. Besides acting as a positive feedback mechanism for endothelial activation, an important effect of mast cell-derived eRNA might also be the stimulation of the expression of adhesion molecules on endothelial cells as was shown for ICAM-1 in vitro [44]—potentially through VEGFR2 or NFκB signaling.

Furthermore, eRNA released by mast cells might also directly influence leukocyte adhesion, transmigration and cytokine/chemokine release such as of TNFα or MCP-1 during arteriogenesis and might thus amplify the budding local inflammatory response. TNFα is a key pro-inflammatory cytokine released by a variety of cell types including granulocytes, macrophages and smooth muscle cells and is able to enhance leukocyte adhesion, coagulation, and endothelial permeability [85–87]. Its ability to promote MCP-1 expression and monocyte extravasation are extremely relevant in arteriogenesis [88], as is its stimulation of neutrophil and T-cell extravasation [60,89–91]. In a murine model of peripheral arteriogenesis, the inhibition of TNFα lead to reduced perfusion recovery and, in a rabbit model, to a decrease in luminal vessel diameter, smooth muscle cell proliferation and leukocyte extravasation [92,93]. MCP-1 has been established as a major trigger of monocyte recruitment and accelerator of collateral growth during arteriogenesis [94–97], and key sources of this chemokine include macrophages, endothelial cells and smooth muscle cells [98–100]. eRNA was found to promote the release of TNFα from monocytes by activating the TNFα converting enzyme (TACE/ADAM17), which releases soluble TNFα from its membrane-bound form [101]. The inhibition of TACE reduced both the eRNA-mediated release of TNFα in vitro and the adhesion of leukocytes following eRNA administration in vivo [14]. This effect of eRNA on TACE activation in macrophages in vitro was found to involve NFκB signaling [102]. The effects of eRNA on TACE activity in arteriogenesis have not yet been explored; however, it would be interesting to see if eRNA released by mast cells could stimulate the release of TNFα via TACE and thus boost the local inflammatory response. Nevertheless, both TNFα and eRNA were demonstrated to have similar effects on cell adhesion to the endothelium in murine cremaster venules in the context of arteriogenesis [3,14]. The stimulatory effect of eRNA on cell adhesion was abolished by pre-treatment with a VEGFR2 inhibitor (Semaxanib), again highlighting that eRNA enhances VEGFR2 activation, whereas the TNFα-mediated effect was not diminished by pre-treatment with Semaxanib [3], since the release of TNFα occurs at a later stage of arteriogenesis following VEGFR2 activation and signaling. The expression of MCP-1, on the other hand, was increased by MV-derived eRNA from mast cells in vitro [44]. eRNA released by mast cells might therefore activate TACE and thus stimulate TNFα and subsequent MCP-1 release in arteriogenesis, thereby enhancing the local inflammatory response and leukocyte transmigration. In addition, NFκB, whose activation can be stimulated by eRNA as previously touched upon, can also induce the expression of pro-inflammatory cytokines such as TNFα [103], suggesting that mast cell-derived eRNA might also promote local inflammation through this avenue of signaling. However, the exact ways through which this second release of eRNA enhances leukocyte extravasation and collateral remodeling during arteriogenesis still have to be confirmed.

At this point, it is interesting to note that eRNA administration in vitro was shown to prompt a shift in macrophage polarization towards the pro-inflammatory M1 phenotype with an upregulation of pro-inflammatory cytokines such as TNFα and a concurrent downregulation of anti-inflammatory cytokines [104]. In the context of arteriogenesis, the pro-inflammatory M1 macrophage phenotype is important during the initial stages of vessel remodeling, which would correlate with the release of eRNA during arteriogenesis and would suggest that the previously described eRNA-induced shift in macrophage polarization could also occur during arteriogenesis, whilst the anti-inflammatory M2 phenotype is more relevant during later stages of vessel remodeling [105].

3. eRNA in Other Forms of Vessel Growth

The role of eRNA in other forms of vessel growth, namely vasculogenesis and angiogenesis, has not been studied in great detail so far. In vasculogenesis, tRNA and rRNA were found to stimulate the formation of new vessels and the leukocyte differentiation of embryonic bodies via increased VEGF signaling and ROS generation [106]. VEGF signaling is crucial in vasculogenesis [107], and upon eRNA exposure, the expression of $VEGF_{165}$, NRP-1 and other hypoxia related factors such as HIF-1α was increased [106]. ROS formation was also enhanced after eRNA administration [106], which is significant, since the interplay between intracellular VEGF signaling and ROS generation is a central issue of embryoid body differentiation [108]. In angiogenesis, the focus has been more on the stimulatory role of endogenous RNases namely of angiogenin, also known as hRNase5, as a strong promoter of endothelial cell proliferation through its effects on rRNA and ribosome synthesis and its regulatory role in translation during cellular stress [109,110].

4. Conclusions

The remodeling of pre-existing arteriolar collaterals during arteriogenesis is a complex process requiring the highly-coordinated interplay of different leukocytes to promote endothelial and smooth muscle cell proliferation and to ultimately establish perfusion. eRNA has been demonstrated to translate fluid shear stress into endothelial activation during arteriogenesis, further stimulating vWF release, PNA formation, mast cell degranulation and leukocyte recruitment, culminating in the beneficial process of arteriogenesis to promote perfusion recovery. In contrast to the beneficial role of eRNA in arteriogenesis, eRNA has been formerly established as a damaging or pathological factor in a variety of cardiovascular diseases based upon its modulation of endothelial cell and leukocyte function, whereby administration of RNase1 was demonstrated to serve as a tissue- and vessel-protective regimen. It remains to be established which particular molecular interactions and binding partners as well as which putative cellular receptors for eRNA appear to be responsible for its either adverse or beneficial functions in the cardiovascular system.

Author Contributions: Writing—Original Draft Preparation, A.-K.K. and A.B.; Writing—Review & Editing, S.F., K.T.P. and E.D.

Funding: This research received no external funding.

Conflicts of Interest: The authors declare no conflict of interest.

Abbreviations

ADAMTS13	A disintegrin and metalloprotease with a thrombospondin type 1 motif, member 13
eRNA	Extracellular RNA
ICAM-1	Intercellular adhesion molecule 1
Mac-1	Macrophage-1 antigen
MCP-1	Monocyte chemoattractant protein 1
MMP	Matrix metalloprotease
MV	Microvesicle
NFkB	Nuclear factor kB
Nox2	NADPH oxidase 2
NRP-1	Neuropilin-1
PECAM-1	Platelet endothelial cell adhesion molecule 1
PLC	Phospholipase C
PNA	Platelet-neutrophil aggregate
ROS	Reactive oxygen species
TACE	TNFa converting enzyme
TNFa	Tumor necrosis factor a
uPA	Urokinase-type plasminogen activator
VE-cadherin	Vascular endothelial cell cadherin
VEGF	Vascular endothelial growth factor
VEGFR2	Vascular endothelial growth factor receptor 2
vWF	Von Willebrand factor

References

1. GBD 2017 Causes of Death Collaborators. Global, regional, and national age-sex-specific mortality for 282 causes of death in 195 countries and territories, 1980-2017: A systematic analysis for the Global Burden of Disease Study 2017. *Lancet* **2018**, *392*, 1736–1788. [CrossRef]
2. Deindl, E.; Schaper, W. The art of arteriogenesis. *Cell Biochem. Biophys.* **2005**, *43*, 1–15. [CrossRef]
3. Lasch, M.; Kleinert, E.C.; Meister, S.; Kumaraswami, K.; Buchheim, J.I.; Grantzow, T.; Lautz, T.; Salpisti, S.; Fischer, S.; Troidl, K.; et al. Extracellular RNA released due to shear stress controls natural bypass growth by mediating mechanotransduction in mice. *Blood* **2019**, *134*, 1469–1479. [CrossRef] [PubMed]
4. Cabrera-Fuentes, H.A.; Ruiz-Meana, M.; Simsekyilmaz, S.; Kostin, S.; Inserte, J.; Saffarzadeh, M.; Galuska, S.P.; Vijayan, V.; Barba, I.; Barreto, G.; et al. RNase1 prevents the damaging interplay between extracellular RNA and tumour necrosis factor-alpha in cardiac ischaemia/reperfusion injury. *Thromb. Haemost.* **2014**, *112*, 1110–1119. [CrossRef] [PubMed]
5. Zhu, L.P.; Zhou, J.P.; Zhang, J.X.; Wang, J.Y.; Wang, Z.Y.; Pan, M.; Li, L.F.; Li, C.C.; Wang, K.K.; Bai, Y.P.; et al. MiR-15b-5p Regulates Collateral Artery Formation by Targeting AKT3 (Protein Kinase B-3). *Arterioscler. Thromb. Vasc. Biol.* **2017**, *37*, 957–968. [CrossRef] [PubMed]
6. Guan, Y.; Cai, B.; Wu, X.; Peng, S.; Gan, L.; Huang, D.; Liu, G.; Dong, L.; Xiao, L.; Liu, J.; et al. microRNA-352 regulates collateral vessel growth induced by elevated fluid shear stress in the rat hind limb. *Sci. Rep.* **2017**, *7*, 6643. [CrossRef] [PubMed]
7. Heuslein, J.L.; McDonnell, S.P.; Song, J.; Annex, B.H.; Price, R.J. MicroRNA-146a Regulates Perfusion Recovery in Response to Arterial Occlusion via Arteriogenesis. *Front. Bioeng. Biotechnol.* **2018**, *6*, 1. [CrossRef]
8. Lei, Z.; van Mil, A.; Brandt, M.M.; Grundmann, S.; Hoefer, I.; Smits, M.; El Azzouzi, H.; Fukao, T.; Cheng, C.; Doevendans, P.A.; et al. MicroRNA-132/212 family enhances arteriogenesis after hindlimb ischaemia through modulation of the Ras-MAPK pathway. *J. Cell. Mol. Med.* **2015**, *19*, 1994–2005. [CrossRef]
9. Stieger, P.; Daniel, J.M.; Tholen, C.; Dutzmann, J.; Knopp, K.; Gunduz, D.; Aslam, M.; Kampschulte, M.; Langheinrich, A.; Fischer, S.; et al. Targeting of Extracellular RNA Reduces Edema Formation and Infarct Size and Improves Survival After Myocardial Infarction in Mice. *J. Am. Heart Assoc.* **2017**, *6*. [CrossRef]
10. Kleinert, E.; Langenmayer, M.C.; Reichart, B.; Kindermann, J.; Griemert, B.; Blutke, A.; Troidl, K.; Mayr, T.; Grantzow, T.; Noyan, F.; et al. Ribonuclease (RNase) Prolongs Survival of Grafts in Experimental Heart Transplantation. *J. Am. Heart Assoc.* **2016**, *5*. [CrossRef]

11. Simsekyilmaz, S.; Cabrera-Fuentes, H.A.; Meiler, S.; Kostin, S.; Baumer, Y.; Liehn, E.A.; Weber, C.; Boisvert, W.A.; Preissner, K.T.; Zernecke, A. Role of extracellular RNA in atherosclerotic plaque formation in mice. *Circulation* **2014**, *129*, 598–606. [CrossRef] [PubMed]
12. Fischer, S.; Gerriets, T.; Wessels, C.; Walberer, M.; Kostin, S.; Stolz, E.; Zheleva, K.; Hocke, A.; Hippenstiel, S.; Preissner, K.T. Extracellular RNA mediates endothelial-cell permeability via vascular endothelial growth factor. *Blood* **2007**, *110*, 2457–2465. [CrossRef] [PubMed]
13. Kannemeier, C.; Shibamiya, A.; Nakazawa, F.; Trusheim, H.; Ruppert, C.; Markart, P.; Song, Y.; Tzima, E.; Kennerknecht, E.; Niepmann, M.; et al. Extracellular RNA constitutes a natural procoagulant cofactor in blood coagulation. *Proc. Natl. Acad. Sci. USA* **2007**, *104*, 6388–6393. [CrossRef] [PubMed]
14. Fischer, S.; Grantzow, T.; Pagel, J.I.; Tschernatsch, M.; Sperandio, M.; Preissner, K.T.; Deindl, E. Extracellular RNA promotes leukocyte recruitment in the vascular system by mobilising proinflammatory cytokines. *Thromb. Haemost.* **2012**, *108*, 730–741. [CrossRef] [PubMed]
15. Pipp, F.; Boehm, S.; Cai, W.J.; Adili, F.; Ziegler, B.; Karanovic, G.; Ritter, R.; Balzer, J.; Scheler, C.; Schaper, W.; et al. Elevated fluid shear stress enhances postocclusive collateral artery growth and gene expression in the pig hind limb. *Arterioscler. Thromb. Vasc. Biol.* **2004**, *24*, 1664–1668. [CrossRef] [PubMed]
16. Deindl, E.; Buschmann, I.; Hoefer, I.E.; Podzuweit, T.; Boengler, K.; Vogel, S.; van Royen, N.; Fernandez, B.; Schaper, W. Role of ischemia and of hypoxia-inducible genes in arteriogenesis after femoral artery occlusion in the rabbit. *Circ. Res.* **2001**, *89*, 779–786. [CrossRef]
17. Busse, R.; Fleming, I. Regulation of endothelium-derived vasoactive autacoid production by hemodynamic forces. *Trends Pharmacol. Sci.* **2003**, *24*, 24–29. [CrossRef]
18. Tzima, E.; Irani-Tehrani, M.; Kiosses, W.B.; Dejana, E.; Schultz, D.A.; Engelhardt, B.; Cao, G.; DeLisser, H.; Schwartz, M.A. A mechanosensory complex that mediates the endothelial cell response to fluid shear stress. *Nature* **2005**, *437*, 426–431. [CrossRef]
19. Shay-Salit, A.; Shushy, M.; Wolfovitz, E.; Yahav, H.; Breviario, F.; Dejana, E.; Resnick, N. VEGF receptor 2 and the adherens junction as a mechanical transducer in vascular endothelial cells. *Proc. Natl. Acad. Sci. USA* **2002**, *99*, 9462–9467. [CrossRef]
20. Carmeliet, P.; Lampugnani, M.G.; Moons, L.; Breviario, F.; Compernolle, V.; Bono, F.; Balconi, G.; Spagnuolo, R.; Oosthuyse, B.; Dewerchin, M.; et al. Targeted deficiency or cytosolic truncation of the VE-cadherin gene in mice impairs VEGF-mediated endothelial survival and angiogenesis. *Cell* **1999**, *98*, 147–157. [CrossRef]
21. Chen, Z.; Rubin, J.; Tzima, E. Role of PECAM-1 in arteriogenesis and specification of preexisting collaterals. *Circ. Res.* **2010**, *107*, 1355–1363. [CrossRef] [PubMed]
22. Gong, Y.; Koh, D.R. Neutrophils promote inflammatory angiogenesis via release of preformed VEGF in an in vivo corneal model. *Cell Tissue Res.* **2010**, *339*, 437–448. [CrossRef] [PubMed]
23. Ramanathan, M.; Giladi, A.; Leibovich, S.J. Regulation of vascular endothelial growth factor gene expression in murine macrophages by nitric oxide and hypoxia. *Exp. Biol. Med.* **2003**, *228*, 697–705. [CrossRef] [PubMed]
24. Morrison, A.R.; Yarovinsky, T.O.; Young, B.D.; Moraes, F.; Ross, T.D.; Ceneri, N.; Zhang, J.; Zhuang, Z.W.; Sinusas, A.J.; Pardi, R.; et al. Chemokine-coupled beta2 integrin-induced macrophage Rac2-Myosin IIA interaction regulates VEGF-A mRNA stability and arteriogenesis. *J. Exp. Med.* **2014**, *211*, 1957–1968. [CrossRef] [PubMed]
25. Lautz, T.; Lasch, M.; Borgolte, J.; Troidl, K.; Pagel, J.I.; Caballero-Martinez, A.; Kleinert, E.C.; Walzog, B.; Deindl, E. Midkine Controls Arteriogenesis by Regulating the Bioavailability of Vascular Endothelial Growth Factor A and the Expression of Nitric Oxide Synthase 1 and 3. *EBioMedicine* **2018**, *27*, 237–246. [CrossRef] [PubMed]
26. Connolly, D.T.; Heuvelman, D.M.; Nelson, R.; Olander, J.V.; Eppley, B.L.; Delfino, J.J.; Siegel, N.R.; Leimgruber, R.M.; Feder, J. Tumor vascular permeability factor stimulates endothelial cell growth and angiogenesis. *J. Clin. Investig.* **1989**, *84*, 1470–1478. [CrossRef] [PubMed]
27. Yuan, F.; Chen, Y.; Dellian, M.; Safabakhsh, N.; Ferrara, N.; Jain, R.K. Time-dependent vascular regression and permeability changes in established human tumor xenografts induced by an anti-vascular endothelial growth factor/vascular permeability factor antibody. *Proc. Natl. Acad. Sci. USA* **1996**, *93*, 14765–14770. [CrossRef]
28. Leung, D.W.; Cachianes, G.; Kuang, W.J.; Goeddel, D.V.; Ferrara, N. Vascular endothelial growth factor is a secreted angiogenic mitogen. *Science* **1989**, *246*, 1306–1309. [CrossRef]

29. Pipp, F.; Heil, M.; Issbrucker, K.; Ziegelhoeffer, T.; Martin, S.; van den Heuvel, J.; Weich, H.; Fernandez, B.; Golomb, G.; Carmeliet, P.; et al. VEGFR-1-selective VEGF homologue PlGF is arteriogenic: Evidence for a monocyte-mediated mechanism. *Circ. Res.* **2003**, *92*, 378–385. [CrossRef]
30. Lloyd, P.G.; Prior, B.M.; Li, H.; Yang, H.T.; Terjung, R.L. VEGF receptor antagonism blocks arteriogenesis, but only partially inhibits angiogenesis, in skeletal muscle of exercise-trained rats. *Am. J. Physiol. Heart Circ. Physiol.* **2005**, *288*, H759–H768. [CrossRef]
31. Toyota, E.; Warltier, D.C.; Brock, T.; Ritman, E.; Kolz, C.; O'Malley, P.; Rocic, P.; Focardi, M.; Chilian, W.M. Vascular endothelial growth factor is required for coronary collateral growth in the rat. *Circulation* **2005**, *112*, 2108–2113. [CrossRef] [PubMed]
32. Koch, S.; Claesson-Welsh, L. Signal transduction by vascular endothelial growth factor receptors. *Cold Spring Harb. Perspect. Med.* **2012**, *2*, a006502. [CrossRef] [PubMed]
33. Lanahan, A.; Zhang, X.; Fantin, A.; Zhuang, Z.; Rivera-Molina, F.; Speichinger, K.; Prahst, C.; Zhang, J.; Wang, Y.; Davis, G.; et al. The neuropilin 1 cytoplasmic domain is required for VEGF-A-dependent arteriogenesis. *Dev. Cell* **2013**, *25*, 156–168. [CrossRef] [PubMed]
34. Lanahan, A.A.; Hermans, K.; Claes, F.; Kerley-Hamilton, J.S.; Zhuang, Z.W.; Giordano, F.J.; Carmeliet, P.; Simons, M. VEGF receptor 2 endocytic trafficking regulates arterial morphogenesis. *Dev. Cell* **2010**, *18*, 713–724. [CrossRef] [PubMed]
35. Fischer, S.; Nishio, M.; Peters, S.C.; Tschernatsch, M.; Walberer, M.; Weidemann, S.; Heidenreich, R.; Couraud, P.O.; Weksler, B.B.; Romero, I.A.; et al. Signaling mechanism of extracellular RNA in endothelial cells. *FASEB J.* **2009**, *23*, 2100–2109. [CrossRef]
36. Landre, J.B.; Hewett, P.W.; Olivot, J.M.; Friedl, P.; Ko, Y.; Sachinidis, A.; Moenner, M. Human endothelial cells selectively express large amounts of pancreatic-type ribonuclease (RNase 1). *J. Cell. Biochem.* **2002**, *86*, 540–552. [CrossRef]
37. Tsui, N.B.; Ng, E.K.; Lo, Y.M. Stability of endogenous and added RNA in blood specimens, serum, and plasma. *Clin. Chem.* **2002**, *48*, 1647–1653.
38. Arras, M.; Ito, W.D.; Scholz, D.; Winkler, B.; Schaper, J.; Schaper, W. Monocyte activation in angiogenesis and collateral growth in the rabbit hindlimb. *J. Clin. Investig.* **1998**, *101*, 40–50. [CrossRef]
39. Hoefer, I.E.; Grundmann, S.; van Royen, N.; Voskuil, M.; Schirmer, S.H.; Ulusans, S.; Bode, C.; Buschmann, I.R.; Piek, J.J. Leukocyte subpopulations and arteriogenesis: Specific role of monocytes, lymphocytes and granulocytes. *Atherosclerosis* **2005**, *181*, 285–293. [CrossRef]
40. Ley, K.; Laudanna, C.; Cybulsky, M.I.; Nourshargh, S. Getting to the site of inflammation: The leukocyte adhesion cascade updated. *Nat. Rev. Immunol.* **2007**, *7*, 678–689. [CrossRef]
41. Hoefer, I.E.; van Royen, N.; Rectenwald, J.E.; Deindl, E.; Hua, J.; Jost, M.; Grundmann, S.; Voskuil, M.; Ozaki, C.K.; Piek, J.J.; et al. Arteriogenesis proceeds via ICAM-1/Mac-1- mediated mechanisms. *Circ. Res.* **2004**, *94*, 1179–1185. [CrossRef] [PubMed]
42. Scholz, D.; Ito, W.; Fleming, I.; Deindl, E.; Sauer, A.; Wiesnet, M.; Busse, R.; Schaper, J.; Schaper, W. Ultrastructure and molecular histology of rabbit hind-limb collateral artery growth (arteriogenesis). *Virchows Arch.* **2000**, *436*, 257–270. [CrossRef] [PubMed]
43. Morigi, M.; Zoja, C.; Figliuzzi, M.; Foppolo, M.; Micheletti, G.; Bontempelli, M.; Saronni, M.; Remuzzi, G.; Remuzzi, A. Fluid shear stress modulates surface expression of adhesion molecules by endothelial cells. *Blood* **1995**, *85*, 1696–1703. [CrossRef] [PubMed]
44. Elsemuller, A.K.; Tomalla, V.; Gartner, U.; Troidl, K.; Jeratsch, S.; Graumann, J.; Baal, N.; Hackstein, H.; Lasch, M.; Deindl, E.; et al. Characterization of mast cell-derived rRNA-containing microvesicles and their inflammatory impact on endothelial cells. *FASEB J.* **2019**, *33*, 5457–5467. [CrossRef] [PubMed]
45. Xia, Y.P.; Li, B.; Hylton, D.; Detmar, M.; Yancopoulos, G.D.; Rudge, J.S. Transgenic delivery of VEGF to mouse skin leads to an inflammatory condition resembling human psoriasis. *Blood* **2003**, *102*, 161–168. [CrossRef] [PubMed]
46. Wang, J.; Wang, S.; Li, M.; Wu, D.; Liu, F.; Yang, R.; Ji, S.; Ji, A.; Li, Y. The Neuropilin-1 Inhibitor, ATWLPPR Peptide, Prevents Experimental Diabetes-Induced Retinal Injury by Preserving Vascular Integrity and Decreasing Oxidative Stress. *PLoS ONE* **2015**, *10*, e0142571. [CrossRef]
47. Numata, T.; Ito, T.; Maeda, T.; Egusa, C.; Tsuboi, R. IL-33 promotes ICAM-1 expression via NF-kB in murine mast cells. *Allergol. Int.* **2016**, *65*, 158–165. [CrossRef]

48. Unthank, J.L.; McClintick, J.N.; Labarrere, C.A.; Li, L.; Distasi, M.R.; Miller, S.J. Molecular basis for impaired collateral artery growth in the spontaneously hypertensive rat: Insight from microarray analysis. *Physiol. Rep.* **2013**, *1*, e0005. [CrossRef]
49. Huang, S.; Pettaway, C.A.; Uehara, H.; Bucana, C.D.; Fidler, I.J. Blockade of NF-kappaB activity in human prostate cancer cells is associated with suppression of angiogenesis, invasion, and metastasis. *Oncogene* **2001**, *20*, 4188–4197. [CrossRef]
50. Hunt, B.J.; Jurd, K.M. Endothelial cell activation. A central pathophysiological process. *Bmj (Clin. Res. Ed.)* **1998**, *316*, 1328–1329. [CrossRef]
51. Wagner, D.D.; Olmsted, J.B.; Marder, V.J. Immunolocalization of von Willebrand protein in Weibel-Palade bodies of human endothelial cells. *J. Cell Biol* **1982**, *95*, 355–360. [CrossRef] [PubMed]
52. McEver, R.P.; Beckstead, J.H.; Moore, K.L.; Marshall-Carlson, L.; Bainton, D.F. GMP-140, a platelet alpha-granule membrane protein, is also synthesized by vascular endothelial cells and is localized in Weibel-Palade bodies. *J. Clin. Investig.* **1989**, *84*, 92–99. [CrossRef] [PubMed]
53. Utgaard, J.O.; Jahnsen, F.L.; Bakka, A.; Brandtzaeg, P.; Haraldsen, G. Rapid secretion of prestored interleukin 8 from Weibel-Palade bodies of microvascular endothelial cells. *J. Exp. Med.* **1998**, *188*, 1751–1756. [CrossRef] [PubMed]
54. Matsushita, K.; Yamakuchi, M.; Morrell, C.N.; Ozaki, M.; O'Rourke, B.; Irani, K.; Lowenstein, C.J. Vascular endothelial growth factor regulation of Weibel-Palade-body exocytosis. *Blood* **2005**, *105*, 207–214. [CrossRef] [PubMed]
55. Vischer, U.M.; Jornot, L.; Wollheim, C.B.; Theler, J.M. Reactive oxygen intermediates induce regulated secretion of von Willebrand factor from cultured human vascular endothelial cells. *Blood* **1995**, *85*, 3164–3172. [CrossRef]
56. Van den Biggelaar, M.; Hernandez-Fernaud, J.R.; van den Eshof, B.L.; Neilson, L.J.; Meijer, A.B.; Mertens, K.; Zanivan, S. Quantitative phosphoproteomics unveils temporal dynamics of thrombin signaling in human endothelial cells. *Blood* **2014**, *123*, e22–e36. [CrossRef]
57. Crawley, J.T.; de Groot, R.; Xiang, Y.; Luken, B.M.; Lane, D.A. Unraveling the scissile bond: How ADAMTS13 recognizes and cleaves von Willebrand factor. *Blood* **2011**, *118*, 3212–3221. [CrossRef]
58. Shim, K.; Anderson, P.J.; Tuley, E.A.; Wiswall, E.; Sadler, J.E. Platelet-VWF complexes are preferred substrates of ADAMTS13 under fluid shear stress. *Blood* **2008**, *111*, 651–657. [CrossRef]
59. Chandraratne, S.; von Bruehl, M.L.; Pagel, J.I.; Stark, K.; Kleinert, E.; Konrad, I.; Farschtschi, S.; Coletti, R.; Gartner, F.; Chillo, O.; et al. Critical role of platelet glycoprotein ibalpha in arterial remodeling. *Arterioscler. Thromb. Vasc. Biol.* **2015**, *35*, 589–597. [CrossRef]
60. Chillo, O.; Kleinert, E.C.; Lautz, T.; Lasch, M.; Pagel, J.I.; Heun, Y.; Troidl, K.; Fischer, S.; Caballero-Martinez, A.; Mauer, A.; et al. Perivascular Mast Cells Govern Shear Stress-Induced Arteriogenesis by Orchestrating Leukocyte Function. *Cell Rep.* **2016**, *16*, 2197–2207. [CrossRef]
61. Page, C.; Pitchford, S. Neutrophil and platelet complexes and their relevance to neutrophil recruitment and activation. *Int. Immunopharmacol.* **2013**, *17*, 1176–1184. [CrossRef] [PubMed]
62. Deindl, E.; Ziegelhoffer, T.; Kanse, S.M.; Fernandez, B.; Neubauer, E.; Carmeliet, P.; Preissner, K.T.; Schaper, W. Receptor-independent role of the urokinase-type plasminogen activator during arteriogenesis. *FASEB J.* **2003**, *17*, 1174–1176. [CrossRef] [PubMed]
63. Brinkmann, V.; Reichard, U.; Goosmann, C.; Fauler, B.; Uhlemann, Y.; Weiss, D.S.; Weinrauch, Y.; Zychlinsky, A. Neutrophil Extracellular Traps Kill Bacteria. *Science* **2004**, *303*, 1532–1535. [CrossRef] [PubMed]
64. Sadler, J.E. Contact—How platelets touch von Willebrand factor. *Science* **2002**, *297*, 1128–1129. [CrossRef] [PubMed]
65. Andrews, R.K.; Gardiner, E.E.; Shen, Y.; Whisstock, J.C.; Berndt, M.C. Glycoprotein Ib-IX-V. *Int. J. Biochem. Cell Biol.* **2003**, *35*, 1170–1174. [CrossRef]
66. Savage, B.; Saldivar, E.; Ruggeri, Z.M. Initiation of platelet adhesion by arrest onto fibrinogen or translocation on von Willebrand factor. *Cell* **1996**, *84*, 289–297. [CrossRef]
67. Goto, S.; Ichikawa, N.; Lee, M.; Goto, M.; Sakai, H.; Kim, J.J.; Yoshida, M.; Handa, M.; Ikeda, Y.; Handa, S. Platelet surface P-selectin molecules increased after exposing platelet to a high shear flow. *Int. Angiol.* **2000**, *19*, 147–151.

68. Moore, K.L.; Patel, K.D.; Bruehl, R.E.; Li, F.; Johnson, D.A.; Lichenstein, H.S.; Cummings, R.D.; Bainton, D.F.; McEver, R.P. P-selectin glycoprotein ligand-1 mediates rolling of human neutrophils on P-selectin. *J. Cell Biol.* **1995**, *128*, 661–671. [CrossRef]
69. Xiao, Z.; Goldsmith, H.L.; McIntosh, F.A.; Shankaran, H.; Neelamegham, S. Biomechanics of P-selectin PSGL-1 bonds: Shear threshold and integrin-independent cell adhesion. *Biophys. J.* **2006**, *90*, 2221–2234. [CrossRef]
70. Dole, V.S.; Bergmeier, W.; Mitchell, H.A.; Eichenberger, S.C.; Wagner, D.D. Activated platelets induce Weibel-Palade-body secretion and leukocyte rolling in vivo: Role of P-selectin. *Blood* **2005**, *106*, 2334–2339. [CrossRef]
71. De Wit, T.R.; van Mourik, J.A. Biosynthesis, processing and secretion of von Willebrand factor: Biological implications. *Best Pract. Res. Clin. Haematol.* **2001**, *14*, 241–255. [CrossRef] [PubMed]
72. Levy, G.G.; Nichols, W.C.; Lian, E.C.; Foroud, T.; McClintick, J.N.; McGee, B.M.; Yang, A.Y.; Siemieniak, D.R.; Stark, K.R.; Gruppo, R.; et al. Mutations in a member of the ADAMTS gene family cause thrombotic thrombocytopenic purpura. *Nature* **2001**, *413*, 488–494. [CrossRef] [PubMed]
73. Feys, H.B.; Anderson, P.J.; Sadler, J.E. Binding of ADAMTS13 to Von Willebrand Factor Under Static Conditions and Under Fluid Shear Stress. *Blood* **2008**, *112*, 258. [CrossRef]
74. Chauhan, A.K.; Motto, D.G.; Lamb, C.B.; Bergmeier, W.; Dockal, M.; Plaimauer, B.; Scheiflinger, F.; Ginsburg, D.; Wagner, D.D. Systemic antithrombotic effects of ADAMTS13. *J. Exp. Med.* **2006**, *203*, 767–776. [CrossRef] [PubMed]
75. Xu, H.; Cao, Y.; Yang, X.; Cai, P.; Kang, L.; Zhu, X.; Luo, H.; Lu, L.; Wei, L.; Bai, X.; et al. ADAMTS13 controls vascular remodeling by modifying VWF reactivity during stroke recovery. *Blood* **2017**, *130*, 11–22. [CrossRef]
76. Lee, M.; Keener, J.; Xiao, J.; Long Zheng, X.; Rodgers, G.M. ADAMTS13 and its variants promote angiogenesis via upregulation of VEGF and VEGFR2. *Cell. Mol. Life Sci.* **2015**, *72*, 349–356. [CrossRef]
77. Tang, H.; Lee, M.; Kim, E.H.; Bishop, D.; Rodgers, G.M. siRNA-knockdown of ADAMTS-13 modulates endothelial cell angiogenesis. *Microvasc. Res.* **2017**, *113*, 65–70. [CrossRef]
78. Wheway, J.; Latham, S.L.; Combes, V.; Grau, G.E. Endothelial microparticles interact with and support the proliferation of T cells. *J.Immunol.* **2014**, *193*, 3378–3387. [CrossRef]
79. Mesri, M.; Altieri, D.C. Endothelial cell activation by leukocyte microparticles. *J. Immunol.* **1998**, *161*, 4382–4387.
80. Baj-Krzyworzeka, M.; Majka, M.; Pratico, D.; Ratajczak, J.; Vilaire, G.; Kijowski, J.; Reca, R.; Janowska-Wieczorek, A.; Ratajczak, M.Z. Platelet-derived microparticles stimulate proliferation, survival, adhesion, and chemotaxis of hematopoietic cells. *Exp. Hematol.* **2002**, *30*, 450–459. [CrossRef]
81. Kunder, C.A.; St John, A.L.; Li, G.; Leong, K.W.; Berwin, B.; Staats, H.F.; Abraham, S.N. Mast cell-derived particles deliver peripheral signals to remote lymph nodes. *J. Exp. Med.* **2009**, *206*, 2455–2467. [CrossRef] [PubMed]
82. Van der Pol, E.; Boing, A.N.; Harrison, P.; Sturk, A.; Nieuwland, R. Classification, functions, and clinical relevance of extracellular vesicles. *Pharmacol. Rev.* **2012**, *64*, 676–705. [CrossRef] [PubMed]
83. Shai, E.; Varon, D. Development, cell differentiation, angiogenesis–microparticles and their roles in angiogenesis. *Arterioscler. Thromb. Vasc. Biol.* **2011**, *31*, 10–14. [CrossRef] [PubMed]
84. Skog, J.; Wurdinger, T.; van Rijn, S.; Meijer, D.H.; Gainche, L.; Sena-Esteves, M.; Curry, W.T., Jr.; Carter, B.S.; Krichevsky, A.M.; Breakefield, X.O. Glioblastoma microvesicles transport RNA and proteins that promote tumour growth and provide diagnostic biomarkers. *Nat. Cell Biol.* **2008**, *10*, 1470–1476. [CrossRef] [PubMed]
85. Bradley, J.R. TNF-mediated inflammatory disease. *J. Pathol.* **2008**, *214*, 149–160. [CrossRef] [PubMed]
86. Bowers, E.; Slaughter, A.; Frenette, P.S.; Kuick, R.; Pello, O.M.; Lucas, D. Granulocyte-derived TNFalpha promotes vascular and hematopoietic regeneration in the bone marrow. *Nat. Med.* **2018**, *24*, 95–102. [CrossRef]
87. Tanaka, H.; Sukhova, G.; Schwartz, D.; Libby, P. Proliferating arterial smooth muscle cells after balloon injury express TNF-alpha but not interleukin-1 or basic fibroblast growth factor. *Arterioscler. Thromb. Vasc. Biol.* **1996**, *16*, 12–18. [CrossRef]
88. Buschmann, I.R.; Hoefer, I.E.; van Royen, N.; Katzer, E.; Braun-Dulleaus, R.; Heil, M.; Kostin, S.; Bode, C.; Schaper, W. GM-CSF: A strong arteriogenic factor acting by amplification of monocyte function. *Atherosclerosis* **2001**, *159*, 343–356. [CrossRef]

89. Griffin, G.K.; Newton, G.; Tarrio, M.L.; Bu, D.X.; Maganto-Garcia, E.; Azcutia, V.; Alcaide, P.; Grabie, N.; Luscinskas, F.W.; Croce, K.J.; et al. IL-17 and TNF-alpha sustain neutrophil recruitment during inflammation through synergistic effects on endothelial activation. *J. Immunol.* **2012**, *188*, 6287–6299. [CrossRef]
90. Stabile, E.; Burnett, M.S.; Watkins, C.; Kinnaird, T.; Bachis, A.; la Sala, A.; Miller, J.M.; Shou, M.; Epstein, S.E.; Fuchs, S. Impaired arteriogenic response to acute hindlimb ischemia in CD4-knockout mice. *Circulation* **2003**, *108*, 205–210. [CrossRef]
91. Stabile, E.; Kinnaird, T.; la Sala, A.; Hanson, S.K.; Watkins, C.; Campia, U.; Shou, M.; Zbinden, S.; Fuchs, S.; Kornfeld, H.; et al. CD8+ T lymphocytes regulate the arteriogenic response to ischemia by infiltrating the site of collateral vessel development and recruiting CD4+ mononuclear cells through the expression of interleukin-16. *Circulation* **2006**, *113*, 118–124. [CrossRef] [PubMed]
92. Hoefer, I.E.; van Royen, N.; Rectenwald, J.E.; Bray, E.J.; Abouhamze, Z.; Moldawer, L.L.; Voskuil, M.; Piek, J.J.; Buschmann, I.R.; Ozaki, C.K. Direct evidence for tumor necrosis factor-alpha signaling in arteriogenesis. *Circulation* **2002**, *105*, 1639–1641. [CrossRef] [PubMed]
93. Grundmann, S.; Hoefer, I.; Ulusans, S.; van Royen, N.; Schirmer, S.H.; Ozaki, C.K.; Bode, C.; Piek, J.J.; Buschmann, I. Anti-tumor necrosis factor-{alpha} therapies attenuate adaptive arteriogenesis in the rabbit. *Am. J. Physiol. Heart Circ. Physiol.* **2005**, *289*, H1497–H1505. [CrossRef] [PubMed]
94. Schirmer, S.H.; Buschmann, I.R.; Jost, M.M.; Hoefer, I.E.; Grundmann, S.; Andert, J.P.; Ulusans, S.; Bode, C.; Piek, J.J.; van Royen, N. Differential effects of MCP-1 and leptin on collateral flow and arteriogenesis. *Cardiovasc. Res.* **2004**, *64*, 356–364. [CrossRef] [PubMed]
95. Ito, W.D.; Arras, M.; Winkler, B.; Scholz, D.; Schaper, J.; Schaper, W. Monocyte chemotactic protein-1 increases collateral and peripheral conductance after femoral artery occlusion. *Circ. Res.* **1997**, *80*, 829–837. [CrossRef] [PubMed]
96. Hoefer, I.E.; van Royen, N.; Buschmann, I.R.; Piek, J.J.; Schaper, W. Time course of arteriogenesis following femoral artery occlusion in the rabbit. *Cardiovasc. Res.* **2001**, *49*, 609–617. [CrossRef]
97. Gunn, M.D.; Nelken, N.A.; Liao, X.; Williams, L.T. Monocyte chemoattractant protein-1 is sufficient for the chemotaxis of monocytes and lymphocytes in transgenic mice but requires an additional stimulus for inflammatory activation. *J. Immunol.* **1997**, *158*, 376–383.
98. Deshmane, S.L.; Kremlev, S.; Amini, S.; Sawaya, B.E. Monocyte chemoattractant protein-1 (MCP-1): An overview. *J. Interferon Cytokine Res.* **2009**, *29*, 313–326. [CrossRef]
99. Kinoshita, M.; Okada, M.; Hara, M.; Furukawa, Y.; Matsumori, A. Mast cell tryptase in mast cell granules enhances MCP-1 and interleukin-8 production in human endothelial cells. *Arterioscler. Thromb. Vasc. Biol.* **2005**, *25*, 1858–1863. [CrossRef]
100. Cushing, S.D.; Berliner, J.A.; Valente, A.J.; Territo, M.C.; Navab, M.; Parhami, F.; Gerrity, R.; Schwartz, C.J.; Fogelman, A.M. Minimally modified low density lipoprotein induces monocyte chemotactic protein 1 in human endothelial cells and smooth muscle cells. *Proc. Natl. Acad. Sci. USA* **1990**, *87*, 5134–5138. [CrossRef]
101. Black, R.A.; Rauch, C.T.; Kozlosky, C.J.; Peschon, J.J.; Slack, J.L.; Wolfson, M.F.; Castner, B.J.; Stocking, K.L.; Reddy, P.; Srinivasan, S.; et al. A metalloproteinase disintegrin that releases tumour-necrosis factor-alpha from cells. *Nature* **1997**, *385*, 729–733. [CrossRef] [PubMed]
102. Fischer, S.; Gesierich, S.; Griemert, B.; Schanzer, A.; Acker, T.; Augustin, H.G.; Olsson, A.K.; Preissner, K.T. Extracellular RNA liberates tumor necrosis factor-alpha to promote tumor cell trafficking and progression. *Cancer Res.* **2013**, *73*, 5080–5089. [CrossRef] [PubMed]
103. Abraham, E. NF-kappaB activation. *Crit. Care Med.* **2000**, *28*, N100–N104. [CrossRef] [PubMed]
104. Cabrera-Fuentes, H.A.; Lopez, M.L.; McCurdy, S.; Fischer, S.; Meiler, S.; Baumer, Y.; Galuska, S.P.; Preissner, K.T.; Boisvert, W.A. Regulation of monocyte/macrophage polarisation by extracellular RNA. *Thromb. Haemost.* **2015**, *113*, 473–481. [CrossRef] [PubMed]
105. Troidl, C.; Jung, G.; Troidl, K.; Hoffmann, J.; Mollmann, H.; Nef, H.; Schaper, W.; Hamm, C.W.; Schmitz-Rixen, T. The temporal and spatial distribution of macrophage subpopulations during arteriogenesis. *Curr. Vasc. Pharmacol.* **2013**, *11*, 5–12. [CrossRef] [PubMed]
106. Sharifpanah, F.; De Silva, S.; Bekhite, M.M.; Hurtado-Oliveros, J.; Preissner, K.T.; Wartenberg, M.; Sauer, H. Stimulation of vasculogenesis and leukopoiesis of embryonic stem cells by extracellular transfer RNA and ribosomal RNA. *Free Radic. Biol. Med.* **2015**, *89*, 1203–1217. [CrossRef] [PubMed]

107. Bekhite, M.M.; Finkensieper, A.; Binas, S.; Muller, J.; Wetzker, R.; Figulla, H.R.; Sauer, H.; Wartenberg, M. VEGF-mediated PI3K class IA and PKC signaling in cardiomyogenesis and vasculogenesis of mouse embryonic stem cells. *J. Cell Sci.* **2011**, *124*, 1819–1830. [CrossRef]
108. Ushio-Fukai, M.; Urao, N. Novel role of NADPH oxidase in angiogenesis and stem/progenitor cell function. *Antioxid. Redox Signal.* **2009**, *11*, 2517–2533. [CrossRef]
109. Lu, L.; Li, J.; Moussaoui, M.; Boix, E. Immune Modulation by Human Secreted RNases at the Extracellular Space. *Front. Immunol.* **2018**, *9*, 1012. [CrossRef]
110. Fett, J.W.; Strydom, D.J.; Lobb, R.R.; Alderman, E.M.; Bethune, J.L.; Riordan, J.F.; Vallee, B.L. Isolation and characterization of angiogenin, an angiogenic protein from human carcinoma cells. *Biochemistry* **1985**, *24*, 5480–5486. [CrossRef]

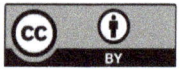

© 2019 by the authors. Licensee MDPI, Basel, Switzerland. This article is an open access article distributed under the terms and conditions of the Creative Commons Attribution (CC BY) license (http://creativecommons.org/licenses/by/4.0/).

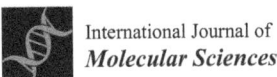

Communication

A Simple and Effective Flow Cytometry-Based Method for Identification and Quantification of Tissue Infiltrated Leukocyte Subpopulations in a Mouse Model of Peripheral Arterial Disease

Konda Kumaraswami [1,2], Natallia Salei [1,2], Sebastian Beck [1,2], Stephan Rambichler [1,2], Anna-Kristina Kluever [1,2], Manuel Lasch [1,2,3], Lisa Richter [4], Barbara U. Schraml [1,2] and Elisabeth Deindl [1,2,*]

1. Walter-Brendel-Centre of Experimental Medicine, University Hospital, LMU Munich, 81377 Munich, Germany; Kumaraswami.Konda@med.uni-muenchen.de (K.K.); Natallia.Salei@med.uni-muenchen.de (N.S.); s.beck1@campus.lmu.de (S.B.); stephan.rambichler@med.uni-muenchen.de (S.R.); annakluever97@gmail.com (A.-K.K.); manuel_lasch@gmx.de (M.L.); barbara.schraml@med.uni-muenchen.de (B.U.S.)
2. Biomedical Center, Institute of Cardiovascular Physiology and Pathophysiology, LMU Munich, 82152 Planegg-Martinsried, Germany
3. Department of Otorhinolaryngology, Head & Neck Surgery, University Hospital, LMU Munich, 81377 Munich, Germany
4. Core Facility Flow Cytometry, Biomedical Centre, LMU Munich, 82152 Planegg-Martinsried, Germany; l.richter@med.uni-muenchen.de
* Correspondence: Elisabeth.Deindl@med.uni-muenchen.de; Tel.: +49-89-2180-76504

Received: 6 May 2020; Accepted: 16 May 2020; Published: 19 May 2020

Abstract: Arteriogenesis, the growth of a natural bypass from pre-existing arteriolar collaterals, is an endogenous mechanism to compensate for the loss of an artery. Mechanistically, this process relies on a locally and temporally restricted perivascular infiltration of leukocyte subpopulations, which mediate arteriogenesis by supplying growth factors and cytokines. Currently, the state-of-the-art method to identify and quantify these leukocyte subpopulations in mouse models is immunohistology. However, this is a time consuming procedure. Here, we aimed to develop an optimized protocol to identify and quantify leukocyte subpopulations by means of flow cytometry in adductor muscles containing growing collateral arteries. For that purpose, adductor muscles of murine hindlimbs were isolated at day one and three after induction of arteriogenesis, enzymatically digested, and infiltrated leukocyte subpopulations were identified and quantified by flow cytometry, as exemplary shown for neutrophils and macrophages (defined as $CD45^+/CD11b^+/Ly6G^+$ and $CD45^+/CD11b^+/F4/80^+$ cells, respectively). In summary, we show that flow cytometry is a suitable method to identify and quantify leukocyte subpopulations in muscle tissue, and provide a detailed protocol. Flow cytometry constitutes a timesaving tool compared to histology, which might be used in addition for precise localization of leukocytes in tissue samples.

Keywords: peripheral arterial disease; arteriogenesis; shear stress; flow cytometry; leukocytes; immunohistology; inflammation; collateral artery growth

1. Introduction

Peripheral occlusive diseases, including atherosclerosis, myocardial infarction and stroke, are a wide spectrum of arterial-based pathologies, reported as one of the leading causes of death worldwide [1]. Currently, the therapeutic options mainly consist of surgical interventions such as balloon dilatation and stent implantation, as well as bypass surgery [2]. However, the body possesses an endogenous mechanism to compensate for stenosis and obstructions by forming natural bypasses. This process is called arteriogenesis [3]. Understanding the mechanisms of arteriogenesis can help to design new therapeutic options to accelerate the process of arteriogenesis in patients with the final aim of minimizing invasive interventions and avoiding amputation.

Previous studies, predominantly performed on murine hindlimb models [4], showed that arteriogenesis essentially depends on the recruitment of leukocytes to the perivascular space, where these cells subsequently supply growth factors for collateral remodeling [5,6]. At present, immunohistochemical (IHC) staining is the technique of choice for analyzing and quantifying the leukocyte subpopulations involved in this process. However, this method is very time-consuming. Analysis by flow cytometry offers an elegant and time-saving alternative to IHC especially in regard to the quantification of leukocytes.

2. Materials

2.1. Mice

C57BL/6J, 8–12 weeks old male mice from Charles River were used. Animal studies were conducted in compliance with ethical standards and with the approval of the Government of Upper Bavaria, Germany. Mice were anesthetized with the standard solution of fentanyl (0.05 mg/kg), midazolam (5 mg/kg) and medetomidine (0.5 mg/kg) applied subcutaneously (s.c.). To antagonize the narcosis, a combination of naloxone (1.2 mg/kg), flumazenile (0.5 mg/kg) and atipamezole (2.5 mg/kg) was applied s.c. To prevent postsurgical pain, mice were treated with buprenorphine (0.05 mg/kg) every 12 h until day 3.

2.2. Reagents

- Fentanyl (CuraMED Pharma, Karlsruhe, Germany)
- Midazolam (Ratiopharm GmbH, Ulm, Germany)
- Medetomidine (Pfizer Pharma, Berlin, Germany)
- Buprenorphine (Reckitt Benckiser Healthcare, London, UK)
- Naloxone (Inresa Arzneimittel GmbH, Freiburg, Germany)
- Flumazenile (Inresa Arzneimittel GmbH, Freiburg, Germany)
- Atipamezole (Zoetis, Berlin, Germany)
- Phosphate buffered saline (PBS, Sigma-Aldrich, Taufkirchen, Germany, cat. D8537)
- 1% fetal bovine serum (FBS, Sigma-Aldrich, Taufkirchen, Germany, cat. F7524)
- Ethylenediaminetetraaceticacid (EDTA, Invitrogen, Waltham, MA, USA, cat. 15575020)
- 0.02% sodium azide (Sigma-Aldrich, Taufkirchen, Germany, cat. 71289)
- Collagenase IV (10,000 U/ml, Worthington, Freehold, NJ, USA, cat. CLS4)
- DNase I (20 mg/ml, Roche, Penzberg, Germany, cat. 11284932001)
- RPMI 1640 medium (Gibco, Dubline, Ireland, cat. 31870-074)
- Percoll (GE Healthcare, Chicago, IL, USA, cat. 17-0891-01)
- Hank's Balanced Salt solution (HBSS, Sigma-Aldrich, Taufkirchen, Germany, cat. H9394-500ML)
- Mounting medium (Thermo Fisher Scientific, Schwerte, Germany, cat. TA-030-FM)
- 4% paraformaldehyde (PFA, Morphisto, Frankfurt am Main, Germany, cat. 1176.00500)

The following antibodies were used for flow cytometry:

- PE/Cy7 anti-mouse CD45.2 (Biolegend, Eching, Germany, cat. 109829, clone: 104, 1/300 dilution)
- BUV737 anti-CD11b (BD Biosciences, Heidelberg, Germany, cat. 564443, clone: M1/70, 1/800 dilution)

- Brilliant Violet 785 anti-mouse F4/80 (Biolegend, Eching, Germany, cat. 123141, clone: BM8, 1/100 dilution)
- PerCP/Cy5.5 anti-mouse Ly6G (Biolegend, Eching, Germany, cat. 127615, clone: 1A8, 1/300 dilution)
- Anti-CD16/32 (BD Biosciences, Heidelberg, Germany, cat. 553142, clone: 2.4G2, 1/300 dilution)
- DAPI (4′, 6-diamidin-2-phenylindole, Sigma-Aldrich, Taufkirchen, Germany, Cat. D9542-5MG, 1/1000 dilution)

The following antibodies were used for immunohistological staining:

- Neutrophils (Ly6G, eBiosciences, San Diego, CA, USA, cat. 16-9668-82, 1/50 dilution)
- Macrophages (CD68-AF488, Abcam, Cambridge, UK, cat. ab201844, 1/100 dilution)
- Endothelial cells (CD31-AF647, BioLegend, cat. 102516, 1/50 dilution)
- Anti-mouse AF546 secondary antibody (Invitrogen, Waltham, MA, USA, cat. A11081, 1/200 dilution)

The following equipment were employed for measurements:

- Bijou sample container (Sigma-Aldrich, Taufkirchen, Germany, cat. Z645338-700EA)
- Scissors (Fine Science Tools, Heidelberg, Germany, cat. 812005-10)
- Falcon tubes 15mL and 50mL (Thermo Fisher Scientific, cat. 10468502/10788561)
- Falcon cell strainer (Thermo Fisher Scientific, cat. 352350)
- 96 well plate (V-bottom, Costar, Schwerte, Germany, cat. 3897)

2.3. Flow Cytometry

Flow cytometry measurements were performed using BD LSRFortessa (BD Biosciences) and analyzed on BD FACSDiva v8.0 and FlowJo-v10 software (BD Biosciences).

2.4. Immunohistochemical Analysis

Images were acquired using a Zeiss epifluorescent microscope (Carl Zeiss Microscopy GmbH, Munic, Germany) and analyzed using AxioVisionRel 4.8 software (Carl Zeiss Microscopy GmbH).

3. Methods

3.1. Reagent Preparation

For flow cytometric cell analysis, the following reagents were prepared: FACS buffer, enzyme solution, and three gradient Percoll solutions.

The FACS buffer was prepared as a solution of PBS, 1% fetal bovine serum, 2.5 mM EDTA and 0.02% sodium azide.

Two-fold concentrated enzyme solution was prepared using a solution of collagenase IV and DNase I at a concentration of 400 U/ml (collagenase IV) and 0.4 mg/mL (DNase I) in RPMI-1640, respectively.

For isotonic Percoll stock solution, 45 mL Percoll and 5 mL 10× PBS were mixed. The solution was then prepared in three concentrations (70%, 37% and 30%). For 70% and 30% Percoll, the prepared Percoll stock solution was diluted with Hank's Balanced Salt solution with phenol red. For 37% Percoll, the prepared Percoll stock solution was diluted with PBS. Different diluents were used for easy recognition of phases.

3.2. Surgical Procedure for Artery Ligation and Tissue Collection

The murine hindlimb ischemia model is a widely used mouse model to study arteriogenesis in detail [7]. The femoral artery of the right leg is ligated, while the left leg is sham operated and serves as an internal control [8]. After femoral artery ligation (FAL), the blood flow is redirected into preexisting arteriolar connections, which thereupon experience increased shear stress [9,10], and results in perivascular recruitment of leukocytes supplying growth factors and cytokines to the growing vessels [5,6].

Depending on the experimental setup, the muscle tissue, in which collaterals are located, can be removed at various time points after arterial occlusion. To analyze the numbers and subpopulations of recruited leukocytes, we have chosen two time points: day 1 and day 3 after femoral artery ligation. For this purpose, the hindlimbs of the mice were perfused with FACS buffer via an aortic catheter (inserted distal to the outlet of the renal arteries). Thereafter, the adductor muscle of the mouse was removed along the dashed line as shown in Figure 1, whereby the femoral artery (FA) and profunda femoris artery (PA) were omitted from isolation. The muscle section was immediately rinsed with FACS buffer and further processed on ice.

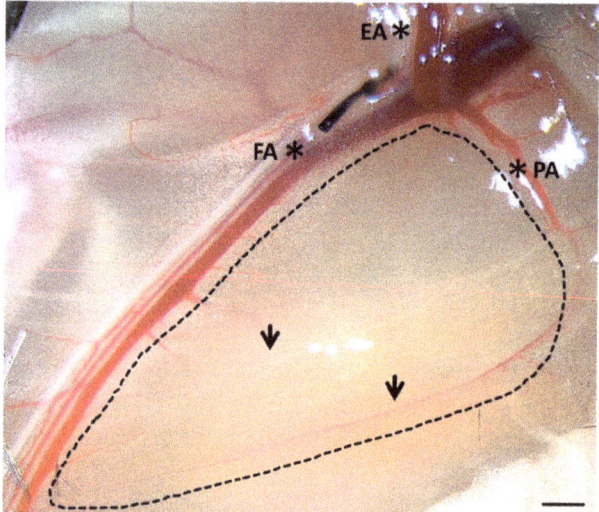

Figure 1. Tissue sampling on the right hindlimb of a C57BL/6J mouse. The part of the M. adductor containing the collaterals (arrows) was extracted along the dashed line. The collaterals connect the profunda femoris artery (PA) to the femoral artery (FA). The epigastric artery (EA) serves as orientation for the ligation. Scale bar 1 mm.

3.3. Stepwise Preparation of a Single Cell Suspension from Collected Tissues

To prepare a single cell suspension for flow cytometric analysis, collected tissue samples were processed using the following protocol:

1. Place the muscle tissue (isolated from one hindlimb) in a bijou vial containing 1 mL of RPMI medium and finely cut the muscle with microsurgical scissors.
2. Add 1 mL of enzyme solution to digest the tissue (final concentration of collagenase IV and DNase I are 200 U/mL and 0.2 mg/mL, respectively).
3. Incubate the tube in a laboratory shaker for 1 h at 37 °C with 120 rpm.
4. Filter the digested tissue through a 70 μm cell strainer and fill up to 50 mL with FACS buffer.
5. Centrifuge the cells for 5 min at 4 °C with 420 g, then carefully discard the supernatant.
6. Resuspend the cell pellet in 4 mL of 70% Percoll.
7. Gently cover the solution with 4 mL of 37% Percoll followed by 1 mL of 30% Percoll.
8. Centrifuge for 30 min at room temperature with 940 g. Centrifuge acceleration and braking should be set to minimum to avoid disintegration of the Percoll gradient.

9. Remove the interphase cells located between the 70% and 37% phases, transfer them to a 15 mL Falcon tube and fill up to 15 mL with the FACS buffer.
10. Centrifuge the cells for 5 min at 4 °C with 420 g, then discard the supernatant.
11. Resuspend the cells in 100 μl FACS buffer for further processing (if the leukocyte subpopulation of interest is not frequent, cells from mice of the same group can be pooled).

3.4. Cell Staining for Flow Cytometry

For cell staining, the single cell suspension that was prepared from collected tissues was processed using the following protocol:

1. Transfer the cell suspension to a 96-well V-bottom plate.
2. Centrifuge the cells for 5 min at 4 °C with 420 g, then discard supernatant by decantation.
3. Resuspend the cells in 50 μL Fc-Block (FACS buffer containing 1.6 μg/mL anti-CD16/32).
4. Incubate for 10 min at 4 °C.
5. Add 50 μL of a two-fold concentrated staining solution (50μL FACS buffer with anti-CD45.2, anti-CD11b, anti-Ly6G and anti-F4/80).
6. Incubate the solution for 20 min at 4 °C in the dark.
7. Centrifuge for 5 min at 4 °C with 420 g, then discard the supernatant.
8. Resuspend the cells twice in 200 μL FACS buffer.
9. Centrifuge for 5 min at 4 °C with 420 g, then discard the supernatant.
10. Resuspend the stained cells in 100 μL FACS buffer.
11. Add 1 μL of 20 μg/mL DAPI in PBS to the cell suspension just before the measurement.
12. Analyze the cell suspension using a flow cytometer.

3.5. Immunohistochemical Staining

Adductor muscle tissue samples were collected after perfusion as previously described [8]. For staining, 10 μm thick frozen sections were used. The following protocol for staining was used:

1. Fix the sections in 4% PFA for 5 min.
2. Wash the sections in PBS for 5 min, repeat twice.
3. Add blocking buffer (1% BSA in PBST) to sections to prevent nonspecific binding.
4. Incubate for 30 min at room temperature.
5. Dilute the primary antibodies against all leukocytes, macrophages, neutrophils and endothelial cells in blocking buffer.
6. Incubate the sections in a humidified dark chamber at 4 °C overnight.
7. Wash the sections in PBS for 5 min, repeat twice.
8. Incubate the sections with anti-mouse AF546 secondary antibody (only for CD45 and Ly6G) for 1 h at room temperature.
9. Wash the sections in PBS for 5 min, repeat twice.
10. Follow the overnight incubation with antibody against endothelial cells.
11. Wash the sections in PBS for 5 min, repeat twice.
12. Incubate the sections with DAPI for 10 min at room temperature.
13. Wash the sections in PBS for 5 min, repeat twice.
14. Fix the sections with mounting medium, then store at 4 °C.

3.6. Statistical Analyses

Statistical analysis was performed using GraphPad Prism v. 8 software. Data are mean ± standard error of the mean (S.E.M.). Significances between two time points were calculated by unpaired student's t-test. $p < 0.05$ was considered statistically significant.

4. Results

Figure 2a shows the gating strategy used for the identification of leukocyte subpopulations, i.e., neutrophils and macrophages. First, we gated on leukocytes based on forward scatter (FSC) and side scatter (SSC) properties and excluded small cell debris. Next, we gated on single cells by plotting the height against the area for forward scatter (FSC-H vs FSC-A), and the width for side scatter against the area for forward scatter (SSC-W vs FSC-A). After doublets exclusion, we distinguished live cells (identified as DAPI negative) CD45.2$^+$ leukocytes. Within live leukocytes we identified CD11b$^+$ and Ly6G$^+$ neutrophils, CD11b$^+$ and F4/80$^+$ macrophages. The proportion of neutrophils and macrophages were quantified on day 1 and 3 after ligation (Figure 2b). IHC staining demonstrated a localization of neutrophils and macrophages in the perivascular space of growing collateral arteries in the adductor muscle of mice as exemplary shown for day 3 after induction of arteriogenesis by FAL (Figure 2c).

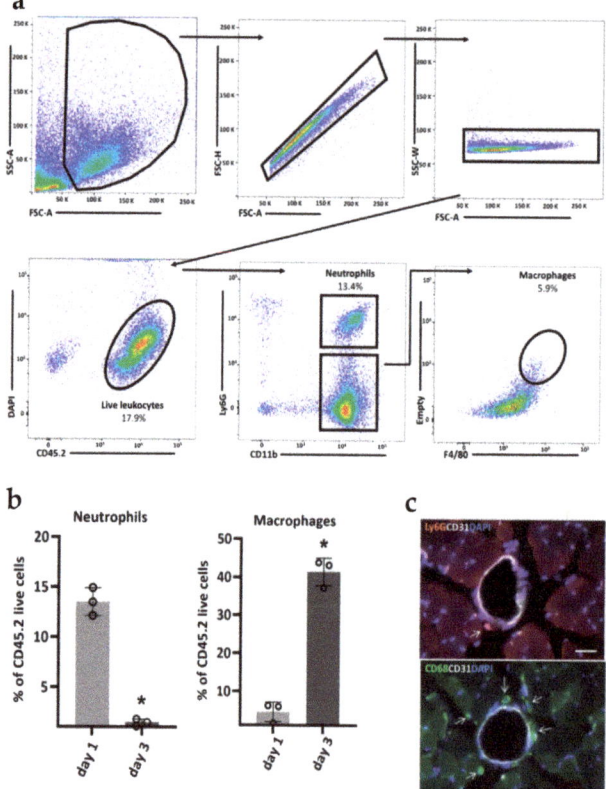

Figure 2. Gating strategy of flow cytometry and immunohistological analyses. (**a**) Sequential gating strategy for the identification of neutrophils (CD45.2$^+$CD11b$^+$Ly6G$^+$) and macrophages (CD45.2$^+$CD11b$^+$F4/80$^+$) in the murine adductor muscle containing growing collateral arteries at day 1 after FAL. (**b**) Bar graphs showing the frequencies of neutrophils and macrophages at day 1 and day 3 after FAL. $n = 3$ mice/group, data are represented as mean ± S.E.M., * $p < 0.05$ from unpaired student's t-test. (**c**) Representative immunohistochemical stains demonstrate the presence of neutrophils (Ly6G$^+$) and macrophages (CD68$^+$) (indicated by arrows) in the perivascular space of growing collaterals in the adductor muscle of a mouse 3 days after FAL. Collaterals were stained with an endothelial marker (CD31) and nuclei with DAPI. Scale bar 20 µm.

5. Conclusions

Flow cytometry is an effective and high-throughput method to analyze and quantify infiltrated leukocyte subpopulations in muscle tissue. If necessary, it can be supplemented by IHC studies on the localization of those leukocytes.

The protocol includes some limitations. Inadequate perfusion of the animals may be associated with residuals of leukocyte in vessels, resulting in inconsistent data. Poor enzymatic muscle digestion may lower the cell yield. In addition, cell preparation that involves washing and centrifugation might lead to cell loss of an unknown extent.

However, when accurately performed, flow cytometry is an elegant method that can be used to complement results obtained from histological analysis, especially those pertaining to cell differentiation and cell counting. Further, flow cytometric analysis gives the possibility to calculate the absolute number of leukocytes per mg muscle tissue by the addition of counting beads to the cell suspension. With the increasing functions of flow cytometers, the further development of tissue extraction methods as well as the capacity to stain various markers on cell surfaces and in the cell interior, the application spectrum of flow cytometry is extremely broad.

Author Contributions: Conceptualization, K.K., N.S., S.B., S.R. and E.D.; methodology, K.K., N.S., S.R. and L.R.; validation, K.K., N.S., S.R., L.R. and B.U.S.; investigation, K.K., N.S., S.R. and L.R.; data curation, K.K.; writing—original draft preparation, K.K., N.S., S.R., and S.B.; writing—review and editing, N.S., S.R., A.-K.K., M.L., L.R., B.U.S. and E.D.; supervision, B.U.S., E.D.; project administration, B.U.S. and E.D.; funding acquisition, B.U.S. and E.D. All authors have read and agreed to the published version of the manuscript.

Funding: This work was supported by the Lehre@LMU program (A.-K.K., E.D.) and the Förderprogramm für Forschung und Lehre (FöFoLe) (S.B., E.D.) from the LMU Munich. The work in the Schraml lab was supported by the German Research Foundation (Emmy Noether grant: Schr 1444/1-1; and project number 360372040—SFB 1335—project 8, to Schraml) and the European Research Council (ERC-2016-STG-715182).

Conflicts of Interest: The authors declare no conflict of interest.

Abbreviations

IHC	immunohistochemical
FACS	Fluorescence Activated Cell Sorting
FA	femoral artery
FAL	femoral artery ligation
PA	profunda femoris artery
EA	epigastric artery
FCS	forward scatter
SSC	side scatter

References

1. WHO. *Global Health Estimates 2016: Disease Burden by Cause, Age, Sex, by Country and by Region, 2000–2016*; World Health Organiozation: Geneva, Switzerland, 2018.
2. Shishehbor, M.H.; Jaff, M.R. Percutaneous Therapies for Peripheral Artery Disease. *Circulation* **2016**, *134*, 2008–2027. [CrossRef] [PubMed]
3. Schaper, W.; Scholz, D. Factors regulating arteriogenesis. *Arterioscler. Thromb. Vasc. Biol.* **2003**, *23*, 1143–1151. [CrossRef] [PubMed]
4. Troidl, C.; Jung, G.; Troidl, K.; Hoffmann, J.; Mollmann, H.; Nef, H.; Schaper, W.; Hamm, C.W.; Schmitz-Rixen, T. The temporal and spatial distribution of macrophage subpopulations during arteriogenesis. *Curr. Vasc. Pharmacol.* **2013**, *11*, 5–12. [CrossRef] [PubMed]
5. Arras, M.; Ito, W.D.; Scholz, D.; Winkler, B.; Schaper, J.; Schaper, W. Monocyte activation in angiogenesis and collateral growth in the rabbit hindlimb. *J. Clin. Investig.* **1998**, *101*, 41–50. [CrossRef] [PubMed]
6. Chillo, O.; Kleinert, E.C.; Lautz, T.; Lasch, M.; Pagel, J.I.; Heun, Y.; Troidl, K.; Fischer, S.; Caballero-Martinez, A.; Mauer, A.; et al. Perivascular Mast Cells Govern Shear Stress-Induced Arteriogenesis by Orchestrating Leukocyte Function. *Cell Rep.* **2016**, *16*, 2197–2207. [CrossRef]

7. Aref, Z.; de Vries, M.R.; Quax, P.H.A. Variations in Surgical Procedures for Inducing Hind Limb Ischemia in Mice and the Impact of These Variations on Neovascularization Assessment. *Int. J. Mol. Sci.* **2019**, *20*, 3704. [CrossRef] [PubMed]
8. Limbourg, A.; Korff, T.; Napp, L.C.; Schaper, W.; Drexler, H.; Limbourg, F.P. Evaluation of postnatal arteriogenesis and angiogenesis in a mouse model of hind-limb ischemia. *Nat. Protoc.* **2009**, *4*, 1737–1746. [CrossRef] [PubMed]
9. Lasch, M.; Nekolla, K.; Klemm, A.H.; Buchheim, J.I.; Pohl, U.; Dietzel, S.; Deindl, E. Estimating hemodynamic shear stress in murine peripheral collateral arteries by two-photon line scanning. *Mol. Cell. Biochem.* **2019**, *453*, 41–51. [CrossRef] [PubMed]
10. Pipp, F.; Boehm, S.; Cai, W.J.; Adili, F.; Ziegler, B.; Karanovic, G.; Ritter, R.; Balzer, J.; Scheler, C.; Schaper, W.; et al. Elevated fluid shear stress enhances postocclusive collateral artery growth and gene expression in the pig hind limb. *Arterioscler. Thromb. Vasc. Biol.* **2004**, *24*, 1664–1668. [CrossRef] [PubMed]

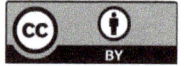

© 2020 by the authors. Licensee MDPI, Basel, Switzerland. This article is an open access article distributed under the terms and conditions of the Creative Commons Attribution (CC BY) license (http://creativecommons.org/licenses/by/4.0/).

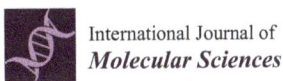

Article

IL10 Alters Peri-Collateral Macrophage Polarization and Hind-Limb Reperfusion in Mice after Femoral Artery Ligation

Alexander M. Götze [1,*], Christian Schubert [2], Georg Jung [3], Oliver Dörr [4], Christoph Liebetrau [5], Christian W. Hamm [5], Thomas Schmitz-Rixen [3], Christian Troidl [4,†] and Kerstin Troidl [2,3,†]

1. Department of Trauma-, Hand- and Reconstructive Surgery, Johann-Wolfgang-Goethe-University, 60590 Frankfurt am Main, Germany
2. Max-Planck Institute for Heart- and Lung-Research, 61231 Bad Nauheim, Germany; christian.schubert@mpi-bn.mpg.de (C.S.); kerstin.troidl@mpi-bn.mpg.de (K.T.)
3. Department of Vascular and Endovascular Surgery, Johann-Wolfgang-Goethe-University, 60590 Frankfurt am Main, Germany; Georg.Jung@kgu.de (G.J.); schmitz-rixen@em.uni-frankfurt.de (T.S.-R.)
4. Department of Cardiology, Justus-Liebig-University, 35392 Gießen, Germany; oliver.doerr@innere.med.uni-giessen.de (O.D.); c.troidl@kerckhoff-fgi.de (C.T.)
5. Department of Cardiology, Kerckhoff Heart and Thorax Center, 61231 Bad Nauheim, Germany; c.liebetrau@kerckhoff-klinik.de (C.L.); c.hamm@kerckhoff-klinik.de (C.W.H.)
* Correspondence: a.goetze@icloud.com; Tel.: +49-172-2363336
† These authors contributed equally to this work.

Received: 31 March 2020; Accepted: 15 April 2020; Published: 17 April 2020

Abstract: Arteriogenesis is a process by which a pre-existing arterioarterial anastomosis develops into a functional collateral network following an arterial occlusion. Alternatively activated macrophages polarized by IL10 have been described to promote collateral growth. This study investigates the effect of different levels of IL10 on hind-limb reperfusion and the distribution of perivascular macrophage activation types in mice after femoral artery ligation (FAL). IL10 and anti-IL10 were administered before FAL and the arteriogenic response was measured by Laser-Doppler-Imaging perioperatively, after 3, 7, and 14 d. Reperfusion recovery was accelerated when treated with IL10 and impaired with anti-IL10. Furthermore, symptoms of ischemia on ligated hind-limbs had the highest incidence after application of anti-IL10. Perivascular macrophages were immunohistologically phenotyped using CD163 and CD68 in adductor muscle segments. The proportion of alternatively activated macrophages ($CD163^+/CD68^+$) in relation to classically activated macrophages ($CD163^-/CD68^+$) observed was the highest when treated with IL10 and suppressed with anti-IL10. This study underlines the proarteriogenic response with increased levels of IL10 and demonstrates an in-vivo alteration of macrophage activation types in the perivascular bed of growing collaterals.

Keywords: arteriogenesis; collateral artery; macrophages; macrophage polarization; M2 macrophages; IL10

1. Introduction

Arteriogenesis is the process by which a pre-existing arterioarterial anastomosis develops into a functional collateral network following an arterial occlusion. The remodeling processes involved in collateral vessel growth are complex and are dependent on mechanical, cellular and molecular factors [1]. Several authors have demonstrated the pertinence of monocytes and macrophages in enhancing collateral vessel growth [1–3]. While there is still debate over whether perivascular macrophages are recruited from circulating monocytes or tissue resident precursors, their proarteriogenic effects, however, are still evident [4–6]. Macrophage activation types have become a growing focus in arteriogenesis research, in particular alternatively activated macrophages [7]. Macrophage heterogeneity and plasticity are reflected by their ability to respond to environmental cues giving rise to a spectrum of distinct functional phenotypes or activation states, fulfilling a variety of functions. The extremes of these functional states are commonly defined as M1, M2, or M2-like polarized macrophages [8]. M1 or classically activated macrophages induced by LPS, IFN-γ, and TNF are associated with inflammation and tumor resistance. They differ from M2 macrophages with regard to their arginine metabolism by exhibiting high levels of iNOS and subsequent NO-synthesis, as well as the production of proinflammatory cytokines and chemoattractant proteins. M2/M2-like or alternatively activated macrophages induced by IL4/IL13, immune complexes, agonists of TLR or IL1R, glucocorticoids and IL10, on the other hand, regulate inflammatory responses and promote tissue remodeling, angiogenesis and tumor progression [9]. They are characterized by their arginase/ornithine production, a precursor of cell proliferation, collagen production and ECM remodeling, and the production of anti-inflammatory cytokines [9,10]. While both M1 and M2 macrophages have been shown to contribute to collateral vessel growth, a systemic modulation of known activators of macrophage differentiation demonstrated a determinate proarteriogenic role of M2 macrophages induced by IL10 [11]. This M2 activation phenotype, also referred to as M2c, not only acts as a regulator of immune responses but also as an effector cell of tissue remodeling and repair [9]. It is important to note that the M1/M2 taxonomy of macrophages only represents a limited attempt to categorize the vast variety of functional states observed in vitro. In vivo, this M1/M2 paradigm undermines the complexity of macrophage plasticity and diversity. Functional and phenotypical characteristics of M1 and M2 activation states are not limited to but may instead be shared by more than one macrophage population, allowing them to cater to situational and tissue specific needs. This dogma change has created the need to explore other classifications that more appropriately reflect macrophage behavior in vivo and are subject of current research [12]. Jetten et al. [6] showed that collateral growth was unaffected in mice with a deletion of the IL10 receptor on myeloid cells (IL10R$^{fl/fl}$/LysMCre$^+$), arguing that the M2c activation phenotype is not required in arteriogenesis. When treated with exogenously polarized M2c macrophages, however, an improved reperfusion of collateral vessels compared to untreated IL10R$^{fl/fl}$/LysMCre$^+$ mice was still observed. As such, this study investigates the in vivo effect of varying levels of IL10 on arteriogenesis as well as the distribution of macrophage activation types around growing collateral vessels.

2. Results

2.1. Modulation of Blood Concentration Levels of IL10 after Pharmacological Stimulation with IL10 and Anti-IL10

To investigate whether blood concentration levels of endogenous IL10 were affected by an intravenous administration of IL10 or anti-IL10 via tail vein injection, a Mouse Magnetic Luminex Assay was used to determine the blood concentration levels of IL10 prior to (baseline, BL) and 24 h (24 h) after the respective treatments. A control group received NaCl 0.9%. At BL, blood concentration levels of IL10 were below the detection limit of 1.59 pg/mL in all groups. At 24 h, elevated blood concentration levels of IL10 were found only in the IL10 treatment group with 6.35 ± 2.20 pg/mL ($p < 0.05$), indicating that an external administration of IL10 leads to a sustainable change in endogenous blood concentration levels of IL10 for at least 24 h when applied via tail vein injection. Blood concentration levels of IL10 in mice treated with anti-IL10 or NaCl 0.9% remained below the detection limit (Figure 1).

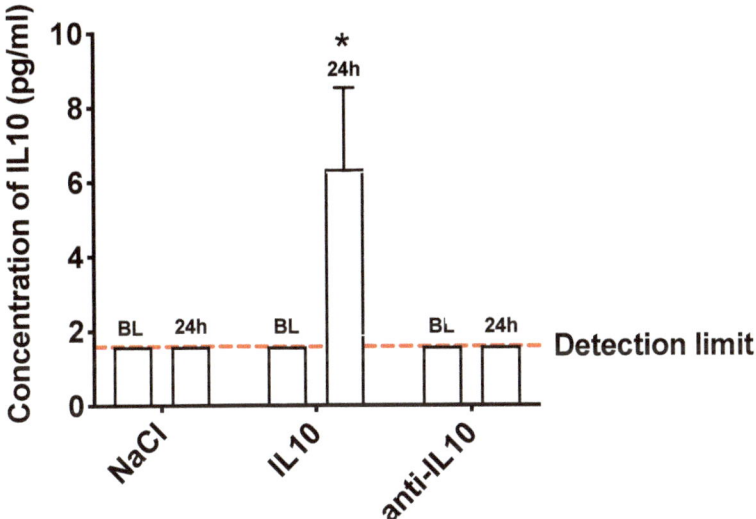

Figure 1. Modulation of blood concentration levels of IL10 after pharmacological stimulation with IL10 and anti-IL10. IL10, anti-IL10, and NaCl were administered via tail vein injection. Blood concentration levels of IL10 were measured before (baseline, BL) and 24 h after pharmacological stimulation. At BL endogenous IL10 levels were below the detection limit of 1.59 pg/mL in all subjects. After an external administration of IL10, blood concentration levels remained significantly increased after 24 h. An effect of anti-IL10 could not be detected, as baseline levels of IL10 remained below the detection limit. * indicates $p < 0.05$; $n = 3$ in each group.

2.2. Alteration of Macrophage Polarization in the Perivascular Bed of Growing Collateral Vessels after Pharmacological Stimulation with IL10 and Anti-IL10

Adductor muscle samples were harvested 3 days (3 d) and 7 d after FAL to analyze the effect of a treatment with IL10 and anti-IL10 on the polarization of macrophages in the perivascular bed of growing collateral vessels. The samples were sectioned and stained using antibodies targeting known macrophage markers CD68 and CD163 [11,13] (Figure 2a). The two largest collateral vessels of each section were selected and the ratio of macrophages of the alternatively activated phenotype $CD163^+/CD68^+$ to the classically activated phenotype $CD163^-/CD68^+$ per visual field was calculated. Mice treated with NaCl had a median ratio of $CD163^+/CD68^+$ to $CD163^-/CD68^+$ macrophages of 0.46 (IQR: 0.37–1.20) on day 3 (3 d) and 0.40 (IQR: 0.37–0.55) 7 d after FAL. When treated with IL10 the ratio is skewed towards the alternatively activated phenotype on both 3 d and 7 d after FAL with a ratio of 1.00 (IQR: 0.45–1.44) and 1.19 (IQR: 0.52–1.69). Contrariwise, the ratio is skewed towards the classically activated phenotype after application of anti-IL10 on both 3 d and 7 d after FAL with a ratio of 0.25 (IQR: 0.18–0.35) and 0.27 (IQR: 0.00–0.53), differing significantly from that of the IL10 treatment group ($p < 0.05$) (Figure 2b).

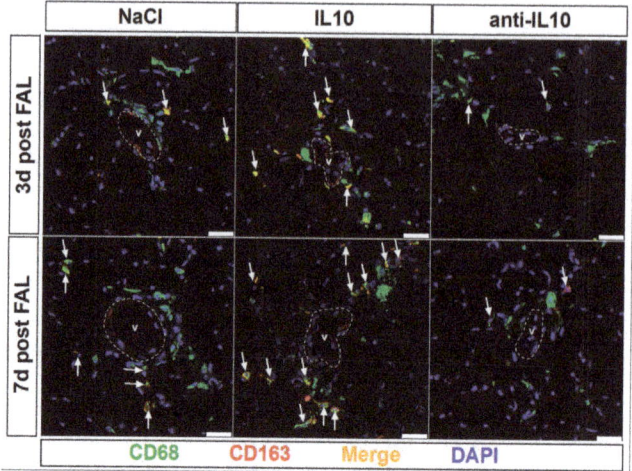

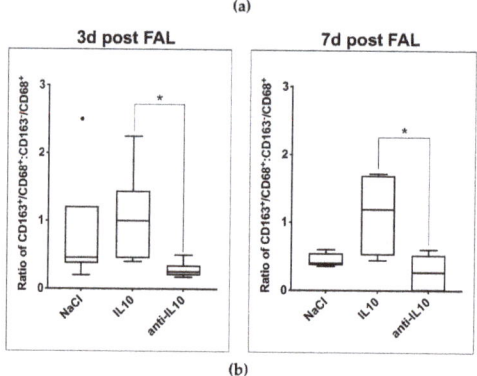

Figure 2. Alteration of macrophage polarization in the perivascular bed of growing collateral vessels after pharmacological stimulation with IL10 and anti-IL10. (**a**) Confocal micrographs of macrophage differentiation subtypes 3 d and 7 d after FAL. Sections of adductor muscles segments containing growing collateral vessels (V) were stained using DAPI and macrophage differentiation markers CD68 and CD163. The ratio of the alternatively (CD163$^+$/CD68$^+$) activated phenotype, indicated by white arrows, and classically (CD163$^-$/CD68$^+$) activated phenotype varies with indicated application. Scale bar: 25μm. (**b**) Quantification of macrophage polarization in the perivascular bed of growing collateral vessels after pharmacological stimulation with IL10 and anti-IL10 3 d and 7 d after FAL. The distribution of macrophage subtypes was skewed towards the alternatively activated phenotype after IL10 application. When anti-IL10 was injected, the opposite effect was observed, and the distribution was skewed towards the classically activated phenotype. * indicates $p < 0.05$; 3 d: $n = 6$ in each group; d7: NaCl and IL10 $n = 4$, anti-IL10: $n = 6$.

2.3. Evaluation of Hind-Limb Perfusion Recovery after FAL and Pharmacological Stimulation with IL10 and Anti-IL10

To assess the effect of varying blood concentration levels of IL10 on growing collateral vessels IL10 and anti-IL10 were externally applied in mice after FAL. Hind-limb perfusion was assessed using Laser-Doppler-Imaging before and shortly after FAL, on 3 d, 7 d, and 14 d and compared to a control group receiving NaCl. Immediately after FAL an acute reduction of hind-limb perfusion was observed in all groups (NaCl: 0.13 ± 0.01, IL10: 0.16 ± 0.03, anti-IL10: 0.13 ± 0.01). Hind-limb reperfusion in the NaCl ($n = 6$) group showed an adequate increase to 0.34 ± 0.04, 0.62 ± 0.07, and 0.62 ± 0.07 on 3 d, 7 d, and 14 d respectively. Elevated blood concentration levels of IL10 led to a significantly higher hind-limb perfusion on 3 d and 14 d ($n = 5$, 3 d: 0.54 ± 0.09, $p < 0.05$, 14 d: 0.83 ± 0.7, $p < 0.05$). Although hind-limb perfusion on 7 d was elevated compared to the control group, the difference was not significant (0.77 ± 0.09, $p = 0.07$) (Figure 3a). Contrariwise, application of anti-IL10 showed a significant impairment of hind-limb perfusion on 7 d ($n = 5$, 0.42 ± 0.4, $p < 0.05$). On 3 d and 14 d, however, no significant difference was observed (3 d: 0.35 ± 0.05, $p = 0.86$, 14d: 0.61 ± 0.07, $p = 0.89$) (Figure 3b).

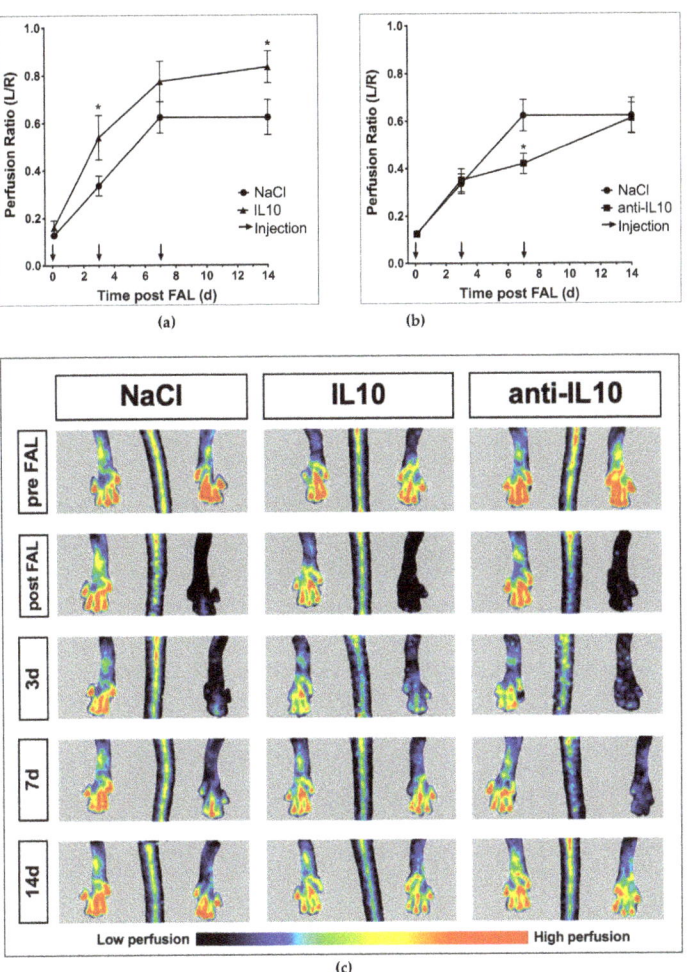

Figure 3. Evaluation of hind-limb perfusion recovery after femoral artery ligation (FAL) and application of IL10 and anti-IL10 (L/R ratio). Hind-limb perfusion was measured prior to and immediately after FAL, on 3 d, 7 d and 14 d. (**a**) IL10 led to a significant acceleration of hind-limb perfusion recovery on 3 d (IL10: 0.54 ± 0.09 vs. NaCl: 0.34 ± 0.04, $p < 0.05$) and 14 d (IL10: 0.83 ± 0.07 vs. NaCl: 0.62 ± 0.07, $p < 0.05$) while (**b**) anti-IL10 led to a brief but significant impairment of hind-limb perfusion recovery on 7 d (anti-IL10: 0.42 ± 0.04 vs. NaCl: 0.62 ± 0.07, $p < 0.05$). (**c**) Representative Laser-Doppler-Images of ligated and non-ligated hind-limbs. *indicates $p < 0.05$; NaCl: $n = 6$, IL10 and anti-IL10: $n = 5$.

2.4. Macroscopic Observations on Ligated Hind-Limbs after FAL and Application of IL10 and Anti-IL10

Ligated hind-limbs were inspected prior to FAL, 3 d and 7 d after FAL. Macroscopic observations associated with an acute ischemia of the affected hind-limb, termed critical ischemic events (CIE), were recorded after FAL and treatment with IL10 and anti-IL10. CIE were categorized as follows: inflamed hind-limb, necrotic digits, necrotic hind-limb and amputation. In total ($n = 115$) CIE occurred in 20%. Necrotic digits were observed most frequently in 65%, followed by a necrotic hind-limb in 17%, an amputation in 13% and an inflamed hind-limb in 4% of CIE. The highest incidence of CIE was observed after application of anti-IL10 (anti-IL10: 37.1% vs. NaCl: 11.1% $p < 0.01$). The incidence of CIE when treated with IL10 was similar to the control group (IL10: 13.6% vs. NaCl: 11.1% $p = 0.73$) (Figure 4).

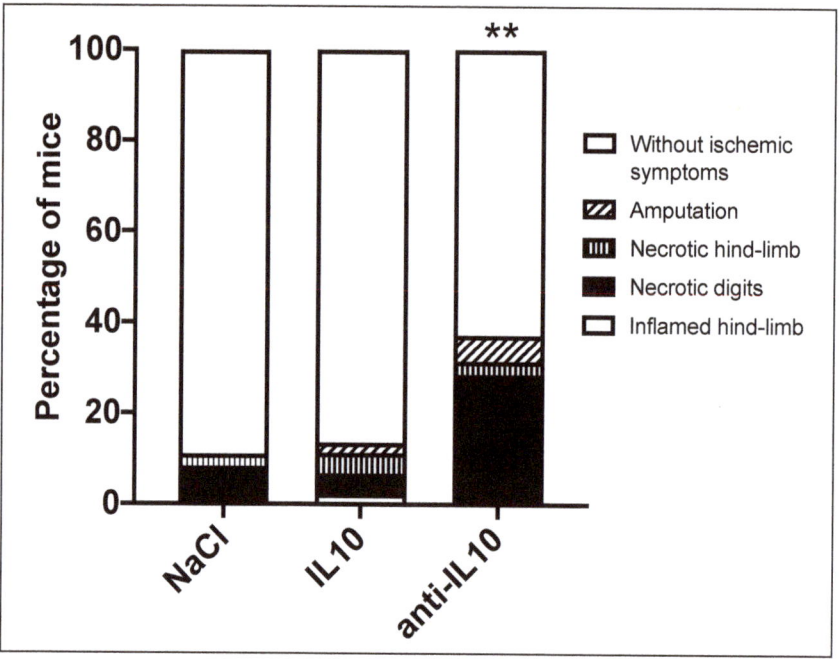

Figure 4. After FAL and pharmacological stimulation with IL10 or anti-IL10 the onset of critical ischemic events (CIE) were recorded. The highest incidence of CIE was observed after application of anti-IL10 (anti-IL10: 37.1% vs. NaCl: 11.1% $p < 0.01$, IL10: 13.6%). **indicates $p < 0.01$; NaCl: $n = 36$, IL10: $n = 44$, anti-IL10: $n = 35$

3. Discussion

In this study we have shown that modulation of IL10, in particular elevated levels of circulating IL10, alters collateral reperfusion after femoral artery ligation (FAL) as well as the distribution of macrophage activation types in the perivascular bed of growing collaterals. Although, the inhibitory effect of an IL10 antibody on circulating IL10 blood levels could not be directly detected due to technical limitations, contrary to elevated levels of circulating IL10, the opposite pertaining to both collateral reperfusion and the distribution of macrophage activation types was observed. The remodeling processes in arteriogenesis involve a controlled destruction of vessel components, activation of endothelial and smooth muscle cell de-differentiation, proliferation and migration, and adventitial restructuring in which monocytes/macrophages were shown to be key orchestrators [1,14]. These seemingly disparate tasks mediated largely by a singular cell type are explained by their heterogeneity and plasticity in response to environmental and situational needs. Previous findings have demonstrated that M1 and M2 macrophages form around growing collateral vessels in a distinct temporal and spatial pattern suggesting a collaborative mechanism of action in collateral artery growth [11]. The M1 phenotype, found proximate to the vessel lumen, is associated with the production of the pro-inflammatory cytokines IL1 and IL6, both described to have autocrine growth effects on vascular smooth muscle cells (VSMC) [15]. Other arteriogenic stimulants expressed by the M1 phenotype include NOS, TNF and MCP-1 [1,2,15,16]. M2 macrophages, on the other hand, are found distal to the vessel lumen [11] and have been ascribed a more prominent role in mediating the growth processes. Takeda et al. [7] showed that improved collateral perfusion after FAL was due to an expansion of the M2 phenotype among tissue-resident macrophages in Phd2 haplodeficient (Phd2$^{+/-}$) mice and that soluble factors secreted by Phd2$^{+/-}$ macrophages in vitro led to increased smooth muscle cell (SMC) proliferation and migration. IL10 is a known activator of the M2c phenotype and we have shown that increased levels of IL10 also led to an improved collateral reperfusion after FAL. Furthermore, an immunohistochemical analysis using the established macrophage polarization marker CD163 [17,18], revealed that perivascular macrophages were proportionally skewed towards the M2 phenotype. The supposed proarteriogenic effects of M2 macrophages induced by IL10 are further supported by the observation that the application of an IL10 antibody led to a transient impairment of collateral reperfusion and was accompanied by an increased onset of ischemic symptoms on ligated hind limbs. Also, the distribution of perivascular macrophages was conversely skewed towards the M1 phenotype. These findings do not undermine the role of M1 macrophages in arteriogenesis. The delayed and transient dip in reperfusion recovery we observed after the application of an IL10 antibody may support the hypothesis, that adluminally located M1 macrophages contribute to collateral vessel growth particularly in early phases through the recruitment of circulating monocytes and expression of arteriogenic relevant cytokines and proteins (IL1, IL6, TNF, NOS, MCP-1). They do, however, highlight the potential role played by M2 macrophages with regard to VSMC differentiation and adventitial restructuring to accommodate the growing collateral vessel. M2 macrophages induced by IL10 secrete high levels of TGFb1, known to stimulate VSMC differentiation and extracellular matrix (ECM) deposition [15,19,20]. They also produce high levels of MMP9 [21], which along with MMP2 was significantly increased in the adventitia of growing coronary collateral vessels [22]. This supports the hypothesis that IL10 induced M2 macrophages may play an active role in the augmentation of adventitial ECM proteolysis and remodeling, thus, facilitating arteriogenic growth. Our findings suggest that varying levels of IL10 in vivo influence collateral reperfusion, which may be explained by a shift in the distribution of macrophages towards the M2 phenotype at the site of collateral growth. From a clinical standpoint, this presents itself as a new therapeutic approach to promote collateral vessel growth in patients suffering from peripheral artery disease. The expression of CD163 on M2 macrophages, however, also poses concerns regarding their use in revascularization therapy. CD163$^+$ macrophages in human atherosclerotic lesions were found to increase plaque instability by promoting angiogenesis within areas of intraplaque hemorrhage, in itself thought to be a result of plaque neovascularization and increased microvessel permeability, resulting in a vicious cycle [23]. Seen as a whole, these observations underline the diversity of macrophage functions and activation states with regard to tissue specific cues and needs. A mere distinction between classically activated M1 and alternatively activated M2 macrophages limited by CD163 as an M2 marker alone will not suffice to fully describe the roles played by the macrophage activation states we observed around growing collateral vessels. Further studies utilizing other macrophage markers will be required to elucidate the underlying mechanism involved in our findings. While these remain hypothetical, the results presented in our study shed light on new therapeutic strategies in promoting collateral vessels growth.

4. Materials and Methods

4.1. Animal Models

Animal handling and all experimental procedures carried out were in full compliance with the Directive 2010/63/EU of the European Parliament on protection of animals used for scientific purposes. Approval was given by the responsible local authority, the hessian governmental council for animal protection and handling (permit reference numbers V54-19c20/15-B2/1152, permit date: 23.05.2017). Throughout this study all mice had access to water and food ad libitum.

4.2. Mouse Model of Hind-Limb Ischemia

To evaluate collateral vessel growth perfusion recovery was measured after femoral artery ligation (FAL) using the model described in [24]. For all experiments 10-14 weeks old male C57BL/6 mice from our own breeding program were used with an approximate bodyweight of 30 g. Prior to each experiment all mice were inspected to ensure a healthy state. Anesthesia was performed by intraperitoneal injection using ketamin hydrochloride (120mg/kg bodyweight) and xylazine hydrochloride (16 mg/kg bodyweight). Pre- and post-operative analgesia was performed by subcutaneous injection with buprenorphine (0.1 mg/kg bodyweight). FAL was carried out on the left hind-limb by ligating the femoral artery immediately distal to the origin of the deep femoral branch to redirect blood flow to the collateral arteries. After termination of experiments the mice were euthanized by an anesthetic overdose using ketamin hydrochloride (180mg/kg bodyweight) and xylazine hydrochloride (16 mg/kg bodyweight) followed by exsanguination.

4.3. Pharmacological Stimulation

FAL was performed on C57BL/6 mice. Mice were randomly allocated to each group receiving either recombinant murine interleukin 10 (IL10) (20 µg/kg bodyweight) or purified anti-mouse IL10 antibody (anti-IL10) (0.5 µg/kg bodyweight) diluted in sodium chloride solution (NaCl 0.9%) immediately after FAL, on day 3 and 7 after FAL. The control group received NaCl 0.9%. The application was carried out via intravenous injection into the tail vein. IL10 was purchased from PeproTech (Hamburg, Germany). Anti-IL10 was purchased from BioLegend (Koblenz, Germany).

4.4. Measurement of Blood Concentration Levels of IL10

Retro orbital blood samples were obtained from mice before and 24 h after pharmacological stimulation with IL10 and anti-IL10 as described above. The control group received NaCl 0.9%. Anesthesia war provided as described above. A Mouse Magnetic Luminex Assay (Thermo Fisher Scientific, Waltham, MA, USA) was used to measure the concentration of endogenous IL10 in the blood samples at baseline and 24 h after pharmacological stimulation.

4.5. Hind-limb Perfusion Measurement after Pharmacological Stimulation and FAL

Hind-limb perfusion was assessed and quantified via erythrocyte motion detection through Laser-Doppler-Imaging using a PeriScan PIM3 System (Perimed Instruments, Järfällä, Sweden, Software: LDPIwin for PIM3 3.1.3) before and immediately after FAL, on day 3, 7 and 14 after FAL. For each measurement mice were positioned on a heating plate at 37 °C for 3min prior to and during each measurement to ensure standardized conditions at a distance of 10 cm and a pixel resolution of 256 × 256. A 2 cm × 3 cm area including both feet was scanned and a region of interest (ROI) of approximately 80 mm^2 containing each foot was defined. Mean perfusion (arbitrary units) was used to calculate hind-limb perfusion and expressed as the ligated limb to non-ligated limb ratio as described in [25]. Follow-up measurements were performed under anesthesia as described above.

4.6. Immunohistochemistry

Mice were perfused with 10 mL vasodilation buffer (100 µg adenosine, 1 µg sodium nitroprusside, 0.05% BSA in PBS, pH 7.4) followed by 10 mL 4% PFA post mortem. Mm. adductores of ligated hind-limbs were harvested on day 3 after FAL and cryosectioned with a thickness of 10 µm. Immunostaining was performed using the following antibodies: RAT ANTI MOUSE CD68: Alexa Fluor 488 Antibody (AbD Serotec, Düsseldorf, Germany), CD163 (M-96) Antibody (Santa Cruz Biotechnology Inc., Dallas, TX, USA), Donkey anti-Rabbit IgG: Alexa Fluor 546 (Thermo Fisher Scientific, Waltham, MA, USA), DAPI. The two largest collateral vessels were selected. Immunopositive cells were classified as classically activated macrophages ($CD68^+/CD163^-$) or alternatively activated macrophages ($CD68^+/CD163^+$). Confocal imaging was carried out using a Leica SP5 (Wetzlar, Germany). Acquired images were processed with ImageJ Software (National Institutes of Health, Maryland, MD, USA) for further analysis.

4.7. Data Analysis

Statistical analysis was performed using Prism (GraphPad Software, San Diego, USA). Data was tested for normality using a D'Agostino–Pearson omnibus normality test. Parametric data is reported as mean ± standard error of mean. Non-parametric data is reported as median (IQR). Unpaired and parametric samples were analyzed using a Student's t-test. Unpaired and non-parametric samples were analyzed using a Mann–Whitney-U test. When more than two groups were compared at different time points, a two-way ANOVA was used for parametric samples followed by a Holm–Sidak's multiple comparison test. For comparison of more than 2 groups with non-parametric samples a Kruskal–Wallis test was used followed by a Dunn's multiple comparison test. Proportions were compared using a Chi-square test. Values of $p < 0.05$ were considered statistically significant.

Author Contributions: Conceptualization, A.M.G., K.T. and C.T.; Data curation, A.M.G.; Formal analysis, A.M.G.; Funding acquisition, C.T.; Investigation, A.M.G., C.S. and K.T.; Methodology, A.M.G., K.T. and C.T.; Project administration, A.M.G.; Resources, K.T. and C.T.; Supervision, K.T. and C.T.; Visualization, A.M.G.; Writing—original draft, A.G.; Writing—review and editing, G.J., O.D., C.L., C.W.H., T.S.-R., K.T., and C.T. All authors have read and agreed to the published version of the manuscript.

Funding: This research was funded by Deutsches Zentrum für Herz-Kreislaufforschung, grant number DZHK FKZ: 81X3200203.

Conflicts of Interest: The authors declare no conflict of interest. The funders had no role in the design of the study; in the collection, analyses, or interpretation of data; in the writing of the manuscript, or in the decision to publish the results.

Abbreviations

FAL	Femoral artery ligation
CIE	Critical ischemic events
VSMC	Vascular smooth muscle cells
SMC	Smooth muscle cells
ECM	Extracellular matrix

References

1. Heil, M.; Schaper, W. Influence of mechanical, cellular, and molecular factors on collateral artery growth (arteriogenesis). *Circ. Res.* **2004**, *95*, 449–458. [CrossRef] [PubMed]
2. Ito, W.D.; Arras, M.; Winkler, B.; Scholz, D.; Schaper, J.; Schaper, W. Monocyte chemotactic protein-1 increases collateral and peripheral conductance after femoral artery occlusion. *Circ. Res.* **1997**, *80*, 829–837. [CrossRef] [PubMed]
3. Buschmann, I.R.; Hoefer, I.E.; Van Royen, N.; Katzer, E.; Braun-Dulleaus, R.; Heil, M.; Kostin, S.; Bode, C.; Schaper, W. GM-CSF: A strong arteriogenic factor acting by amplification of monocyte function. *Atherosclerosis* **2001**, *159*, 343–356. [CrossRef]

4. Ziegelhoeffer, T.; Fernandez, B.; Kostin, S.; Heil, M.; Voswinckel, R.; Helisch, A.; Schaper, W. Bone marrow-derived cells do not incorporate into the adult growing vasculature. *Circ. Res.* **2004**, *94*, 230–238. [CrossRef] [PubMed]
5. Khmelewski, E.; Becker, A.; Meinertz, T.; Ito, W.D. Tissue resident cells play a dominant role in arteriogenesis and concomitant macrophage accumulation. *Circ. Res.* **2004**, *95*, e56–e64. [CrossRef] [PubMed]
6. Jetten, N.; Donners, M.M.P.C.; Wagenaar, A.; Cleutjens, J.P.M.; Van Rooijen, N.; De Winther, M.P.J.; Post, M.J. Local delivery of polarized macrophages improves reperfusion recovery in a mouse hind limb ischemia model. *PLoS ONE* **2013**, *8*, e68811. [CrossRef]
7. Takeda, Y.; Costa, S.; Delamarre, E.; Roncal, C.; Leite De Oliveira, R.; Squadrito, M.L.; Finisguerra, V.; Deschoemaeker, S.; Bruyere, F.; Wenes, M.; et al. Macrophage skewing by Phd2 haplodeficiency prevents ischaemia by inducing arteriogenesis. *Nature* **2011**, *479*, 122–126. [CrossRef]
8. Mantovani, A.; Biswas, S.K.; Galdiero, M.R.; Sica, A.; Locati, M. Macrophage plasticity and polarization in tissue repair and remodelling. *J. Pathol.* **2013**, *229*, 176–185. [CrossRef]
9. Mantovani, A.; Sica, A.; Sozzani, S.; Allavena, P.; Vecchi, A.; Locati, M. The chemokine system in diverse forms of macrophage activation and polarization. *Trends Immunol.* **2004**, *25*, 677–686. [CrossRef]
10. Mills, C.D.; Ley, K. M1 and M2 macrophages: The chicken and the egg of immunity. *J. Innate Immun.* **2014**, *6*, 716–726. [CrossRef]
11. Troidl, C.; Jung, G.; Troidl, K.; Hoffmann, J.; Mollmann, H.; Nef, H.; Schaper, W.; Hamm, C.W.; Schmitz-Rixen, T. The temporal and spatial distribution of macrophage subpopulations during arteriogenesis. *Curr. Vasc. Pharmacol.* **2013**, *11*, 5–12. [CrossRef] [PubMed]
12. Italiani, P.; Boraschi, D. From monocytes to M1/M2 macrophages: Phenotypical vs. functional differentiation. *Front. Immunol.* **2014**, *5*, 514. [CrossRef] [PubMed]
13. Komohara, Y.; Jinushi, M.; Takeya, M. Clinical significance of macrophage heterogeneity in human malignant tumors. *Cancer Sci.* **2014**, *105*, 1–8. [CrossRef] [PubMed]
14. Schaper, W.; Ito Wulf, D. Molecular mechanisms of coronary collateral vessel growth. *Circ. Res.* **1996**, *79*, 911–919. [CrossRef]
15. Berk, B.C. Vascular smooth muscle growth: Autocrine growth mechanisms. *Physiol. Rev.* **2001**, *81*, 999–1030. [CrossRef] [PubMed]
16. Schaper, W. Collateral circulation: Past and present. *Basic Res. Cardiol.* **2009**, *104*, 5–21. [CrossRef]
17. Micklem, K.; Rigney, E.; Cordell, J.; Simmons, D.; Stross, P.; Turley, H.; Seed, B.; Mason, D. A human macrophage-associated antigen (CD68) detected by six different monoclonal antibodies. *Br. J. Haematol.* **1989**, *73*, 6–11. [CrossRef]
18. Buechler, C.; Ritter, M.; Orsó, E.; Langmann, T.; Klucken, J.; Schmitz, G. Regulation of scavenger receptor CD163 expression in human monocytes and macrophages by pro-and antiinflammatory stimuli. *J. Leukoc. Biol.* **2000**, *67*, 97–103. [CrossRef]
19. O'rourke, S.A.; Dunne, A.; Monaghan, M.G. The Role of macrophages in the infarcted myocardium: Orchestrators of ECM remodeling. *Front. Cardiovasc. Med.* **2019**, *6*, 101. [CrossRef]
20. Royen, N.V.; Hoefer, I.; Buschmann, I.; Heil, M.; Kostin, S.; Deindl, E.; Vogel, S.; Korff, T.; Augustin, H.; Bode, C.; et al. Exogenous application of transforming growth factor beta 1 stimulates arteriogenesis in the peripheral circulation. *FASEB J.* **2002**, *16*, 432–434. [CrossRef]
21. Krzyszczyk, P.; Schloss, R.; Palmer, A.; Berthiaume, F. The role of macrophages in acute and chronic wound healing and interventions to promote pro-wound healing phenotypes. *Front. Physiol.* **2018**, *9*, 419. [CrossRef] [PubMed]
22. Cai, W.-J.; Koltai, S.; Kocsis, E.; Scholz, D.; Kostin, S.; Luo, X.; Schaper, W.; Schaper, J. Remodeling of the adventitia during coronary arteriogenesis. *Am. J. Physiol. Heart Circ. Physiol.* **2003**, *284*, H31–H40. [CrossRef]
23. Guo, L.; Akahori, H.; Harari, E.; Smith, S.L.; Polavarapu, R.; Karmali, V.; Otsuka, F.; Gannon, R.L.; Braumann, R.E.; Dickinson, M.H.; et al. CD163+ macrophages promote angiogenesis and vascular permeability accompanied by inflammation in atherosclerosis. *J. Clin. Investig.* **2018**, *128*, 1106–1124. [CrossRef] [PubMed]

24. Limbourg, A.; Korff, T.; Napp, L.C.; Schaper, W.; Drexler, H.; Limbourg, F.P. Evaluation of postnatal arteriogenesis and angiogenesis in a mouse model of hind-limb ischemia. *Nat. Protoc.* **2009**, *4*, 1737–1748. [CrossRef] [PubMed]
25. Heil, M.; Ziegelhoeffer, T.; Pipp, F.; Kostin, S.; Martin, S.; Clauss, M.; Schaper, W. Blood monocyte concentration is critical for enhancement of collateral artery growth. *Am. J. Physiol. Heart Circ. Physiol.* **2002**, *283*, H2411–H2419. [CrossRef]

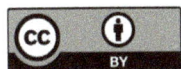

© 2020 by the authors. Licensee MDPI, Basel, Switzerland. This article is an open access article distributed under the terms and conditions of the Creative Commons Attribution (CC BY) license (http://creativecommons.org/licenses/by/4.0/).

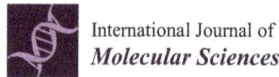

Communication

The Phosphatase SHP-2 Activates HIF-1α in Wounds In Vivo by Inhibition of 26S Proteasome Activity

Yvonn Heun [1,2], Katharina Grundler Groterhorst [1,3], Kristin Pogoda [1,2], Bjoern F Kraemer [3], Alexander Pfeifer [4], Ulrich Pohl [1,2] and Hanna Mannell [1,2,5,*]

1. Walter Brendel Centre of Experimental Medicine, University Hospital, Ludwig-Maximilians-University, Marchioninistr. 27, 81377 Munich, Germany
2. Biomedical Center, Ludwig-Maximilians-University, Großhaderner Str. 9, 82152 Planegg, Germany
3. Medizinische Klinik und Poliklinik I, Klinikum der Universität München, LMU, Marchioninistrasse 15, 81377 Munich, Germany
4. Institute of Pharmacology and Toxicology, Biomedical Center University of Bonn, Sigmund-Freud-Straße 25, 53105 Bonn, Germany
5. Hospital Pharmacy, Klinikum der Universität München, LMU, Marchioninistrasse 15, 81377 Munich, Germany
* Correspondence: hanna.mannell@med.uni-muenchen.de; Tel.: +49-89-4400-44560

Received: 27 July 2019; Accepted: 5 September 2019; Published: 7 September 2019

Abstract: Vascular remodeling and angiogenesis are required to improve the perfusion of ischemic tissues. The hypoxic environment, induced by ischemia, is a potent stimulus for hypoxia inducible factor 1α (HIF-1α) upregulation and activation, which induce pro-angiogenic gene expression. We previously showed that the tyrosine phosphatase SHP-2 drives hypoxia mediated HIF-1α upregulation via inhibition of the proteasomal pathway, resulting in revascularization of wounds in vivo. However, it is still unknown if SHP-2 mediates HIF-1α upregulation by affecting 26S proteasome activity and how the proteasome is regulated upon hypoxia. Using a reporter construct containing the oxygen-dependent degradation (ODD) domain of HIF-1α and a fluorogenic proteasome substrate in combination with SHP-2 mutant constructs, we show that SHP-2 inhibits the 26S proteasome activity in endothelial cells under hypoxic conditions in vitro via Src kinase/p38 mitogen-activated protein kinase (MAPK) signalling. Moreover, the simultaneous expression of constitutively active SHP-2 (E76A) and inactive SHP-2 (CS) in separate hypoxic wounds in the mice dorsal skin fold chamber by localized magnetic nanoparticle-assisted lentiviral transduction showed specific regulation of proteasome activity in vivo. Thus, we identified a new additional mechanism of SHP-2 mediated HIF-1α upregulation and proteasome activity, being functionally important for revascularization of wounds in vivo. SHP-2 may therefore constitute a potential novel therapeutic target for the induction of angiogenesis in ischemic vascular disease.

Keywords: SHP-2; tyrosine phosphatase; HIF-1; 26S proteasome; hypoxia; vascular remodeling; angiogenesis

---

1. Introduction

The transcription factor hypoxia inducible factor 1α (HIF-1α) is involved in vascular remodeling and angiogenesis [1]. Ischemic cardiovascular disease is characterized by reduced tissue perfusion and reduced tissue oxygen partial pressure (hypoxia), which represent a strong stimulus for HIF-1α activation [2]. HIF-1α induces the expression of several angiogenic genes, such as vascular endothelial growth factor (VEGF), platelet derived growth factor (PDGF) or matrix metalloprotease 2 (MMP-2), which are potent inducers of angiogenesis and arteriogenesis [1,3]. It has therefore been the target of therapeutic strategies to increase tissue perfusion in ischemic limbs [4,5] and to improve wound healing [6,7]. During normoxic conditions, HIF-1α is hydroxylated on prolyl residues within its oxygen-dependent degradation (ODD) domain, leading to von-Hippel-Lindau protein (pVHL) dependent ubiquitinylation and subsequent degradation by the proteasome [8,9]. Hypoxia inhibits the proteasomal degradation of HIF-1α by inhibition of the prolyl hydroxylation domain containing enzymes (PHD), resulting in stabilization of HIF-1α and subsequent accumulation within the cell [8,9]. Additionally, it has been shown that HIF-1α may be degraded by the protease calpain [10].

The tyrosine phosphatase SHP-2 has been demonstrated by us to positively influence angiogenesis in vitro and in vivo [11–13] and may constitute an interesting future therapeutic target within this context. In an earlier study we demonstrated that SHP-2 is important for HIF-1α stabilisation and activity during hypoxia, resulting in enhanced hypoxia induced HIF-1α dependent revascularisation of wounds in vivo [12]. Further, we showed that SHP-2 activates the Src kinase upon hypoxia, which in turn influenced HIF-1α prolyl hydroxylation [12]. Finally, we found that the impaired HIF-1α accumulation observed upon SHP-2 inactivation could be rescued by treatment with a PHD inhibitor as well as the proteasome inhibitors MG132 and Epoxomicin [12]. However, while our data indicated that SHP-2 influences HIF-1α accumulation during hypoxia by affecting the activity of the PHD, thus determining the proteasomal degradation of HIF-1α, we did not investigate whether the effect may additionally be caused by regulation of proteasome activity.

The 26S proteasome is responsible for the degradation of ubiquitinylated proteins and consists of a 20S core particle and two 19S regulatory particles [14]. The 20S core particle exhibits three peptidase activities (caspase-like; C-L, trypsin-like; T-L and chymotrypsin-like; CT-L), which are responsible for the cleavage of protein substrates. Ubiquitinylated proteins are recognized and bind to the 19S regulatory particle, which is in addition responsible for the ATP-dependent unfolding of the substrate protein and the opening of the 20S core particle, where degradation occurs [14]. The activity of the 26S proteasome has been shown to be regulated by phosphorylations via threonine/serine kinases as well as tyrosine kinases on several subunits of the 19S and 20S particles [15]. However, not very much is known regarding the role of phosphatases in regulating 26S proteasome activity. Moreover, its regulation during hypoxia still needs to be investigated.

In this study, we investigated the activity of the 26S proteasome during hypoxia and the connection to SHP-2 in endothelial cells in vitro and in hypoxic wounds in vivo. We found SHP-2 to inhibit the 26S proteasome activity in hypoxic cells, as assessed by measuring 26S peptidase activity as well as the accumulation of a HIF-1-ODD-Luc reporter construct. Importantly, we demonstrated that SHP-2 regulates 26S proteasome activity in hypoxic wounds in vivo.

2. Results

2.1. SHP-2 Inactivation Leads to Increased Proteasome Dependent HIF-1α Degradation during Hypoxia

As HIF-1α has been shown to be degraded by the proteasome as well as calpain [10], we first investigated whether this is also true in endothelial cells upon hypoxia. Treatment with the specific proteasome inhibitor epoxomicin or the calpain inhibitor MG101, respectively, resulted in an increase in HIF-1α protein accumulation (Figure 1A). We previously observed that SHP-2 inactivation impaired HIF-1α accumulation [12], which was rescued by treatment with proteasome inhibitors. We now additionally investigated the involvement of calpain. As seen in Figure 1B, overexpression of a dominant negative SHP-2 (SHP-2 CS) impaired HIF-1α accumulation under hypoxic conditions compared to cells overexpressing SHP-2 wildtype (WT). Treatment with the calpain inhibitor MG101 could not rescue this effect. Having observed a proteasome dependent [12] but calpain independent degradation of HIF-1α upon SHP-2 inactivation, we next investigated 26S proteasome activity in endothelial cells under hypoxia. For this, we induced the lentiviral expression of a construct containing the oxygen-dependent degradation (ODD) domain of HIF-1α [16], which guides its proteasomal degradation upon ubiquitinylation [3], fused to a luciferase gene (HIF1-ODD-Luc) with simultaneous expression of mCherry, in endothelial cells. The expression of HIF1-ODD-Luc thus inversely correlates with 26S proteasome activity and has been used as a measure of proteasome activity before [16]. First, to test its function in endothelial cells, luciferase activity upon treatment with proteasome inhibitors or hypoxia was measured 72 h after transduction with HIF1-ODD-Luc. As seen in Figure 1C, treatment with the proteasome inhibitors Bortezomib and MG132 as well as hypoxic exposure (4 h) significantly increased the accumulation of HIF1-ODD-Luc, reflecting the inhibition of the 26S proteasome. The transduction of endothelial cells with a control reporter construct lacking the HIF-1α ODD (Ctrl-Luc) showed a strong constitutive expression of luciferase, as expected, which did not differ between normoxic and hypoxic conditions (Figure S1). Expression of dominant negative SHP-2 (CS) impaired HIF1-ODD-Luc accumulation compared to SHP-2 WT expressing cells upon hypoxia, thus demonstrating an increase in 26S proteasome activity (Figure 1D).

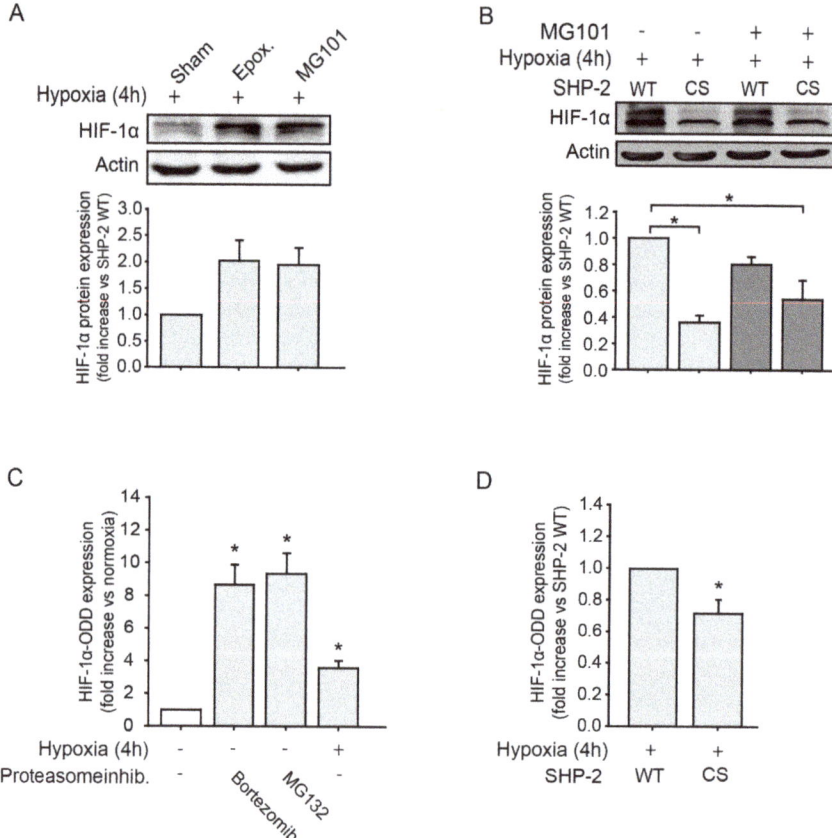

Figure 1. SHP-2 inactivation enhances proteasome dependent hypoxia inducible factor 1α (HIF-1α) degradation in endothelial cells during hypoxia. (**A**) HIF-1α protein levels were increased during hypoxia upon inhibition of the 26S proteasome (Epoxomicin, 10 µM) as well as calpain (MG101, 5 µM) (n = 3). Graph underneath blot shows the protein band densities normalized to β-actin. (**B**) Expression of dominant negative SHP-2 (CS) prevents hypoxic HIF-1α protein upregulation, which could not be rescued by calpain inhibition (MG101, 5 µM; * $p < 0.05$; n = 3). Graph underneath blot shows the protein band densities normalized to β-actin. (**C**) The reporter construct HIF1-ODD-Luc accumulated upon inhibition of the proteasome (Bortezomib 64 nM; MG132 10 µM) during normoxia as well as under only hypoxia (* $p < 0.05$; n = 16–25), confirming the specificity of the reporter constructs. (**D**) Expression of dominant negative SHP-2 (CS) increased HIF-1α degradation by the proteasomal pathway, as detected by lower expression of HIF1-ODD-Luc (* $p < 0.05$, n = 17).

2.2. SHP-2 Regulates Proteasomal Degradation of HIF-1α in Hypoxic Wounds In Vivo

As we previously found SHP-2 inactivation to prevent HIF-1α accumulation and activity in endothelial cells upon hypoxia, resulting in impaired wound healing angiogenesis in vivo [12] and, as we now observed that SHP-2 inactivation increases 26S proteasomal activity under hypoxia in endothelial cells in vitro, we investigated the proteasomal activity in vivo. For this, HIF1-ODD-Luc or Ctrl-Luc were expressed in wounds of the dorsal skin of mice by localized magnetic nanoparticles-assisted lentiviral transduction (Figure S3). By using lentiviruses (LV) coupled to magnetic nanoparticles (MNP) and the application of an external magnetic field, the simultaneous transduction of three individual wounds in the same animal can be achieved [12]. As seen in Figure 2A and Figure S2B, HIF1-ODD-Luc only accumulated in the malperfused wound and not after transduction of healthy tissue, confirming that the wound is hypoxic and that proteasome activity is higher in normoxic tissues. As a positive control, wounds were transduced with Ctrl-Luc, which causes a continuous strong expression of luciferase, as this construct does not contain the HIF-1α ODD domain. Next, we performed co-transductions of individual wounds in the same animal with HIF1-ODD-Luc and the different SHP-2 constructs, to investigate the influence of SHP-2 on proteasome activity in vivo. Whereas the expression of inactive SHP-2 CS in hypoxic wounds significantly inhibited HIF1-ODD-Luc accumulation via increased proteasome activity, introduction of the constitutively active SHP-2 E76A (Glu76 to Ala76) enhanced the HIF1-ODD-Luc protein accumulation compared to SHP-2 WT expressing wounds (Figure 2B and Figure S2C). This indicates that SHP-2 regulates HIF-1α stabilization and accumulation in hypoxic wounds by decreasing 26S proteasome activity.

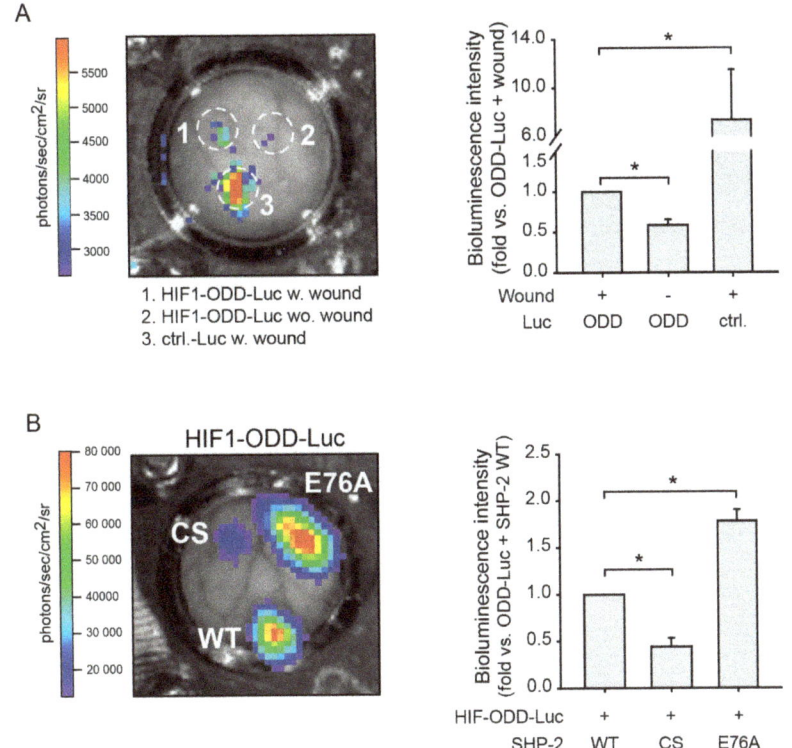

Figure 2. SHP-2 inactivation induces HIF-1α degradation via the proteasome pathway in hypoxic wounds in vivo. (**A**) Wounds in the same dorsal skin fold chamber in mice were simultaneously transduced with HIF1-ODD-Luc or Ctrl-Luc lacking HIF1-ODD using site directed lentiviral magnetic

targeting [12]. HIF1-ODD-Luc was expressed in wounds (1) but was degraded by the proteasome in healthy tissue (2), demonstrating the specificity of the lentiviral constructs and that the wounds are hypoxic (* $p < 0.05$; n = three animals). (3) Ctrl-Luc lacking the HIF-ODD domain was therefore constitutively expressed in the wound (* $p < 0.05$; n = three animals). (**B**) Wounds in the same dorsal skin fold chamber in mice were simultaneously co-transduced with HIF1-ODD-Luc and different SHP-2 constructs. While HIF1-ODD-Luc accumulated in hypoxic wounds upon transduction with SHP-2 WT, expression of dominant negative SHP-2 (CS) impaired this, demonstrating an increased 26S proteasomal activity (* $p < 0.05$; n = 3–4 animals). Expression of constitutively active SHP-2 (E76A) further enhanced HIF1-ODD-Luc accumulation, demonstrating enhanced inhibition of 26S proteasome activity (* $p < 0.05$; n = 3–4 animals). Wounding was performed the day after implantation of the dorsal skin fold chamber. Transduction of wounds was performed 24h after wounding and measurements of luciferase activity were performed eight days after transduction (see also Figure S2A).

2.3. The Proteasomal Degradation of HIF-1α is Dependent on Src Kinase and p38 MAPK Activation

In a former study, we could show that SHP-2 induces HIF-1α expression via a Src kinase dependent mechanism in endothelial cells upon hypoxia [12]. We thus hypothesized that the observed effect of SHP-2 on 26S proteasome activity and HIF-1α stabilization in this study may be mediated by Src as well. To test this, endothelial cells were transduced with the HIF1-ODD-Luc reporter construct and treated with the pharmacological Src inhibitor PP2 upon hypoxia. Whereas hypoxia induced the stabilization, and thus accumulation, of HIF1-ODD-Luc, representing a decrease in proteasome activity, Src inhibition significantly impaired this response (Figure 3A). Src kinases have been demonstrated to induce the activation of p38 MAPK during hypoxia [17]. Thus, we next explored whether this was the case in endothelial cells. The hypoxia induced HIF-1α accumulation was prevented upon inhibition of p38 MAPK (Figure 3B). Moreover, hypoxia induced the phosphorylation and thus activation of p38 MAPK and this was abrogated when treating cells with the Src kinase inhibitor PP2 (Figure 3C). Moreover, treatment with the p38 MAPK inhibitor SB203580 increased proteasome activity, reflected by reduced HIF1-ODD-Luc accumulation (Figure 3D). Finally, the phosphorylation of p38 MAPK was impaired in endothelial cells expressing SHP-2 CS and enhanced in cells expressing the constitutively active SHP-2 E76A compared to the expression of SHP-2 WT upon hypoxia (Figure 3E).

2.4. SHP-2 Activity Inhibits the Chymotrypsin-Like Activity of the 26S Proteasome upon Hypoxia

As previously published data from our group showed that treatment with epoxomicin and MG132, which are both inhibitors of the CT-L activity of the 26S proteasome [18], rescued the low HIF-1α protein level caused by SHP-2 inactivation [12], we next detected the 26S CT-L proteolytic activity in endothelial cells under hypoxia. We used experimental conditions optimized to investigate proteolytic protease activity of the 26S proteasome as previously described [19]. For this, cells expressing SHP-2 WT were exposed to hypoxia and the chymotrypsin-like (CT-L) activity of the 26S proteasome was assessed by a specific fluorogenic proteasome substrate (Suc-LLVY-AMC). Hypoxia significantly reduced CT-L activity (Figure 4A and Figure S4), and endothelial cells expressing constitutively active SHP-2 E76A exhibited an even lower 26S CT-L activity upon hypoxia compared to SHP-2 WT expressing cells (Figure 4B), indicating a downregulation of the CT-L proteolytic activity of the 26S proteasome.

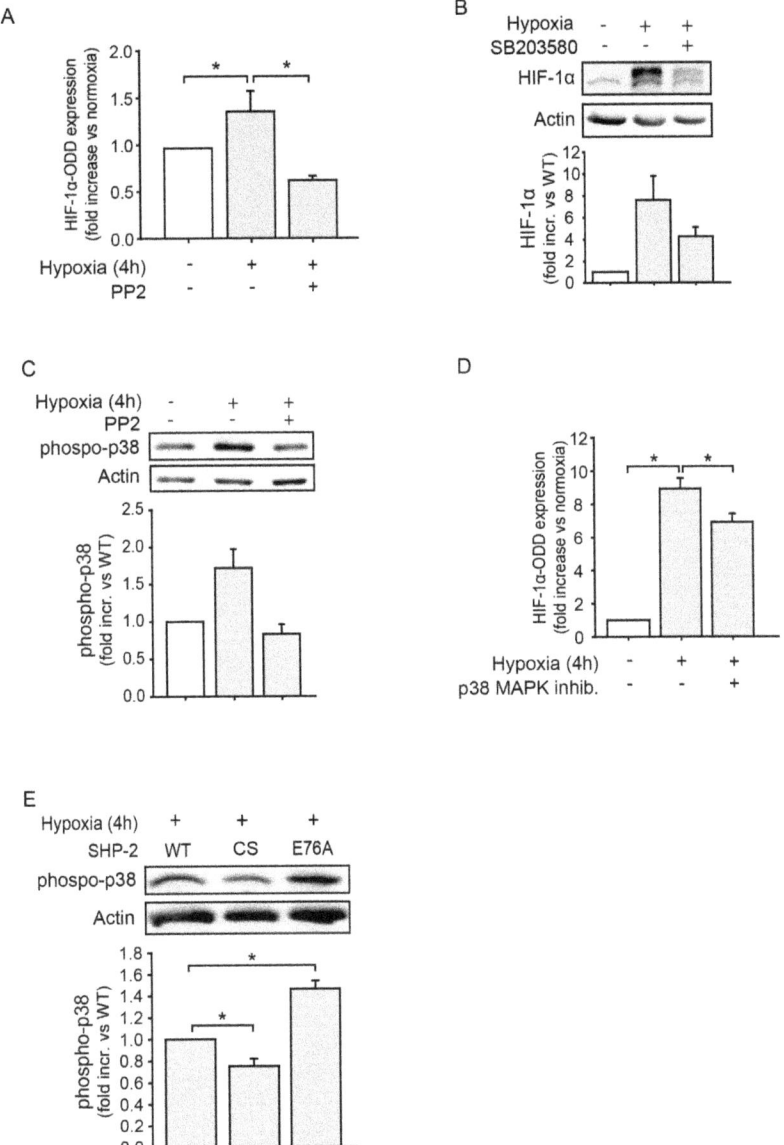

Figure 3. The proteasomal HIF-1α degradation is dependent on Src kinase and p38 mitogen-activated protein kinase (MAPK) signaling. (**A**) Whereas hypoxia inhibited 26S proteasome activity in endothelial cells, as seen by increased expression of HIF1-ODD-Luc, inhibition of Src kinase (PP2, 100 nM) reversed this (* $p < 0.05$; $n = 9$). (**B**) Inhibition of p38 MAPK (SB203580, 10 μM) in endothelial cells impaired hypoxia induced HIF-1α expression ($n = 6$). (**C**) Src kinase inhibition (PP2, 100 nM) reduced hypoxia induced p38 MAPK activation ($n = 2$). (**D**) p38 MAPK inhibition (SB203580, 10 μM) increased 26S proteasome activity, as measured by a lower level of HIF1-ODD-Luc reporter expression (* $p < 0.05$; $n = 4$). (**E**) Expression of dominant negative SHP-2 (CS) impaired hypoxia induced p38 MAPK phosphorylation, whereas expression of constitutively active SHP-2 (E76A) enhanced this compared to SHP-2 WT (* $p < 0.05$; $n = 4$). Graphs underneath blots show the protein band densities normalized to β-actin.

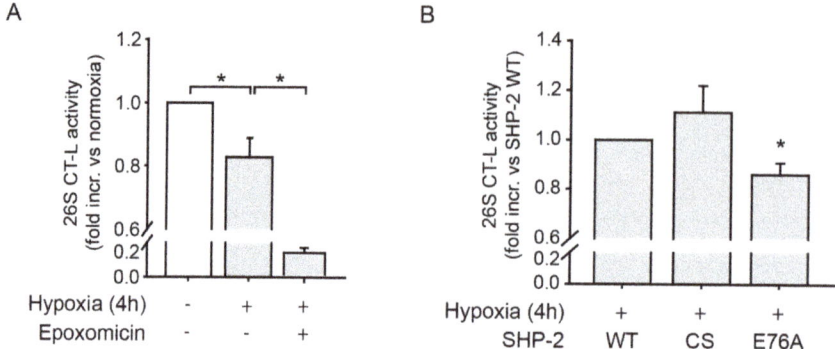

Figure 4. SHP-2 inhibits 26S chymotrypsin-like (CT-L) proteasomal activity during hypoxia. (**A**) The CT-L activity of the 26S proteasome was decreased upon hypoxia (* $p < 0.05$, $n = 11$), as measured by the fluorogenic substrate Suc-LLVY-AMC. Treatment with epoxomicin (10 µM) was used as a positive control and effectively inhibited the CT-L proteolytic activity of the 26S proteasome (* $p < 0.05$; $n = 3$). (**B**) Expression of constitutively active SHP-2 (E76A) also significantly impaired the CT-L activity of the 26S proteasome compared to SHP-2 WT during hypoxia (* $p < 0.05$, $n = 9$), whereas the expression of dominant negative SHP-2 (CS) showed a tendency towards increased CT-L activity ($n = 9$).

3. Discussion

Vascular remodeling and angiogenesis are important for maintaining tissue perfusion upon ischemia [2]. We previously demonstrated that the tyrosine phosphatase SHP-2 drives hypoxia mediated HIF-1α upregulation, resulting in revascularization of wounds in vivo [12]. Here, we show that this is achieved by SHP-2 dependent inhibition of 26S proteolytic activity via Src kinase/p38 MAPK signalling.

In a former study, we demonstrated that SHP-2 promotes HIF-1α stabilization and activity in endothelial cells during hypoxia as well as revascularization of hypoxic wounds in vivo by increasing HIF-1α activity, resulting in higher expression of VEGF, MMP-2 and PDGF [12]. Moreover, we showed SHP-2 to negatively influence the proteasomal degradational pathway, as the impaired HIF-1α expression seen upon SHP-2 inactivation was rescued by inactivation of the proteasome as well as the PHD [12]. While these results indicate that SHP-2 influences the prolylhydroxylation of HIF-1α and in this way its proteasomal degradation, we further investigated here the mechanisms of SHP-2 and its regulation of proteasomal activity. The data obtained in this study confirm our previous findings and additionally reveal a second mechanism of promoting HIF-1α upregulation by directly affecting 26S proteasomal activity. Inactivation of SHP-2 prevented the cellular accumulation of HIF1-ODD-Luc, which inversely correlated with 26S proteasomal activity, in endothelial cells in vitro. The in vivo relevance of SHP-2 mediated proteasome regulation was confirmed in hypoxic wounds of intact animals using co-transduction of HIF1-ODD-Luc and SHP-2 constructs. Of note, expression of constitutively active SHP-2 further enhanced HIF1-ODD-Luc levels, demonstrating an increased inhibition of the 26S proteasome. This correlates well with the impaired 26S CT-L proteolytic activity measured in cells with constitutive SHP-2 activation. Thus, we conclude that SHP-2 activity negatively affects proteasomal activity during wound healing under hypoxic conditions in vivo.

As we previously found SHP-2 dependent Src kinase activation to be involved in HIF-1α upregulation during hypoxia [12], we now investigated if it is also important for proteasomal activity. Indeed, Src integrity was crucial for 26S proteasomal activity and in addition, was important for activation of the p38 MAPK upon hypoxia. p38 MAPK, in turn, positively affected HIF-1α upregulation while negatively influencing 26S proteasomal activity, a mechanism which was promoted by SHP-2. These results are not only in accordance with but additionally extend the study from Lee et al.

performed in HeLa cells, demonstrating that p38 MAPK negatively affects 26S proteolytic activity also in endothelial cells [20]. This inhibition was further shown to be due to the phosphorylation of Thr-273 on the subunit Rpn2 in the 19S regulatory particle [20]. Whether this is the case during hypoxia, remains to be investigated. Posttranslational phosphorylation of the 26S proteasome has repeatedly been shown to regulate its enzymatic activities [15]. Several stimuli, such as stress, metabolic changes, and growth factor signalling have been demonstrated to induce its phosphorylation [15]. Here, we identified hypoxia as a novel stimulus of 26S proteasomal inactivation, particularly the CT-L activity. In addition, we found the caspase-like (C-L) activity to be deprived upon hypoxia (Figure S4). Intriguingly, we measured an increased trypsin-like (T-L) activity during hypoxia, suggesting that the different proteolytic activities of the 26S proteasome may be differentially regulated. One may hypothesize that the differential regulation of activities is involved in substrate specificity of proteasomal degradation. However, more investigations are needed to elucidate the mechanisms behind this. The observed reduction in CT-L and C-L activity, however, is supported by the fact that the 26S proteasome relies on the activity of ATPases in the 19S regulatory particle for substrate de-ubiquitinylation, unfolding and 20S gate opening and activation [15], which do not function upon ATP deprivation, as is the case during hypoxia. Moreover, we observed that inhibition of Src kinase/p38 MAPK signalling rescued proteasomal activation. Additionally, an inhibition of 26S proteasomal activity via direct dephosphorylation of subunits by SHP-2 was not investigated here and has to be the focus of further studies. However, this is per se possible, as Zong et al. demonstrated the phosphatase PP2A to negatively affect 20S proteolytic activity via dephosphorylation [21]. Nevertheless, this is to our knowledge the first study to report a regulation of 26S proteolytic activity by SHP-2.

In summary, we were able to further characterize the mechanism behind the regulation of hypoxia mediated HIF-1α upregulation by SHP-2, which is essential for revascularisation of malperfused wounds. Moreover, we demonstrate for the first time that the 26S proteasomal activity is regulated by SHP-2 during hypoxia in vitro and is functionally relevant in vivo. We show that SHP-2 not only inhibits the proteasomal degradation pathway by influencing HIF-1α prolylhydroxylation [12] but in addition by directly inhibiting 26S proteolytic activity via p38 MAPK (for a summary of our findings, see Figure 5). We thus believe that SHP-2 is important for HIF-1α upregulation in vitro and in wounds in vivo by inhibition of the proteasomal pathway via activation of Src kinase/p38 MAPK signalling. Together with our previous results, this regulation may be achieved by redundant and or additive pathways, involving external regulators of the proteasome (PHD and pVHL activation), and directly via the CT-L activity of the 26S proteasome. Finally, our findings confirm SHP-2 to be essential for hypoxic HIF-1α upregulation in vivo. SHP-2 may therefore constitute a novel therapeutic target in ischemic vascular disease, aiming for the revascularization of ischemic tissues.

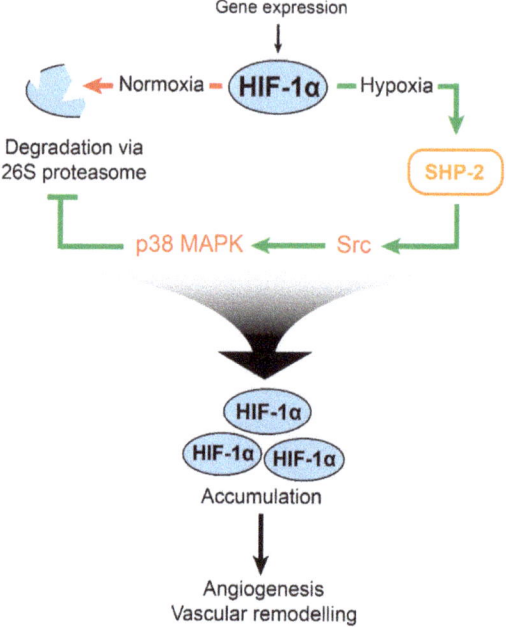

Figure 5. Illustration of 26S proteasome regulation and HIF-1α accumulation by SHP-2 in hypoxia. HIF-1α is constitutively expressed but degraded by the proteasomal pathway during hypoxia (left). Upon hypoxia (right), the degradation of HIF-1α is inhibited. In our previous study, we found SHP-2 to influence the prolyl hydroxylation of HIF-1α, which targets it for degradation [12]. In this study, we found a second mechanism of SHP-2 mediated HIF-1α upregulation: SHP-2 positively affects Src kinase and p38 MAPK activity during hypoxia, which in turn negatively influences the activity of the 26S proteasome. As a consequence, HIF-1α is stabilized and accumulates in the cell, promoting hypoxic angiogenesis and vascular remodeling.

4. Materials and Methods

4.1. Antibodies and Chemicals

Rabbit phospho-p38 MAPK (Thr180/Tyr182) (D3F9) XP™ (#4511) and β-Actin (13E5) antibodies were from Cell Signaling Technology, Frankfurt am Main, Germany. HIF-1α clone H1α67, HIF-1α clone EP1215Y, anti-mouse and -rabbit horseradish peroxidase-conjugated secondary antibodies were from Merck Millipore, Darmstadt, Germany. Src-Inhibitor PP2 was purchased from Sigma-Aldrich (#P0042), Darmstadt, Germany. p38 MAPK inhibitor (SB203580), MG132 and MG101 were from Tocris, Wiesbaden-Nordenstadt, Germany. Bortezomib and Epoxomicin were from Calbiochem. All other chemicals were from Sigma-Aldrich, Darmstadt, Germany.

4.2. Human Microvascular Endothelial Cell (HMEC) Culture

Human dermal microvascular endothelial cells (HMEC) [22] were cultivated as described earlier [23]. In detail, HMEC were cultivated in DMEM (Sigma-Aldrich, Darmstadt, Germany) containing 10% fetal calf serum (Biochrom, Berlin, Germany) and 1% Penicillin-Streptomycin (Sigma-Aldrich, Darmstadt, Germany) and kept in an incubator with 5% CO_2 at 37 °C.

4.3. Lentiviral Constructs and Transductions

Wild type (WT) SHP-2 and catalytically inactive mutant SHP-2 CS (Cys459 to Ser459) plasmid vectors were kind gifts from the Bennett laboratory [24]. The constitutively active SHP-2 E76A (Glu76 to Ala) was generated as previously described [12]. The lentiviral constructs containing the above mentioned cDNAs were generated as described earlier [12] and lentiviral particles were produced as described elsewhere [25]. Flow cytometry of transduced HEK293T cells was used to determine the biological titer as previously described [25]. The FUW-ODD-Luc-mCherry lentiviral plasmid (referred to as HIF1-ODD-Luc in this manuscript) and the control vector FUW-Luc-mCherry (referred to as Ctrl-Luc in this manuscript) were kindly provided by Kimbrel et al. [16] and packaged into lentiviral particles as previously described [25]. The ODD-Luc insert encodes a reporter fusion protein consisting of the oxygen-dependent domain (ODD) from hypoxia-inducible factor 1a (HIF-1a) and firefly luciferase, inversely reflecting proteasomal activity, with simultaneous expression of mCherry after a self-cleavage 2A site. Lentiviral transduction of HMECs was carried out using a multiplicity of infection (MOI) of five. Lentiviral particles were diluted in Hank's solution and applied onto subconfluent HMEC. After incubation for 4–6 h at 37 °C, culture medium was added. The next day the medium was changed, and cells were left 72 h before assaying.

4.4. Hypoxia Treatment

For hypoxia treatment, HMECs were incubated in cultivation media in a hypoxia chamber (Cell Systems, Troisdorf, Germany) at pO_2 8 ± 2 mmHg equivalent to a O_2 concentration of 1 ± 0.2% for 4 h as previously described [26]. To reach these experimental hypoxic conditions, the chamber was flooded for four minutes with 15–20 L/min with an anoxic gas mixture (5% CO_2, 95% N_2). After hypoxia, the media was discarded, and cells quickly washed once with phosphate buffered saline and lysed for further processing.

4.5. In Vitro 26S Proteasome Activity

The 26S CT-L proteasome activity was measured as previously described [19]. In detail, HMEC were subjected to hypoxia (4 h), rinsed with cold phosphate buffered saline supplemented with calcium (PBS+) and lysed at 4 °C with lysis buffer (1mM DTT, 1× Roche PhosphoStop Tablet in homogenizing buffer containing 20 mM HEPES, 1 mM $MgCl_2$, 150 mM NaCl, and 0.5 mM EDTA). 10 µg protein in assay buffer containing 1mM DTT, 50 µM ATP and 100 µM Suc-LLVY-AMC (R&D systems, Wiesbaden, Germany) in homogenizing buffer was measured at 37 °C with excitation wavelength 339 nm and emission wavelength 439 nm for 2 h.

4.6. In Vitro Luciferase Assay

HMEC were seeded in 24-well plates and transduced the following day. Indicated inhibitor treatments and hypoxia was performed 72 h post transduction and cells were lysed on ice for 30 min (250 mM Tris base pH7.8, 0.1% Triton-X). Then, 10 µL of cell lysate were transferred to a black 96-well plate in triplicates and 100 µL luciferin assay buffer (60 mM DTT, 10 mM $MgSO_4$, 1 mM ATP, 25 mM Glycil-Glycin, 0.3 mM D-Luciferin) were added to each well. Bioluminescence was detected using the Spectrafluor (Tecan, Männedorf, Switzerland) with a one-second integration time and normalized to protein concentrations.

4.7. In Vivo Transduction and Luciferase Imaging

Animal studies were conducted in accordance with the German animal protection law and approved by the district government of upper Bavaria (Regierung von Oberbayern, approval reference number AZ55.2-1-54-2532-172-13). The investigation conforms to the Guide for the Care and Use of Laboratory Animals published by the US National Institutes of Health (NIH Publication No. 85-23, revised 1996). 16–20-week old male and female C57 BL6/J mice (Charles River) were anesthetized

(5 mg/kg midazolam, 0.5 mg/kg medetomidin, and 0.05 mg/kg fentanyl) and the dorsal skinfold chamber was implanted as described before [27]. Wounds were introduced using a hot probe as previously described 24 h after dorsal skinfold chamber implantation [12]. Proteasomal activity in avascular wounds in the dorsal skin of mice was detected by localized magnetic nanoparticles-assisted transduction of individual wounds in the same animal with HIF1-ODD-Luc (FUW-ODD-Luc-mCherry) and Ctrl-Luc (FUW-Luc-mCherry) lentiviral vectors as well as co-transductions of with the ODD-Luc vector and SHP-2 WT, CS and E76A lentiviral vectors, respectively, as previously described [12]. Luciferase activity was detected eight days after transduction by application of 3 mg/mL D-Luciferin directly to the imaging window of the dorsal skinfold chamber. Bioluminescence was imaged using the IVIS® spectrum in vivo imaging system from PerkinElmer at medium binning and exposure times between five and 10 minutes. Signal intensities were quantified using the Fiji software.

4.8. Immunoblotting

Cell lysates were prepared and subjected to SDS-PAGE followed by western blotting as previously described [28]. Protein band intensities were measured using the Hokawo software (Hamamatsu, Herrsching, Germany) and normalized to the respective β-Actin protein bands, which was used as equal loading control.

4.9. Statistical Analysis

Data are presented as means ± SEM. Statistical analyses were performed with Sigma Plot 10.0. The Student's t-test was used for comparisons between two groups of normal distributed data, rank-sum test was performed for comparisons of two groups of not normally distributed data. The one-way analysis of variance (one-way ANOVA) was performed for multiple comparisons. Differences were considered significant at an error probability level of $p < 0.05$.

Supplementary Materials: Supplementary materials can be found at http://www.mdpi.com/1422-0067/20/18/4404/s1.

Author Contributions: Conceptualization, supervision and project administration: H.M.; Investigation: Y.H., K.G.G., K.P., H.M.; Methodology: A.P., Y.H., H.M.; Visualization: H.M., Y.H. Writing–original draft preparation: H.M., B.F.K., U.P., A.P.; Funding Acquisition: H.M., Y.H.

Funding: This research was funded by *Dr. Kleist-Stiftung* and *Friedrich Baur Stiftung*.

Acknowledgments: The authors would like to thank Andrew Kung at Harvard Medical School, Boston, USA for kindly providing us with the lentiviral constructs HIF1-ODD-Luc (FUW-ODDLuc-mCherry) and Ctrl-luc (FUW-wtLuc-mCherry) [16].

Conflicts of Interest: The authors declare no conflict of interest and the funders had no role in the design of the study; in the collection, analyses, or interpretation of data; in the writing of the manuscript, or in the decision to publish the results.

Abbreviations

Ctrl-Luc	Lentiviral control luciferase reporter construct lacking the HIF-1α ODD
HIF1-ODD-Luc	Lentiviral construct containing the oxygen-dependent degradation (ODD) domain of HIF-1α fused to luciferase
HMEC	Human microvascular endothelial cells
SHP-2	Src homology domain containing tyrosine phosphatase 2
SHP-2 WT	SHP-2 wildtype construct
SHP-2 CS	Dominant negative SHP-2 construct where Cys459 was exchanged to Ser459
SHP-2 E76A	Constitutively active SHP-2 construct where Glu76 was exchanged to Ala76

References

1. Semenza, G.L. Targeting hypoxia-inducible factor 1 to stimulate tissue vascularization. *J. Investig. Med. Off. Publ. Am. Fed. Clin. Res.* **2016**, *64*, 361–363. [CrossRef] [PubMed]
2. Rey, S.; Semenza, G.L. Hypoxia-inducible factor-1-dependent mechanisms of vascularization and vascular remodelling. *Cardiovasc. Res.* **2010**, *86*, 236–242. [CrossRef] [PubMed]
3. Krock, B.L.; Skuli, N.; Simon, M.C. Hypoxia-induced angiogenesis: Good and evil. *Genes Cancer* **2011**, *2*, 1117–1133. [CrossRef] [PubMed]
4. Sarkar, K.; Fox-Talbot, K.; Steenbergen, C.; Bosch-Marce, M.; Semenza, G.L. Adenoviral transfer of HIF-1alpha enhances vascular responses to critical limb ischemia in diabetic mice. *Proc. Natl. Acad. Sci. USA* **2009**, *106*, 18769–18774. [CrossRef] [PubMed]
5. Patel, T.H.; Kimura, H.; Weiss, C.R.; Semenza, G.L.; Hofmann, L.V. Constitutively active HIF-1alpha improves perfusion and arterial remodeling in an endovascular model of limb ischemia. *Cardiovasc Res.* **2005**, *68*, 144–154. [CrossRef] [PubMed]
6. Botusan, I.R.; Sunkari, V.G.; Savu, O.; Catrina, A.I.; Grunler, J.; Lindberg, S.; Pereira, T.; Yla-Herttuala, S.; Poellinger, L.; Brismar, K.; et al. Stabilization of HIF-1alpha is critical to improve wound healing in diabetic mice. *Proc. Natl. Acad. Sci. USA* **2008**, *105*, 19426–19431. [CrossRef] [PubMed]
7. Mace, K.A.; Yu, D.H.; Paydar, K.Z.; Boudreau, N.; Young, D.M. Sustained expression of Hif-1α in the diabetic environment promotes angiogenesis and cutaneous wound repair. *Wound Repair Regen.* **2007**, *15*, 636–645. [CrossRef]
8. Walshe, T.E.; D'Amore, P.A. The role of hypoxia in vascular injury and repair. *Annu Rev. Pathol.* **2008**, *3*, 615–643. [CrossRef]
9. Bilton, R.L.; Booker, G.W. The subtle side to hypoxia inducible factor (HIFalpha) regulation. *Eur. J. Biochem.* **2003**, *270*, 791–798. [CrossRef]
10. Zhou, J.; Kohl, R.; Herr, B.; Frank, R.; Brune, B. Calpain mediates a von Hippel-Lindau protein-independent destruction of hypoxia-inducible factor-1alpha. *Mol. Biol. Cell* **2006**, *17*, 1549–1558. [CrossRef]
11. Mannell, H.; Hellwig, N.; Gloe, T.; Plank, C.; Sohn, H.Y.; Groesser, L.; Walzog, B.; Pohl, U.; Krötz, F. Inhibition of the tyrosine phosphatase SHP-2 suppresses angiogenesis in vitro and in vivo. *J. Vasc. Res.* **2008**, *45*, 153–163. [CrossRef] [PubMed]
12. Heun, Y.; Pogoda, K.; Anton, M.; Pircher, J.; Pfeifer, A.; Woernle, M.; Ribeiro, A.; Kameritsch, P.; Mykhaylyk, O.; Plank, C.; et al. HIF-1alpha Dependent Wound Healing Angiogenesis In Vivo Can Be Controlled by Site-Specific Lentiviral Magnetic Targeting of SHP-2. *Mol. Ther.* **2017**, *25*, 1616–1627. [CrossRef] [PubMed]
13. Rieck, S.; Heun, Y.; Heidsieck, A.; Mykhaylyk, O.; Pfeifer, A.; Gleich, B.; Mannell, H.; Wenzel, D. Local anti-angiogenic therapy by magnet-assisted downregulation of SHP2 phosphatase. *J. Control. Release* **2019**, *305*, 155–164. [CrossRef]
14. Jang, H.H. Regulation of Protein Degradation by Proteasomes in Cancer. *J. Cancer Prev.* **2018**, *23*, 153–161. [CrossRef] [PubMed]
15. Guo, X.; Huang, X.; Chen, M.J. Reversible phosphorylation of the 26S proteasome. *Protein Cell* **2017**, *8*, 255–272. [CrossRef] [PubMed]
16. Kimbrel, E.A.; Davis, T.N.; Bradner, J.E.; Kung, A.L. In vivo pharmacodynamic imaging of proteasome inhibition. *Mol. Imaging* **2009**, *8*, 140–147. [CrossRef]
17. Thobe, B.M.; Frink, M.; Choudhry, M.A.; Schwacha, M.G.; Bland, K.I.; Chaudry, I.H. Src family kinases regulate p38 MAPK-mediated IL-6 production in Kupffer cells following hypoxia. *Am. J. Physiol.* **2006**, *291*, C476–C482. [CrossRef]
18. Wojcik, C.; Di Napoli, M. Ubiquitin-proteasome system and proteasome inhibition: New strategies in stroke therapy. *Stroke* **2004**, *35*, 1506–1518. [CrossRef]
19. Grundler, K.; Rotter, R.; Tilley, S.; Pircher, J.; Czermak, T.; Yakac, M.; Gaitzsch, E.; Massberg, S.; Krotz, F.; Sohn, H.Y.; et al. The proteasome regulates collagen-induced platelet aggregation via nuclear-factor-kappa-B (NFkB) activation. *Thromb. Res.* **2016**, *148*, 15–22. [CrossRef]
20. Lee, S.H.; Park, Y.; Yoon, S.K.; Yoon, J.B. Osmotic stress inhibits proteasome by p38 MAPK-dependent phosphorylation. *J. Biol. Chem.* **2010**, *285*, 41280–41289. [CrossRef]

21. Zong, C.; Gomes, A.V.; Drews, O.; Li, X.; Young, G.W.; Berhane, B.; Qiao, X.; French, S.W.; Bardag-Gorce, F.; Ping, P. Regulation of murine cardiac 20S proteasomes: Role of associating partners. *Circ. Res.* **2006**, *99*, 372–380. [CrossRef] [PubMed]
22. Ades, E.W.; Candal, F.J.; Swerlick, R.A.; George, V.G.; Summers, S.; Bosse, D.C.; Lawley, T.J. HMEC-1: Establishment of an immortalized human microvascular endothelial cell line. *J. Investig. Derm.* **1992**, *99*, 683–690. [CrossRef] [PubMed]
23. Mannell, H.K.; Pircher, J.; Chaudhry, D.I.; Alig, S.K.; Koch, E.G.; Mettler, R.; Pohl, U.; Krötz, F. ARNO regulates VEGF-dependent tissue responses by stabilizing endothelial VEGFR-2 surface expression. *Cardiovasc. Res.* **2012**, *93*, 111–119. [CrossRef] [PubMed]
24. Kontaridis, M.I.; Liu, X.; Zhang, L.; Bennett, A.M. Role of SHP-2 in fibroblast growth factor receptor-mediated suppression of myogenesis in C2C12 myoblasts. *Mol. Cell. Biol.* **2002**, *22*, 3875–3891. [CrossRef] [PubMed]
25. Hofmann, A.; Wenzel, D.; Becher, U.M.; Freitag, D.F.; Klein, A.M.; Eberbeck, D.; Schulte, M.; Zimmermann, K.; Bergemann, C.; Gleich, B.; et al. Combined targeting of lentiviral vectors and positioning of transduced cells by magnetic nanoparticles. *Proc. Natl. Acad. Sci. USA* **2009**, *106*, 44–49. [CrossRef] [PubMed]
26. Alig, S.K.; Stampnik, Y.; Pircher, J.; Rotter, R.; Gaitzsch, E.; Ribeiro, A.; Wornle, M.; Krötz, F.; Mannell, H. The Tyrosine Phosphatase SHP-1 Regulates Hypoxia Inducible Factor-1alpha (HIF-1alpha) Protein Levels in Endothelial Cells under Hypoxia. *PLoS ONE* **2015**, *10*, e0121113. [CrossRef] [PubMed]
27. Mannell, H.; Pircher, J.; Fochler, F.; Stampnik, Y.; Räthel, T.; Gleich, B.; Plank, C.; Mykhaylyk, O.; Dahmani, C.; Wornle, M.; et al. Site directed vascular gene delivery in vivo by ultrasonic destruction of magnetic nanoparticle coated microbubbles. *Nanomedicine* **2012**, *8*, 1309–1318. [CrossRef]
28. Krötz, F.; Engelbrecht, B.; Buerkle, M.A.; Bassermann, F.; Bridell, H.; Gloe, T.; Duyster, J.; Pohl, U.; Sohn, H.Y. The tyrosine phosphatase, SHP-1, is a negative regulator of endothelial superoxide formation. *J. Am. Coll. Cardiol.* **2005**, *45*, 1700–1706.

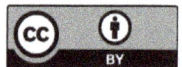

© 2019 by the authors. Licensee MDPI, Basel, Switzerland. This article is an open access article distributed under the terms and conditions of the Creative Commons Attribution (CC BY) license (http://creativecommons.org/licenses/by/4.0/).

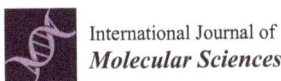

Communication

Insulin Treatment Forces Arteriogenesis in Diabetes Mellitus by Upregulation of the Early Growth Response-1 (Egr-1) Pathway in Mice

Senthilkumar Thulasingam [1], Sundar Krishnasamy, David Raj C. [1], Manuel Lasch [2,3], Srinivasan Vedantham [1,†] and Elisabeth Deindl [3,*,†]

1. School of Chemical and Biotechnology, SASTRA Deemed to be University, Thanjavur 613401, India
2. Department of Otorhinolaryngology, Head & Neck Surgery, University Hospital, LMU Munich, 81377 Munich, Germany
3. Walter-Brendel-Centre of Experimental Medicine, University Hospital, LMU Munich, 81377 Munich, Germany
* Correspondence: Elisabeth.Deindl@med.uni-muenchen.de; Tel.: +49-89-2180-76504
† These authors contributed equally to this work.

Received: 30 May 2019; Accepted: 3 July 2019; Published: 5 July 2019

Abstract: The process of arteriogenesis is severely compromised in patients with diabetes mellitus (DM). Earlier studies have reported the importance of *Egr-1* in promoting collateral outward remodeling. However, the role of *Egr-1* in the presence of DM in outward vessel remodeling was not studied. We hypothesized that *Egr-1* expression may be compromised in DM which may lead to impaired collateral vessel growth. Here, we investigated the relevance of the transcription factor *Egr-1* for the process of collateral artery growth in diabetic mice. Induction of arteriogenesis by femoral artery ligation resulted in an increased expression of Egr-1 on mRNA and protein level but was severely compromised in streptozotocin-induced diabetic mice. Diabetes mellitus mice showed a significantly reduced expression of *Egr-1* endothelial downstream genes Intercellular Adhesion Molecule-1 (*ICAM-1*) and urokinase Plasminogen Activator (*uPA*), relevant for extravasation of leukocytes which promote arteriogenesis. Fluorescent-activated cell sorting analyses confirmed reduced leukocyte recruitment. Diabetes mellitus mice showed a reduced expression of the proliferation marker Ki-67 in growing collaterals whose luminal diameters were also reduced. The Splicing Factor-1 (SF-1), which is critical for smooth muscle cell proliferation and phenotype switch, was found to be elevated in collaterals of DM mice. Treatment of DM mice with insulin normalized the expression of *Egr-1* and its downstream targets and restored leukocyte recruitment. SF-1 expression and the diameter of growing collaterals were normalized by insulin treatment as well. In summary, our results showed that Egr-1 signaling was impaired in DM mice; however, it can be rescued by insulin treatment.

Keywords: arteriogenesis; endothelial cells; smooth muscle cells; diabetes mellitus; Egr-1; streptozotocin; collateral arteries; insulin

---

1. Introduction

Peripheral artery disease (PAD) is one of the common vascular complications in diabetes mellitus [1]. Patients with PAD exhibit poor lower extremity function and develop critical limb ischemia and ulceration, ultimately leading to limb amputation [2–4]. Moreover, compared to healthy individuals, diabetic patients with PAD exhibit cardiovascular co-morbidities, neuropathy, and higher mortality [5–8]. Patients with PAD show poorer outcomes after leg bypass surgery with higher incidence of restenosis, longer hospitalization, and reduced amputation-free survival [8–11].

Arteriogenesis, which is an endothelial dependent process [12], is characterized by outward remodeling of pre-existing anastomoses in conducting arteries, and through this process, the blood flow to peripheral tissues can largely be restored. The process of collateral artery growth is strongly dependent on perivascular recruitment and accumulation of leukocytes, particularly macrophages, which supply growth factors and cytokines to the growing vessel [13]. In addition, lymphocytes accumulate in the perivascular space [14]; however, little is known about their function. It is well established that the presence of DM limits the process of arteriogenesis [15]. Indeed, it has been previously shown by van Weel et al. [16] that reperfusion recovery after femoral artery ligation (FAL) was significantly reduced in streptozotocin (STZ)-induced diabetic mice, as shown by laser Doppler perfusion measurements. The exact mechanisms through which impairment of arteriogenesis in DM occurs are not clear. Elevated vasomotor function attenuating the sensing of shear stress and defects in downstream monocyte signaling are reported as major contributors to the vascular impairments seen in arteriogenesis [17].

Early growth response-1 (*Egr-1*) is a zinc finger transcription factor, which is expressed after exposure of cells to mediators associated with growth and differentiation [18]. Several studies have shown a link between the activation of *Egr-1* through hypoxia, ischemia/reperfusion, mechanical stress, shear stress, emphysema, atherosclerosis, and acute vascular injury [19]. Early growth response-1 has been reported to play a critical role in a hind limb ischemia model [20], and in a separate study, it was shown that adenoviral-mediated *Egr-1* delivery improved perfusion recovery [21]. Early growth response-1 is important for leukocyte recruitment and vascular cell proliferation during arteriogenesis in vivo in mice subjected to FAL [22]. Thus, with increased *Egr-1* expression playing a critical role in both arteriogenesis and regulation under hyperglycemic conditions, the present study was performed to understand the influence of DM on *Egr-1* expression and its consequent biological events. We hypothesized that *Egr-1* expression may be compromised in DM which may lead to impaired collateral vessel growth. In the present study, we investigated the role of *Egr-1* in collateral artery growth in vivo in streptozotocin-induced diabetic mice employing a hind limb model in which arteriogenesis was induced by FAL.

2. Results

C57Bl6J mice were made diabetic using streptozotocin. The diabetic mice showed a significant rise in blood glucose levels (328 ± 38 mg/dL) compared to non-diabetic mice (144 ± 10 mg/dl) 24 h post-ligation. In accordance with this, diabetic mice treated with insulin showed a significant decrease in glucose levels (216 ± 35 mg/dL) compared to the diabetic group (Table 1) at the same timepoint.

Table 1. Plasma glucose levels measured 24 h post-Femoral Artery Ligation prior to sacrifice ($n = 7$ in each group).

Group	Random Plasma Glucose (mg/dL)
Control	144 ± 10
Streptozotocin	328 ± 38 *
Streptozotocin + Insulin	216 ± 35 **

* $p < 0.05$ compared to Control group, ** $p < 0.05$ compared to Streptozotocin group.

2.1. Reduced Upregulation of Egr-1 in Growing Collaterals of Diabetic Mice

The Egr-1 mRNA expression levels were significantly increased in growing collaterals of control mice, diabetic mice, and diabetic mice treated with insulin compared to resting collaterals isolated from the sham-operated side (Figure 1a). However, the increase in the expression levels of *Egr-1* was significantly less pronounced in diabetic mice compared to non-diabetic mice and control mice 24 h post-FAL ($2^{-\Delta\Delta CT}$, 3.19 ± 0.172 versus 22 ± 0.25, $p < 0.05$) (Figure 1a). Treatment of diabetic mice with insulin significantly increased *Egr-1* expression compared to the diabetic mice (3.45 ± 0.25) (Figure 1a), resulting in similar levels as in the control group. Western blot analyses revealed a significantly lower expression of Egr-1 protein in the diabetic group compared to both the non-diabetic control group and the insulin treated group (Figure 1b) 24 h after the surgical procedure.

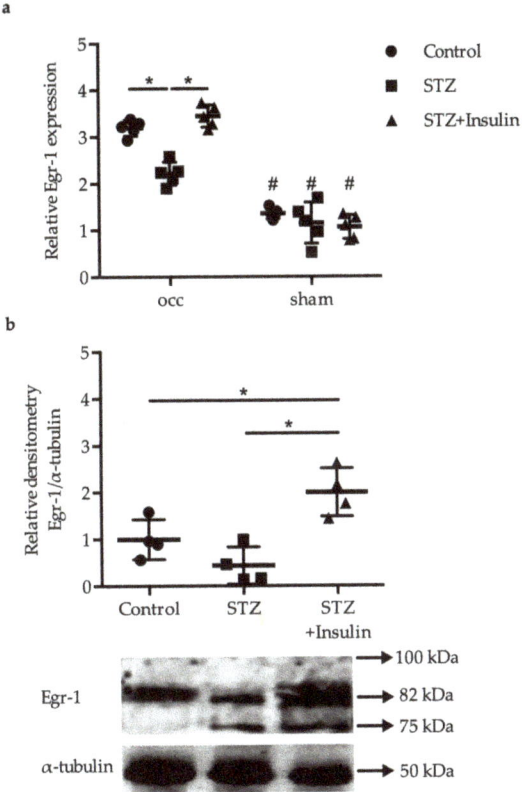

Figure 1. Gene expression studies of (**a**) mRNA levels and (**b**) protein levels of collateral arteries obtained from occluded and sham-operated mice 24 h after the surgical procedure. (**a**) Dot plots representing the results of qRT-PCR analyses ($n = 5$ per group, * $p < 0.05$ (each group compared to each other group), # $p < 0.05$ compared to corresponding occ group from one-way ANOVA with Bonferroni's multiple comparison test). Results were normalized to the expression level of the 18S rRNA. (**b**) Quantitative analyses (upper panel) and corresponding representative pictures of a Western blot (lower panel) showing the protein expression of Egr-1 as well as of α-tubulin, which was used for normalization, 24 h post-FAL ($n = 4$ per group, * $p < 0.05$ (each group compared to each other group) from one-way ANOVA with Bonferroni's multiple comparison test).

2.2. Expression of Egr-1 Downstream Genes in Collaterals of Diabetic Mice Was Restored by Insulin Treatment

The mRNA expression levels of Egr-1 downstream target genes, namely, Intercellular Adhesion Molecule-1 (ICAM-1), urokinase Plasminogen Activator (uPA), and Monocyte Chemoattractant Protein-1 (MCP-1) [18,23,24], were measured via qRT-PCR. Our results revealed decreased expression of ICAM-1 (Figure 2a) and uPA (Figure 2b) in the diabetic group compared to the non-diabetic control group (1.49 ± 0.49 versus 2.84 ± 0.49 and 1.53 ± 0.64 versus 3.2 ± 0.60, respectively). Mice treated with insulin showed a significant rise in ICAM-1 (2.35 ± 0.34) and uPA (3.56 ± 0.10) expression compared to the diabetic group. The expression of *MCP-1* decreased in diabetic mice (2.34 ± 0.15); however, its expression levels did not significantly rise upon treatment with insulin (2.65 ± 0.29) (Figure 2c). As previous results have shown that the transcriptional repressor Splicing Factor-1 (SF-1), which controls smooth muscle cell proliferation, is upregulated in growing collaterals during the process of arteriogenesis [22], we also investigated the expression level of the corresponding transcript. Our data showed a significant upregulation of SF-1 in the diabetic group (2.25 ± 0.36) compared to the non-diabetic group (1.15 ± 0.26), but its expression level was normalized again by insulin treatment (0.72 ± 0.04) (Figure 2d).

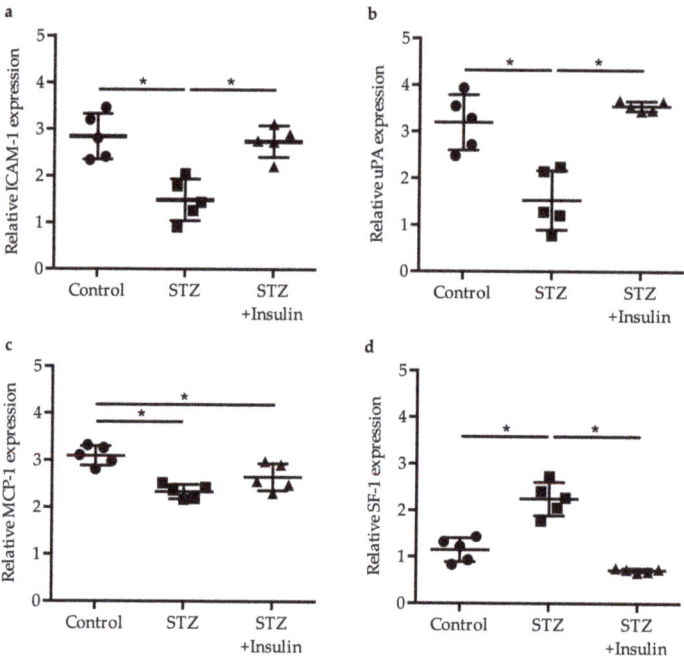

Figure 2. Gene expression of downstream targets of *Egr-1* in collateral tissues obtained from mice after induction of arteriogenesis was performed by qRT-PCR ($n = 5$ in each group, * $p < 0.05$ (each group compared to each other group) using a one-way ANOVA with Bonferroni's multiple comparison test). The relative expression is represented as 2^{-ddCT}. The relative expressions of (**a**) ICAM-1, (**b**) uPA, (**c**) MCP-1, and (**d**) SF-1 were normalized to the expression level of the 18S rRNA.

2.3. Insulin Treatment Restored Vessel Growth in Diabetic Mice

The luminal collateral vessel diameter, which was measured 7 days post-FAL, was found to be significantly decreased in the diabetic group (23.61 ± 2.1 µm) compared to the control group (30.76 ± 2.5 µm); however, it was restored to control levels by insulin treatment (29.58 ± 1.8 µm) (Figure 3a). Moreover, qRT-PCR results on the cell proliferation marker Ki-67 revealed significantly reduced Ki-67 mRNA expression in the diabetic group (1.36 ± 0.37) compared to the non-diabetic control group (2.35 ± 0.50); however, Ki-67 expression levels increased when STZ mice were treated with insulin (3.02 ± 0.15) (Figure 3b).

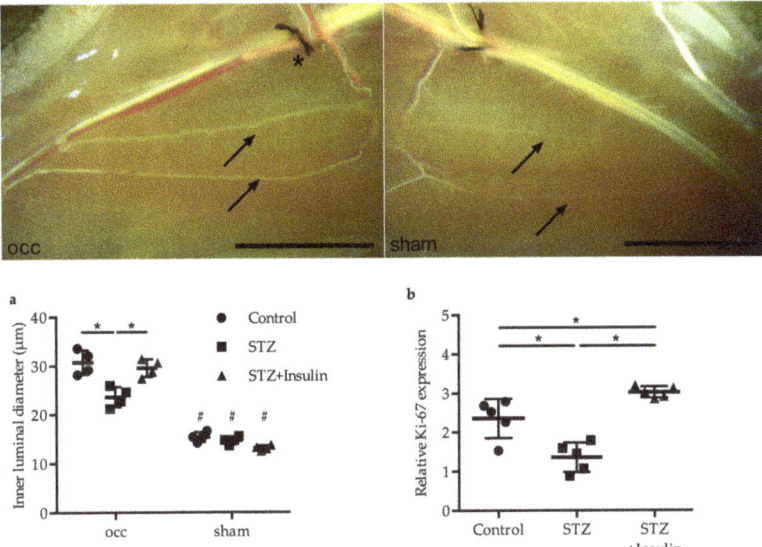

Figure 3. Upper panel: pictures of superficial collateral arteries of STZ-treated mice 7 days after femoral artery ligation (FAL, occ, left picture) or sham operation (right picture). Arrows indicate pre-existing (resting) collaterals of the sham-operated site or growth-induced collaterals of the experimental site. The ligation (*) of the femoral artery was executed downstream of the profound artery. Scale bars: 5 mm. Lower panel: (**a**) dot plots represent the inner luminal vessel diameter measured 7 days post-FAL ($n = 4$ per group, at least two collateral arteries per mouse and two sections were evaluated, * $p < 0.05$ (each group compared to each other group), # $p < 0.05$ compared to the corresponding occ group using a one-way ANOVA with Bonferroni's multiple comparison test). (**b**) Dot plots show the expression level of the proliferation marker Ki-67 in collaterals of control, STZ, and STZ + insulin-treated mice 24 h after FAL. Results were normalized to the expression level of the 18S rRNA ($n = 5$ per group, * $p < 0.05$ (each group compared to each other group) using a one-way ANOVA with Bonferroni's multiple comparison test).

2.4. Diminished Leukocyte Infiltration Was Improved in Diabetic Mice by Insulin Treatment

Fluorescent-activated cell sorting (FACS) studies from blood collected from non-ligated mice showed significantly increased levels of $CD11b^+$ cells in diabetic (55%) and insulin-treated groups (77%) compared to the non-diabetic control group (33%) with respect to $CD45^+$ cells, whereas the levels of $CD19^+$ or $CD3^+$ cells decreased in both the diabetic (10% and 14%, respectively) and the insulin-treated group (7% and 30%, respectively) (Figure 4a). There were no significant changes in leukocyte count in the adductor muscle of sham-operated mice in STZ-treated and STZ and insulin-treated mice compared to control mice (data not shown). However, in diabetic mice, there was a significant decrease in $CD11b^+$ (27% versus 13%), $CD19^+$ (45% versus 18%), and $CD3^+$ (55% versus 33%) cells three days post-ligation compared to control mice. Interestingly, insulin treatment increased the number of leukocytes in STZ-induced DM mice (Figure 4b).

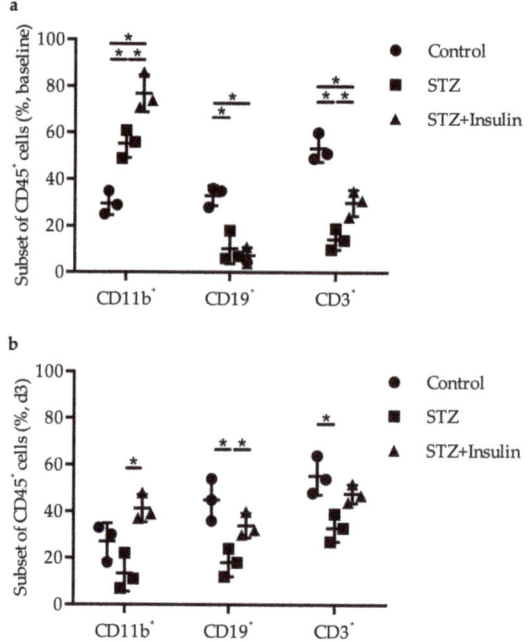

Figure 4. Dot plots represent the results of FACS analyses on CD11b[+], CD19[+], and CD3[+] cells performed on (**a**) whole blood of control, STZ, and STZ + insulin-treated mice without any surgical treatment and on (**b**) adductor muscles isolated from mice 3 days post-FAL (**a**,**b**: $n = 3$ per group, each group compared to each other group using a two-way ANOVA with Bonferroni's multiple comparison test).

3. Discussion

PAD is one of the common complications of DM that inflicts substantial damage to the lower limbs and has a very poor outcome. In mice, it was shown that impaired arteriogenesis is a major problem in hypercholesterolemia and DM [16]. While in the study by van Weel et al. [16], the influence of DM on perfusion recovery was less compared to that of hypercholesterolemia, our study showed a more pronounced impact of ligation on collateral vessel growth in DM. This may be due to the different experimental setup, age groups of animals under study, timepoints measured, and animal strains used. The mechanism by which impaired arteriogenesis occurs in DM is not fully understood. Earlier, Pagel et al. [22] reported the importance of *Egr-1* in promoting collateral outward remodeling through augmenting leukocyte infiltration and endothelial cell proliferation. In the present study, we report that there was a decreased expression of Egr-1 at the transcript and protein levels in collaterals of mice rendered diabetic by administration of streptozotocin. The decreased expression of *Egr-1* correlated with decreased collateral artery diameter in the diabetic mice. Important downstream targets of *Egr-1*, namely, *ICAM-1* and *uPA*, were found to be decreased, too. ICAM-1 plays a critical role in endothelial monocyte adhesion, which is essential for arteriogenesis. An earlier study identified an upregulation of ICAM-1 mRNA in growing collateral arteries after induction of arteriogenesis by femoral artery ligation [25]. Moreover, it was shown that the process of arteriogenesis is reduced in ICAM-1 deficient mice [26]. Treatment of the diabetic mice with insulin improved the expression of *Egr-1*, increased the collateral artery diameter, and normalized the expression of downstream targets of *Egr-1*. A proposed model is shown in Figure 5.

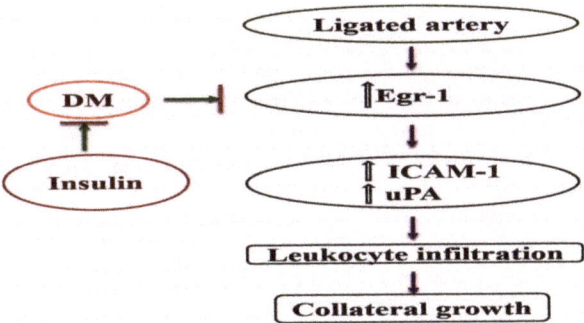

Figure 5. Graphical representation showing the mechanisms by which Egr-1 controls leukocyte recruitment, and hence, the process of collateral artery growth. While this process is impaired in DM due to the reduced *Egr-1* expression, it can be rescued by insulin treatment.

Earlier studies have clearly shown that induction of arteriogenesis in C57Bl6 mice by FAL resulted in an increased expression of *Egr-1* at the transcript and the protein levels in growing collaterals [22]. Interestingly, *Egr-1* deficient mice have been shown to have increased basal levels of CD11b$^+$ monocytes in the peripheral blood; however, levels of collateral perivascular macrophages as well as CD3$^+$ T cells and CD19$^+$ B cells in adductor muscles harvesting growing collaterals were reduced. Moreover, FAL in Egr-1−/− mice was associated with poor leukocyte recruitment and reduced collateral artery growth [22]. Our results showed that induction of DM, which was associated with reduced expression levels of *Egr-1*, also resulted in increased systemic levels of CD11b$^+$ cells, and after induction of arteriogenesis, in reduced levels of CD11b$^+$, CD3$^+$, and CD19$^+$ cells. Interestingly enough, treatment with insulin rescued perivascular leukocyte counts.

Decreased expression of *Egr-1* in DM mice in our study may support earlier findings showing that *Egr-1* is critical for collateral vessel development and that functional regulation of *Egr-1* may be compromised in DM. Evidence of induction and expression of *Egr-1* by elevated levels of glucose in murine glomerular endothelial cells and aortic smooth muscle cells have been reported. Exposure to insulin or high concentrations of D-glucose increased the expression of Egr-1 on the mRNA and protein level in glomerular endothelial cells and increased its promoter activity irrespectively of the concentration of insulin [27,28]. TNF-α is downstream of *Egr-1* and induces the expression of *MCP-1*. However, in arteriogenesis, increased levels of TNF-α, relevant for *MCP-1* expression, are dependent on mast cell activation [14]. Vedantham et. al. demonstrated a novel mechanism linking glucose metabolism to increased inflammatory and prothrombotic signaling in diabetic atherosclerosis via activation and post-translational modification of *Egr-1*. Hyperglycemia-induced hyper-acetylation of Egr-1 in endothelial cells was reported to be an important event linking diabetes to accelerated atherosclerosis [29]. Though acetylation of Egr-1 was not studied, it will be interesting to pursue future studies to understand the role of Egr-1 in the pathophysiology of arteriogenesis. Our observations in this study are contrary to those observed in diabetic atherosclerosis. There may be a possibility of additional regulation of Egr-1, as indicated by the shift in bands of Egr-1. Post-translational modifications of Egr-1 such as acetylation and phosphorylation have been reported to play an important role in the transcriptional activity and stability of Egr-1 [17,30]. Phosphorylation/dephosphorylation events may act as regulators for restricting the function of Egr-1. Furthermore, *SP-1* has been reported to compete for DNA binding sites of *Egr-1* [17]. Recently, a splice form of *Egr-1* was reported which lacks the N-terminal activation domain between amino acids 141 and 278 [31]. It will be interesting to further understand the mechanism through which hyperglycemia interferes with *Egr-1* upregulation during the process of arteriogenesis.

Leukocyte infiltration mediated through downstream target genes of *Egr-1*, namely, *ICAM-1*, *uPA* and *MCP-1*, was found to be decreased during collateral artery growth in diabetic mice. Endothelial uPA is vital for neutrophil adherence to the endothelial cells [32]. Neutrophils accumulate around day 1 after FAL in the perivascular space of growing collaterals and have a relevant function in the recruitment of macrophages and lymphocytes, which appear at day 3 [14]. Indeed, it has been shown that *uPA* deficiency is associated with reduced perivascular leukocyte accumulation and results in reduced collateral artery growth after induction of arteriogenesis via FAL [33]. These data comply with reported findings that *Egr-1* mediates leukocyte infiltration through activation of the abovementioned genes in arteriogenesis [21]. Furthermore, the expression of the cell proliferation marker Ki-67 was found to be decreased in the growing collaterals of diabetic mice, highlighting the fact that, indeed, there was a decrease in the proliferation of vascular cells. SF-1, an important transcriptional repressor critical for smooth muscle proliferation and phenotype switch [33], was found to be elevated in our study in support of an earlier report demonstrating that Egr-1−/− mice exhibited increased expression of SF-1 in growing collateral arteries [21]. One of the interesting findings of our study as the beneficial effect of insulin on collateral artery growth in DM mice. SF-1 regulates gene expression of pro-inflammatory cytokines in smooth muscle cells [33] and antagonizes platelet-derived growth factor BB (PDGF-BB)-induced growth and differentiation of vascular cells [34]. Several earlier reports have shown a regulation of *Egr-1* by insulin. Furthermore, Gousseva et al. [28] have reported an insulin-mediated increase in *Egr-1* promoter activity and cell proliferation in bovine aortic smooth muscle cells. Egr-1 has a role in adipocyte insulin resistance through activation of the MAPK-ERK pathway [35]. Our studies clearly show that diabetic mice treated with insulin show an increased expression of *Egr-1*, accompanied by an augmented expression of *Egr-1* downstream target genes relevant for leukocyte recruitment. Indeed, our results show that insulin treatment, moreover, goes along with increased numbers of leukocytes—relevant for the process of arteriogenesis—in collateral harboring muscles.

In summary, *Egr-1* expression decreased after induction of arteriogenesis in growing collaterals of streptozotocin-induced diabetic mice compared to control mice. Decreased *Egr-1* expression led to poor collateral growth. Insulin treatment, however, normalized the *Egr-1* expression, thereby promoting arteriogenesis. Though this was an observational study, this study assumes significance as it is the first time associating *Egr-1* with impaired arteriogenesis in DM. It will be interesting to see whether the same processes occur in patients with DM. Further investigations exploring the mechanism by which hyperglycemia suppresses *Egr-1* expression during the process of arteriogenesis will lead to better understanding of impaired arteriogenesis in DM.

4. Materials and Methods

4.1. Animal Studies

All studies with mice were performed after approval by the Institutional and Local Animal Ethics Committee (CPCSEA Approval number: H01/SASTRA/IAEC/RPP-23/12/15). Male C57B6NTac (Taconic Biosciences, USA) mice were procured through Vivo Biotech Ltd., Telangana, India and were maintained in an air-conditioned room (25 °C) with a 12 h light/12 h dark cycle. Feed and water were provided ad libitum to all the animals. Mice were rendered diabetic by treating them with STZ according to published protocols [36]. Briefly, eight-week-old male mice were made diabetic by administration of 50 mg/kg STZ dissolved in fresh citrate buffer (0.05 mol/L, pH 4.5) i.p. per day for five consecutive days. Those mice displaying blood glucose levels ≥ 250 mg/dL were considered diabetic (DM mice). The non-diabetic (NDM mice) control mice received citrate buffer alone. One group of mice received insulin after confirmation of hyperglycemia. Insulin was administered subcutaneously at a daily dose of 0.20 mL/100 g (4–5 U) until the end of the experiment.

4.2. Femoral Artery Ligation and Collection of Collaterals

Femoral artery ligation was performed as published earlier [37]. In brief, using a silk braided suture (0/7) the right femoral artery was ligated distally from the origin of the profunda femoris branching, while the left leg was sham operated. Adductor muscles and collateral arteries were collected as previously described [20]. To carry out fluorescent-activated cell sorting (FACS) analyses, adductor muscles were collected 3 days after the surgical procedure and for histological analysis, the adductor muscles were harvested 7 days after FAL. Gene expression studies on RNA and protein levels were performed with collateral arteries isolated 24 h after induction of arteriogenesis.

4.3. RNA Isolation and Quantitative Real-Time PCR Studies

Gene expression studies were performed using quantitative real time PCR (qRT-PCR). Total RNA was isolated using the RNeasy kit (TaKaRA). After DNase I (Qiagen, Hilden, Germany) digestion, one microgram of total RNA was reverse transcribed by random hexamers and Superscript RT-PCR System (Invitrogen, Carlsbad, CA, USA). After purification, the cDNA was used for qRT-PCR using specific primers for Egr-1, MCP-1, ICAM-1, SF-1, and Ki-67 [21]. Results were normalized to the expression level of the 18S rRNA.

4.4. FACS Analyses of Blood and Muscle Tissue

Whole blood withdrawn from the left ventricle 3 days post-ligation was analyzed by flow cytometry analyses (BD FACS Aria III, CA, USA) according to standard protocols. Furthermore, the adductor muscles from C57B6NTac mice were perfused with PBS (phosphate buffered saline) to eliminate the blood, harvested, and placed in small cell culture dishes. The tissue was cut into small pieces and digested 45 min at 37 °C using PBS buffer (50 mL) containing collagenase II (1 mg/mL), hyaluronidase (0.5 mg/mL) (both Sigma, St. Louis, MO, USA), dispase (1 mg/mL) (Gibco, Invitrogen, Carlsbad, CA, USA), and BSA (bovine serum albumin) (0.6 mg/mL) (Sigma). The suspension was then filtered with PBS/2%BSA through a 70 µm cell strainer (BD Falcon™), spun 10 min at 95 g, and the pellet finally resuspended in 100 µL PBS/2%BSA. The resulting cell suspension was analyzed by FACS using a panel of monoclonal antibodies against CD3 (T cells); (BioLegend Cat. No. 100201), CD11b (neutrophils, monocytes) (BioLegend Cat. No. 305902), CD19 (B cells) (BioLegend Cat. No. 115501), and CD45 (pan-leukocytes marker) (BioLegend Cat. No. 103101). Leukocyte populations were identified by fluorescence and scatter light characteristics. Cells from both peripheral blood and tissue were gated based on forward scatter (FSC-A)/side scatter (SSC-A). Leukocytes were identified by their positive staining with CD45. The final gating was based on CD45+/CD11b+, CD45+/CD19+, and CD45+/CD3+ cells (14).

4.5. Histological Analyses

Histological analyses were performed on adductor muscles (harboring collateral arteries) isolated from C57B6NTac mice as described earlier [20]. Briefly, 7 days after the surgical procedure both hind limbs were perfused with PBS containing 0.1% adenosine and 0.05% BSA (Sigma), then 4 min with fixing solution (4% buffered paraformaldehyde) via cannulation of the aorta. Thereafter, tissue samples were paraffin-embedded, cut in cross-sections, and H&E staining was performed to measure luminal collateral artery diameters.

4.6. Western Blot

Western blot analysis was performed on protein extracts, which were isolated from collaterals 24 h after femoral artery ligation or sham operation of DM and NDM mice according to standard procedures. Briefly, 30 µg of protein from all the tissue lysates was loaded onto a 10% sodium dodecyl sulfate (SDS) gel and ran at a power of 110 V. The protein in the gel was shifted to an immune-blot polyvinylidene difluoride (PVDF) membrane (1620112, Bio-Rad, USA) at 100 V for 1 h using Trans-Blot Turbo Transfer System (Bio-Rad). The blots were probed for Egr-1 protein (Egr-1 antibody (588)-Santa Cruz BioTechnology Cat.no #sc110). α-Tubulin served as a housekeeping protein (alpha tubulin antibody (B-7): Santa Cruz Biotechnology Cat.no. #sc-5286). The density of Egr-1 to α-tubulin was measured through the Quant-One software (Bio-Rad). The immunoblots are a representation of at least three independent experiments.

4.7. Statistical Analysis

All values are expressed as means ± SD unless mentioned. Statistical analyses were conducted as indicated in the figure legends using GraphPad software PRISM6 (GraphPad Software, USA). The limit of statistical significance was set at $p < 0.05$.

Author Contributions: S.V. and E.D. conceived the research idea, executed the study, and prepared the manuscript. S.T. and S.K. performed the experiments. M.L. contributed in the transfer of technology and helped in manuscript preparation. D.R.C. assisted in animal surgery.

Funding: This research was funded by Indo-German co-operation in health grant funded by ICMR-BMBF [50/6/2013/BMS] to S.V. and E.D.

Acknowledgments: The authors would like to acknowledge ICMR-BMBF (50/6/2013/BMS) and SASTRA Deemed to be University for supporting the research funding and facility, respectively. Moreover, we would like to thank Anna-Kristina Kluever for editing the manuscript.

Conflicts of Interest: The authors declare no conflict of interest.

Abbreviations

SF-1	Splicing Factor 1
DM	Diabetes Mellitus
NDM	Non-Diabetes Mellitus
Egr-1	Early growth response-1
uPA	urokinase Plasminogen Activator
MCP-1	Monocyte Chemoattractant Protein-1
ICAM-1	Intercellular Adhesion Molecule-1
FAL	Femoral Artery Ligation
STZ	Streptozotocin
PAD	Peripheral Artery Disease

References

1. American Diabetes Association. Peripheral Arterial Disease in People with Diabetes. *Diabetes Care* **2003**, *26*, 3333–3341. [CrossRef] [PubMed]
2. Dolan, N.C.; Liu, K.; Criqui, M.H.; Greenland, P.; Guralnik, J.M.; Chan, C.; Schneider, J.R.; Mandapat, A.L.; Martin, G.; McDermott, M.M. Peripheral artery disease, diabetes, and reduced lower extremity functioning. *Diabetes Care* **2002**, *25*, 113–120. [CrossRef] [PubMed]
3. Prompers, L.; Schaper, N.; Apelqvist, J.; Edmonds, M.; Jude, E.; Mauricio, D.; Uccioli, L.; Urbancic, V.; Bakker, K.; Holstein, P.; et al. Prediction of outcome in individuals with diabetic foot ulcers: Focus on the differences between individuals with and without peripheral arterial disease. The EURODIALE Study. *Diabetologia* **2008**, *51*, 747–755. [CrossRef] [PubMed]
4. Shu, J.; Santulli, G. Update on peripheral artery disease: Epidemiology and evidence-based facts. *Atherosclerosis* **2018**, *275*, 379–381. [CrossRef] [PubMed]
5. Beckman, J.A.; Creager, M.A.; Libby, P. Diabetes and atherosclerosis: Epidemiology, pathophysiology, and management. *JAMA* **2002**, *287*, 2570–2581. [CrossRef] [PubMed]
6. Lanzer, P. Topographic distribution of peripheral arteriopathy in non-diabetics and type 2 diabetics. *Z. Kardiol.* **2001**, *90*, 99–103. [CrossRef] [PubMed]
7. Eberhardt, R.T.; Coffman, J.D. Cardiovascular morbidity and mortality in peripheral arterial disease. *Curr. Drug Targets Cardiovasc. Haematol. Disord.* **2004**, *4*, 209–217. [CrossRef]
8. Faglia, E.; Clerici, G.; Clerissi, J.; Gabrielli, L.; Losa, S.; Mantero, M.; Caminiti, M.; Curci, V.; Quarantiello, A.; Lupattelli, T.; et al. Long-term prognosis of diabetic patients with critical limb ischemia: A population-based cohort study. *Diabetes Care* **2009**, *32*, 822–827. [CrossRef]

9. Kamalesh, M.; Shen, J. Diabetes and peripheral arterial disease in men: Trends in prevalence, mortality, and effect of concomitant coronary disease. *Clin. Cardiol.* **2009**, *32*, 442–446. [CrossRef]
10. Malmstedt, J.; Leander, K.; Wahlberg, E.; Karlstrom, L.; Alfredsson, L.; Swedenborg, J. Outcome after leg bypass surgery for critical limb ischemia is poor in patients with diabetes: A population-based cohort study. *Diabetes Care* **2008**, *31*, 887–892. [CrossRef]
11. Currie, C.J.; Morgan, C.L.; Peters, J.R. The epidemiology and cost of inpatient care for peripheral vascular disease, infection, neuropathy, and ulceration in diabetes. *Diabetes Care* **1998**, *21*, 42–48. [CrossRef] [PubMed]
12. Moraes, F.; Paye, J.; Mac Gabhann, F.; Zhuang, Z.W.; Zhang, J.; Lanahan, AA.; Simons, M. Endothelial cell-dependent regulation of arteriogenesis. *Circ. Res.* **2013**, *113*, 1076–1086. [CrossRef] [PubMed]
13. Arras, M.; Ito, W.D.; Scholz, D.; Winkler, B.; Schaper, J.; Schaper, W. Monocyte activation in angiogenesis and collateral growth in the rabbit hindlimb. *J. Clin. Invest.* **1998**, *101*, 41–50. [CrossRef] [PubMed]
14. Chillo, O.; Kleinert, E.C.; Lautz, T.; Lasch, M.; Pagel, J.I.; Heun, Y.; Troidl, K.; Fischer, S.; Caballero-Martinez, A.; Mauer, A.; et al. Perivascular Mast Cells Govern Shear Stress-Induced Arteriogenesis by Orchestrating Leukocyte Function. *Cell Rep.* **2016**, *23*, 2197–2207. [CrossRef] [PubMed]
15. De Vivo, S.; Palmer-Kazen, U.; Kalin, B.; Wahlberg, E. Risk factors for poor collateral development in claudication. *Vasc. Endovasc. Surg.* **2005**, *39*, 519–524. [CrossRef] [PubMed]
16. Van Weel, V.; de Vries, M.; Voshol, P.J.; Verloop, R.E.; Eilers, P.H.; van Hinsbergh, V.W.; van Bockel, J.H.; Quax, P.H. Hypercholesterolemia reduces collateral artery growth more dominantly than hyperglycemia or insulin resistance in mice. *Arterioscler. Thromb. Vasc. Biol.* **2006**, *26*, 1383–1390. [CrossRef] [PubMed]
17. Lambiase, P.D.; Edwards, R.J.; Anthopoulos, P.; Rahman, S.; Meng, Y.G.; Bucknall, C.A.; Redwood, S.R.; Pearson, J.D.; Marber, M.S. Circulating humoral factors and endothelial progenitor cells in patients with differing coronary collateral support. *Circulation* **2004**, *109*, 2986–2992. [CrossRef] [PubMed]
18. Gashler, A.; Sukhatme, V. Egr-1: Prototype of a zinc finger family of transcription factors. *Prog. Nucleic Acid. Res. Mol Biol.* **1995**, *50*, 191–224.
19. Yan, S.F.; Harja, E.; Andrassy, M.; Fujita, T.; Schmidt, A.M. Protein kinase C beta/early growth response-1 pathway: A key player in ischemia, atherosclerosis, and restenosis. *J. Am. Coll. Cardiol.* **2006**, *48*, A47–A55. [CrossRef]
20. Sarateanu, C.S.; Retuerto, M.A.; Beckmann, J.T.; McGregor, L.; Carbray, J.; Patejunas, G.; Nayak, L.; Milbrandt, J.; Rosengart, T.K. An Egr-1 master switch for arteriogenesis: Studies in Egr-1 homozygous negative and wild-type animals. *J. Thorac. Cardiovasc. Surg.* **2006**, *131*, 138–145. [CrossRef]
21. Lee, J.S.; Lee, J.Y.; Li Kim, K.; Shin, I.S.; Suh, W.; Choi, J.H.; Jeon, E.S.; Byun, J.; Kim, D.K. Adenoviral-mediated delivery of early growth response factor-1 gene increases tissue perfusion in a murine model of hindlimb ischemia. *Mol. Ther.* **2005**, *12*, 328–336. [CrossRef] [PubMed]
22. Pagel, J.I.; Ziegelhoeffer, T.; Heil, M.; Fischer, S.; Fernández, B.; Schaper, W.; Preissner, K.T.; Deindl, E. Role of early growth response 1 in arteriogenesis: Impact on vascular cell proliferation and leukocyte recruitment in vivo. *Thromb. Haemost.* **2012**, *107*, 562–574. [PubMed]
23. McMahon, S.B.; Monroe, J.G. The role of early growth response gene 1 (egr-1) in regulation of the immune response. *J. Leukoc. Biol.* **1996**, *60*, 159–166. [CrossRef] [PubMed]
24. Yan, SF.; Fujita, T.; Lu, J.; Okada, K.; Shan Zou, Y.; Mackman, N.; Pinsky, DJ.; Stern, DM. Egr-1, a master switch coordinating upregulation of divergent gene families underlying ischemic stress. *Nat. Med.* **2000**, *6*, 1355–1361. [CrossRef] [PubMed]
25. Scholz, D.; Ito, W.; Fleming, I.; Deindl, E.; Sauer, A.; Babiak, A.; Bühler, A.; Wiesnet, M.; Busse, R.; Schaper, J.; et al. Ultrastructure and molecular histology of rabbit hindlimb collateral artery growth (arteriogenesis). *Virchows. Arch.* **2000**, *436*, 257–270. [CrossRef] [PubMed]
26. Hoefer, I.E.; van Royen, N.; Rectenwald, J.E.; Deindl, E.; Hua, J.; Jost, M.; Grundmann, S.; Voskuil, M.; Ozaki, C.K.; et al. Arteriogenesis proceeds via ICAM-1/Mac-1- mediated mechanisms. *Circ. Res.* **2004**, *94*, 1179–1185. [CrossRef] [PubMed]
27. Hasan, R.N.; Phukan, S.; Harada, S. Differential regulation of early growth response gene-1 expression by insulin and glucose in vascular endothelial cells. *Arterioscler. Thromb. Vasc. Biol.* **2003**, *23*, 988–993. [CrossRef] [PubMed]
28. Gousseva, N.; Kugathasan, K.; Chesterman, C.N.; Khachigian, L.M. Early growth response factor-1 mediates insulin-inducible vascular endothelial cell proliferation and regrowth after injury. *J. Cell. Biochem.* **2001**, *81*, 523–534. [CrossRef]

29. Vedantham, S.; Thiagarajan, D.; Ananthakrishnan, R.; Wang, L.; Rosario, R.; Zou, S.; Goldberg, I.J.; Yan, S.F.; Schmidt, A.M.; Ramasamy, R. Aldose Reductase drives hyperacetylation of Egr-1 in hyperglycemia and consequent upregulation of proinflammatory and prothrombotic signals. *Diabetes* **2014**, *63*, 761–774. [CrossRef]
30. Aliperti, V.; Sgueglia, G.; Aniello, F.; Vitale, E.; Fucci, L.; Donizetti, A. Identification, Characterization, and Regulatory Mechanisms of a Novel EGR-1 Splicing Isoform. *Int. J. Mol. Sci.* **2019**, *20*, 1548. [CrossRef]
31. Reichel, C.A.; Uhl, B.; Lerchenberger, M.; Puhr-Westerheide, D.; Rehberg, M.; Liebl, J.; Khandoga, A.; Schmalix, W.; Zahler, S.; Deindl, E.; et al. Urokinase-type plasminogen activator promotes paracellular transmigration of neutrophils via Mac-1, but independently of urokinase-type plasminogen activator receptor. *Circulation* **2011**, *124*, 1848–1859. [CrossRef] [PubMed]
32. Deindl, E.; Ziegelhöffer, T.; Kanse, S.M.; Fernandez, B.; Neubauer, E.; Carmeliet, P.; Preissner, K.T.; Schaper, W. Receptor-independent role of the urokinase-type plasminogen activator during arteriogenesis. *FASEB J.* **2003**, *17*, 1174–1176. [CrossRef] [PubMed]
33. Cattaruzza, M.; Schafer, K.; Hecker, M. Cytokine-induced down-regulation of zfm1/splicing factor-1 promotes smooth muscle cell proliferation. *J. Biol. Chem.* **2002**, *277*, 6582–6589. [CrossRef]
34. Cattaruzza, M.; Nogoy, N.; Wojtowicz, A.; Hecker, M. Zinc finger motif-1 antagonizes PDGF-BB-induced growth and dedifferentiation of vascular smooth muscle cells. *FASEB J.* **2012**, *26*, 4864–4875. [CrossRef] [PubMed]
35. Yu, X.; Shen, N.; Zhang, M.L.; Pan, F.Y.; Wang, C.; Jia, W.P.; Liu, C.; Gao, Q.; Gao, X.; Xue, B.; et al. Egr-1 decreases adipocyte insulin sensitivity by tilting PI3K/Akt and MAPK signal balance in mice. *EMBO J.* **2011**, *30*, 3754–3765. [CrossRef] [PubMed]
36. Jawerbaum, A.; White, V. Animal models in diabetes and pregnancy. *Endocr. Rev.* **2010**, *31*, 680–701. [CrossRef]
37. Limbourg, A.; Korff, T.; Napp, L.C.; Schaper, W.; Drexler, H.; Limbourg, F.P. Evaluation of postnatal arteriogenesis and angiogenesis in a mouse model of hind-limb ischemia. *Nat. Protoc.* **2009**, *4*, 1737–1746. [CrossRef]

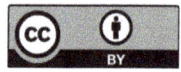

© 2019 by the authors. Licensee MDPI, Basel, Switzerland. This article is an open access article distributed under the terms and conditions of the Creative Commons Attribution (CC BY) license (http://creativecommons.org/licenses/by/4.0/).

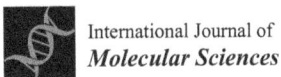

Review

Applications of Ultrasound to Stimulate Therapeutic Revascularization

Catherine M. Gorick [1], John C. Chappell [2] and Richard J. Price [1,*]

1. Department of Biomedical Engineering, University of Virginia, Charlottesville, VA 22908, USA; cmg6ae@virginia.edu
2. Fralin Biomedical Research Institute at Virginia Tech Carilion School of Medicine, Roanoke, VA 24016, USA; jchappell@vtc.vt.edu
* Correspondence: rprice@virginia.edu; Tel.: +1-434-924-0020

Received: 29 May 2019; Accepted: 21 June 2019; Published: 24 June 2019

Abstract: Many pathological conditions are characterized or caused by the presence of an insufficient or aberrant local vasculature. Thus, therapeutic approaches aimed at modulating the caliber and/or density of the vasculature by controlling angiogenesis and arteriogenesis have been under development for many years. As our understanding of the underlying cellular and molecular mechanisms of these vascular growth processes continues to grow, so too do the available targets for therapeutic intervention. Nonetheless, the tools needed to implement such therapies have often had inherent weaknesses (i.e., invasiveness, expense, poor targeting, and control) that preclude successful outcomes. Approximately 20 years ago, the potential for using ultrasound as a new tool for therapeutically manipulating angiogenesis and arteriogenesis began to emerge. Indeed, the ability of ultrasound, especially when used in combination with contrast agent microbubbles, to mechanically manipulate the microvasculature has opened several doors for exploration. In turn, multiple studies on the influence of ultrasound-mediated bioeffects on vascular growth and the use of ultrasound for the targeted stimulation of blood vessel growth via drug and gene delivery have been performed and published over the years. In this review article, we first discuss the basic principles of therapeutic ultrasound for stimulating angiogenesis and arteriogenesis. We then follow this with a comprehensive cataloging of studies that have used ultrasound for stimulating revascularization to date. Finally, we offer a brief perspective on the future of such approaches, in the context of both further research development and possible clinical translation.

Keywords: arteriogenesis; therapeutic revascularization; ultrasound; microbubbles; biomaterials; drug and gene delivery

---

1. Therapeutic Vascular Remodeling

The vascular system facilitates the transport of oxygen and essential nutrients to all tissues, aids in maintaining body temperature and tissue fluid levels, and removes metabolic waste byproducts, regulating each process through specific mechanisms for different physiological states. In the case of disease pathology, the vasculature can be driven from quiescence and can actively alter its structure, engaging in processes such as vasculogenesis (de novo vessel formation), angiogenesis (new vessels sprouting from existing vessels), arteriogenesis (collateral artery growth), and vessel regression (disassembly of vascular structures). Alzheimer's disease, atherosclerosis (leading to peripheral arterial disease and myocardial ischemia), and osteoporosis are prominent examples of conditions characterized or influenced by insufficient vascularization or vessel regression [1]. Insight into the complex and highly integrated cellular, molecular, and genetic mechanisms underlying the aforementioned vascular growth and remodeling processes is steadily increasing through worldwide research efforts. In turn, there has been an expansion in the potential of clinically relevant therapies that seek to augment angiogenesis or arteriogenesis in states of vascular deficiency or regression.

Many current treatments for vascular disorders involve invasive surgical procedures that risk severe complications and are not available to all patients [2–6]. Therefore, with the goal of minimizing invasiveness and undesired side effects, novel cell-, molecule-, and gene-based interventions for therapeutic revascularization are being explored in a wide range of studies, all seeking the potential development of clinically relevant therapies. For instance, adult stem cells, i.e., adipose-derived cells, bone marrow-derived cells (BMDCs), and circulating endothelial progenitor cells (EPCs), have been investigated for their ability to promote enhanced vascular growth and remodeling in tissues afflicted by an ischemic injury [7–10]. Vascular growth factors and cytokines like vascular endothelial growth factor-A (VEGF-A) [11–13], platelet-derived growth factor-BB (PDGF-BB) [14,15], and granulocyte-macrophage colony-stimulating factor (GM-CSF) [16–18], and genes encoding various pro-angiogenic and pro-arteriogenic molecules [19–21], have also been explored in the context of tissue ischemia. Furthermore, our emerging understanding of the roles of various epigenetic factors (e.g., DNA methylation [22] and non-coding RNAs [23,24]) in regulating vascular growth and remodeling now offers opportunities for new therapeutic targets [25].

However, considerable limitations exist not only in designing revascularization therapies that influence only the intended molecular targets, but also in physically delivering the therapeutic agents only to the disease site in a way where unrelated tissues are not affected. For instance, adsorption from the gut to the bloodstream (i.e., oral administration) may pose risks to systemic tissues and organs, and intravenous injection and catheter-based administration methods face similar difficulties. Implanting controlled release devices can involve an invasive procedure and also present the risk of infection or an adverse biomaterial response. Direct injection of a therapeutic agent into and/or near ischemic tissue is perhaps the most commonly used mode of delivery for revascularization, but this invasive approach often lacks a sustained vascular remodeling response and can yield the poor dispersion of therapeutic agents away from injection site(s). Thus, in the context of therapeutic revascularization, substantial opportunities remain for developing more efficient delivery approaches that offer high spatial accuracy and minimal invasiveness.

2. Ultrasound Technology: Basic Principles and Contrast Agents

One minimally-invasive technology that has the potential to both achieve high spatial accuracy and yield wide therapeutic dispersion through tissue for revascularization is therapeutic ultrasound (US). Before discussing how ultrasound may be applied therapeutically for revascularization, we provide here a brief background on the basic principles that govern US and its potentially beneficial effects on tissue. An US waveform is transmitted into a region of interest when specific piezoelectric elements positioned on the face of a transducer are activated by an appropriate electrical signal. The generated acoustic energy propagates through the tissue, encountering regions of varying acoustic (i.e., mechanical) impedance. These mechanical heterogeneities modify the ultrasound beam through attenuation and diffraction as well as reflection and scattering. In diagnostic ultrasound imaging, reflected and scattered energy returns to the transducer, which now behaves as a receiver, converting the mechanical acoustic energy into electrical energy. A meaningful image can then be displayed when these electrical signals are processed appropriately.

After many years of use as a minimally invasive imaging modality, it was discovered that US in conjunction with gas-filled contrast agent microbubbles (which enhance blood echogenicity and, consequently, the contrast between tissues during an US exam) could also be used for other applications. These microbubbles (MBs) circulating within the bloodstream can be destroyed by US, facilitating the assessment of tissue perfusion by its correlation to MB replenishment in a given region [26,27]. Concerns about the possible deleterious bioeffects from ultrasonic MB destruction have fueled investigations into the impact of this phenomenon on surrounding tissues. Observations from these studies have shown that localized regions of microvessels experienced increases in permeabilization as indicated by red blood cell (RBC) extravasation from sites of intravascular US + MB interactions [28–31]. Based on these findings, significant interest was generated in possibly exploiting these US + MB-induced bioeffects for beneficial purposes including the direct stimulation of vascular remodeling through the bioeffects of ultrasonic MB activation as well as the targeted delivery of therapeutic agents.

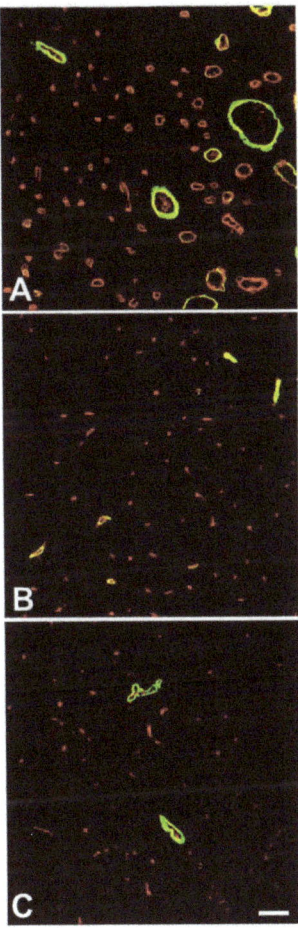

Figure 1. Activation of microbubbles with ultrasound can elicit arteriogenesis. Confocal micrographs illustrating the expression of SM α-actin (green fluorescence) in relation to microvessels, as labeled with BS-I lectin (red fluorescence). Images were taken 14 days after muscles were exposed to US-MB treatment (**A**) or sham treatment (**B**). Panel (**C**) represents the untreated muscle. Note the increased number and caliber of SM α-actin+ vessels with US + MB treatment (**A**). Bar = 30 µm. Adapted from Song et al. [32].

3. Ultrasound Activation of Microbubbles to Facilitate Angiogenesis and Arteriogenesis

Interactions between relatively low-power US and circulating MBs elicit a range of bioeffects through mechanisms that remain only partially understood [33,34]. In addition to the increase in microvascular permeability discussed in the previous sections [29,30], hemolysis (i.e., RBC destruction) [35–38] and arterial vasospasms [39] have been shown to occur near sites of US + MB interactions. Additionally, cavitation of MBs by US may cause free radical production [40–42], heating [43–45], shockwave emanation resulting in microstreaming [46–48], and bubble fragmentation producing microjets [34,49]. These effects may individually or collaboratively impact the surrounding microenvironment to elicit the tissue level consequences (e.g., capillary disruptions, wound healing pathways, hemostasis, inflammation signaling pathways). Components of these pathways are known to be involved in modulating vascular remodeling; thus, it was postulated that selectively instigating these pathways, among others, through the targeted destruction of MBs with US might result in a localized neovascularization response in treated tissues.

Indeed, this hypothesis was verified by an exploration of the vascular remodeling response in the gracilis muscle of a rat hindlimb exposed to low-power US and intravascular MBs [32]. Here, the application of 1-MHz pulsed US following intravenous injection of MBs induced capillary disruption sites as visualized by RBC extravasation. This elicited an arteriogenic response (Figure 1), which, in turn, enhanced blood flow in the hindlimb skeletal muscle. Furthermore, a follow-up study demonstrated the ability of this US + MB treatment scheme to significantly augment the vascular remodeling response of, and subsequently restore the perfusion to, a rat hindlimb affected by an arterial occlusion [50]. The experimental procedures from the rat studies were recapitulated in normal mice [51], in part to lay the foundation for studies addressing possible mechanisms behind the US + MB-induced neovascular adaptations. This transition to a mouse model provided a platform that was also advantageous for both mechanistic experiments involving genetic and/or cellular alterations and for experiments in a model of hindlimb ischemia. Although transient and failing to match the duration and extent of the response observed in the rat study, mouse hindlimb skeletal muscle exposed to a comparable US + MB treatment indeed exhibited a significant increase in neovascularization in comparison to the sham-treated muscles.

An investigation into the method by which these therapeutic vascular remodeling responses occur in the ischemic mouse and rat hindlimb revealed that the recruitment of CD18+ (integrin beta chain-2+) BMDCs is necessary for angiogenesis, arteriogenesis, and CD11b+ monocyte recruitment, as animals with CD18$^{-/-}$ BMDCs did not exhibit vascular remodeling [52]. A separate study demonstrated that treatment with US + MBs induced the recruitment of CD45+ leukocytes including macrophages and T-lymphocytes to the treated tissue. Both of these cell types produce VEGF-A, and VEGF-A levels were elevated in the treated muscle, corresponding to increased capillary density, surface vascularity, blood flow, and functional improvement in the previously-ischemic skeletal muscle [53].

The selected parameters of the US + MB application have been shown to play a role in the ensuing vascular responses. For example, the influence of raising peak US rarefactional pressure to 3.8 MPa (in contrast to the previously described studies, which used pressures as high as 1.4 MPa), which ensures collapse of 100% of all MBs within the US focal region, has been tested. Animals treated at this high US pressure exhibited a marked decrease in capillary density immediately following treatment as well as clear evidence of hemorrhage. While capillary density increased somewhat in the weeks following treatment, it only reached 70% of baseline by 27 days post-treatment, suggesting that 100% MB collapse by high pressure US causes capillary destruction from which normal rats cannot recover [54]. Further study by this group explored the effects of different concentrations of MBs at a lower US pressure (0.7 MPa), and found that increased concentrations of MBs were associated with a greater degree of vascular permeability and VEGF expression [55].

While the majority of studies investigating the role of US activation of MBs to promote vascular remodeling have been in the context of skeletal muscle, several other tissues have also been investigated. US + MBs have been used to stimulate revascularization in the myocardium following acute myocardial infarction. In a mouse model, US activation of MBs resulted in increased microvascular density and reduced scar size, along with a transient up-regulation of VEGF-A and IGF-1 in the myocardium and improved left ventricular function [56]. Recently, there has been increased interest in the potential application of US and MBs to induce remodeling of brain vasculature. Focused US (FUS) in combination with MBs can be used to temporarily open the blood–brain barrier (BBB) at specific sites in the brain [57–60], consistent with the increased vascular permeability observed in other tissues. It has been observed that following disruption of the BBB by FUS and MBs, there is an acute upregulation of proinflammatory cytokine genes as well as angiogenesis-related genes in microvessels [61]. Further investigation of this phenomenon revealed that the transcriptional changes did in fact correspond with functional responses—following FUS activation of MBs in the hippocampus, there was a transient increase in blood vessel density as well as increased newborn endothelial cell density and frequency of small blood vessel segments [62].

4. Ultrasound and Microbubbles to Deliver Genes, Molecules, or Cells to Facilitate Angiogenesis and Arteriogenesis

As described previously, observations that US-mediated destruction of MBs could enhance blood vessel permeability have spurred interest in using these phenomena to facilitate the targeted delivery of therapeutic agents. The general premise is to co-administer a therapeutic agent, either freely circulating in the bloodstream alongside MBs, or physically associated with the MBs (i.e., bound/tethered to their surface or contained within the MB (Figure 2)) into the bloodstream while the MBs are circulating. Following US-induced cavitation of the MBs, there is increased permeability of the vessels at the site of US exposure, allowing for increased extravasation or uptake of the therapeutic agent in the circulation (Figure 2). Demonstrating this targeted delivery concept, Price et al. delivered polymer microspheres into the interstitium of rat spinotrapezius muscle via microvessel disruptions caused by ultrasonic MB destruction [31]. One of the first studies to show successful US + MB-targeted gene delivery involved the transfer of the P-galactosidase gene into rat myocardium through echocardiographic MB destruction [63]. While gene delivery to the myocardium with this US + MB technique has been investigated in several other studies [36,53,64–68], the potential treatment of various pathologies using US + MB-mediated gene transfer has also been explored in numerous other tissues including skeletal muscle [69–74], liver [75–83], and brain [84–97].

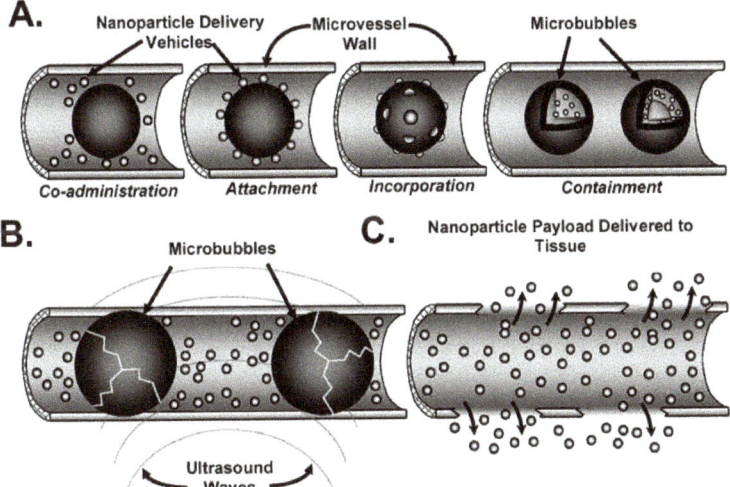

Figure 2. Overview of approaches to US + MB-mediated drug and/or gene delivery. (**A**) The therapeutic agent (nanoparticles in this example) may be co-administered with contrast agent microbubbles, attached to microbubble shells, incorporated into the microbubble shell, and/or contained within the microbubble. (**B**) The application of US activates the oscillation of microbubbles. At high enough peak-negative acoustic pressures, microbubbles can be fragmented. In some approaches, microbubble activation may lead to dissociation of a bound therapeutic from the microbubble. (**C**) Ultrasound–microbubble interactions simultaneously act to permeabilize the surrounding microvasculature, facilitating delivery of the therapeutic via diffusion and/or convection from the bloodstream to the ultrasound-targeted tissue. Adapted from Chappell and Price. [98].

Using US + MBs to facilitate nucleic acid delivery to specifically modulate vascular remodeling remains a relatively underexplored technology. The delivery of a VEGF-A gene to the rat myocardium has been demonstrated using US-targeted MB destruction. After treatment, increased levels of VEGF-A mRNA and protein were evident as well as increased capillary and arteriolar density within the myocardium [65]. The VEGF-A gene is also delivered to skeletal muscle in rats following a hindlimb ischemia surgery. In this study, the authors noted increased levels of the VEGF-A mRNA shortly after US + MB treatment as well as enhanced tissue perfusion, which was attributed to an observed increase in arteriolar density [73]. Moreover, it has been shown that genes may be delivered in a highly-targeted manner to hindlimb skeletal muscle using ultrasound in combination with non-viral gene nanocarriers (Figure 3) [70]. Although not yet utilized in a therapeutic revascularization capacity, this nanocarrier approach offers enticing options for technology development in this space going forward.

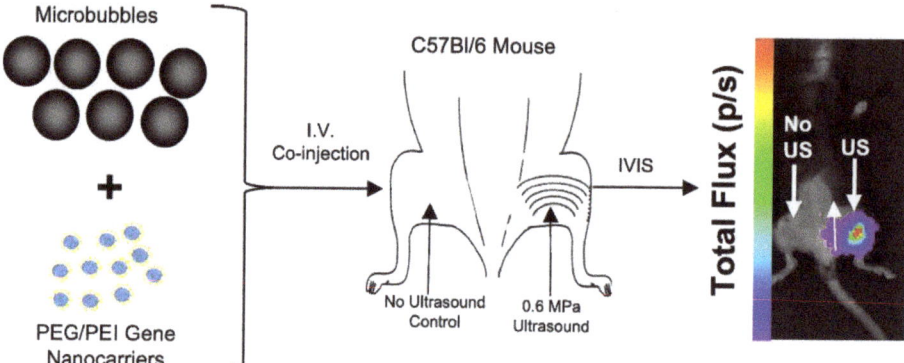

Figure 3. Overview of the strategy for eliciting ultrasound-targeted transfection of hindlimb adductor muscles via the delivery of non-viral gene nanocarriers. (**Left**) Contrast agent microbubbles are intravenously co-injected with gene-bearing nanocarriers. (**Middle**) Pulsed ultrasound is then applied to the adductor muscle group, which activates microbubble oscillation and facilitates nanocarrier delivery to the muscle tissue. (**Right**) Reporter gene expression is evident only where ultrasound has been applied. Adapted from Burke et al. [70].

US and MB interactions have also been used to stimulate vascular remodeling in tissues other than skeletal muscle. One particularly interesting example entails the use of ultrasound to deliver a VEGF-A gene to the placental basal plate in a pregnant baboon to stimulate uterine artery remodeling [99]. Meanwhile, myocardium obviously also represents an important target for therapeutic revascularization. Delivery of a hepatocyte growth factor (HGF) plasmid to the myocardium in a canine model of myocardial infarction resulted in increased capillary density as well as reduced infarct size and scar tissue formation [100]. An HGF plasmid has also been delivered with US + MBs in a rat model of myocardial infarction. This treatment resulted in reduced left ventricular hypertrophy and scar formation as well as increased capillary and arterial density in the US-treated region [68]. Additionally, recent studies have explored the potential of the US + MB approach to deliver therapeutic genes to the brain. Following evidence that VEGF-A delivery to the brain promotes angiogenesis and functional recovery after ischemic stroke [101–103], US + MBs were employed to deliver a VEGF-A plasmid to the peri-ischemic region of the brain after infarction. The VEGF-A treatment reduced infarct size and apoptosis, and increased vessel density through stimulation of angiogenesis [92].

While not within the strict definition of "vascular remodeling" as applied in this review article (i.e., vasculogenesis, angiogenesis, and arteriogenesis), a few groups have investigated the use of US for targeted delivery in the context of neointimal hyperplasia, and such studies may offer insight into therapeutic revascularization strategies. In a handful of studies, US + MB-mediated approaches have been utilized to deliver an NFκB cis-element 'decoy' to inhibit neointimal hyperplasia development in arterial injury models. Delivery of this decoy in a rat carotid artery injury model was found to prevent the upregulation of intercellular adhesion molecule 1 (ICAM-1) and vascular cell adhesion molecule 1 (VCAM-1) in the neointimal area otherwise activated by arterial injury as well as the influx of macrophages and T-lymphocytes into the intima and media [104]. Similar observations were made following delivery of the 'decoy' in murine [105] or porcine [106] arterial injury models, suggesting the potential of this approach for minimizing neointimal hyperplasia following angioplasty or other coronary interventions. In addition, US + MB delivery of an siRNA against ICAM-1 has also been shown to suppress the development of neointimal formation following a murine arterial injury, and inhibit the accumulation of T cells within the injured artery [107].

The US + MB-targeted delivery method can be used to deliver more than just nucleic acids to stimulate therapeutic revascularization. Intramuscular injections of bone marrow mononuclear cells (BM-MNCs) have been demonstrated to promote angiogenesis and functional recovery of ischemic muscle in both animals [108] and humans [109], motivating the development of a noninvasive delivery system for these cells. In a rat model of hindlimb ischemia, intravenous injection of BM-MNCs immediately after US activation of MBs resulted in a significant enhancement in blood flow recovery, increased capillary and arteriolar density, and augmented collateral vessel formation [110]. US + MBs have also been used to deliver BM-MNCs to the myocardium in a hamster model of cardiomyopathy. US-mediated delivery of the BM-MNCs resulted in increased capillary density as well as expression of VEGF-A and FGF-2 by the myocardial tissue. The BM-MNCs were found to adhere to the US-targeted vascular endothelium within the myocardium, and endothelial progenitors within the BM-MNC population were shown to trans-differentiate into endothelial-like cells to repair US-stimulated endothelium and supply angiogenic factors (VEGF-A and FGF-2) to promote neovessel formation. The authors also observed reduced fibrosis and improved cardiac function and blood flow in the US + MB + BM-MNC treated group relative to the controls [111].

US can also be used to deliver proteins. VEGF-A was delivered to the heart with US + MBs as early as 2000, although functional impacts on angiogenesis and arteriogenesis were not investigated [112]. In 2007, US + MBs were used in conjunction with granulocyte colony-stimulating factor (G-CSF) in the ischemic hindlimb muscles of mice. Here, instead of utilizing an intravenous injection strategy, G-CSF was injected subcutaneously. Specifically, mice were pre-treated with either a single or repeated subcutaneous injection of G-CSF after hindlimb ischemia surgery. One day following the final injection, the hindlimb muscle was targeted with US + MBs. Animals that received the G-CSF and US + MBs exhibited increased capillary density and collateral growth relative to animals that received only the G-CSF (no US) or just the US + MBs (no G-CSF) [113]. In 2008, we made use of an intravascular co-injection strategy, rather than pre-treatment. We first demonstrated the ability of US + MB interactions to facilitate the delivery of intra-arterially injected nanoparticles to the hindlimb skeletal muscle (Figure 4). Next, we injected nanoparticles containing FGF-2 intraarterially along with the MBs, and then used US to activate the MBs in the ischemic gracilis muscle of mice following hindlimb ischemia surgery. The therapy increased both the number and maximum intraluminal diameter of collateral arterioles (stimulating arteriogenesis, but not apparent angiogenesis) (Figure 5) [114].

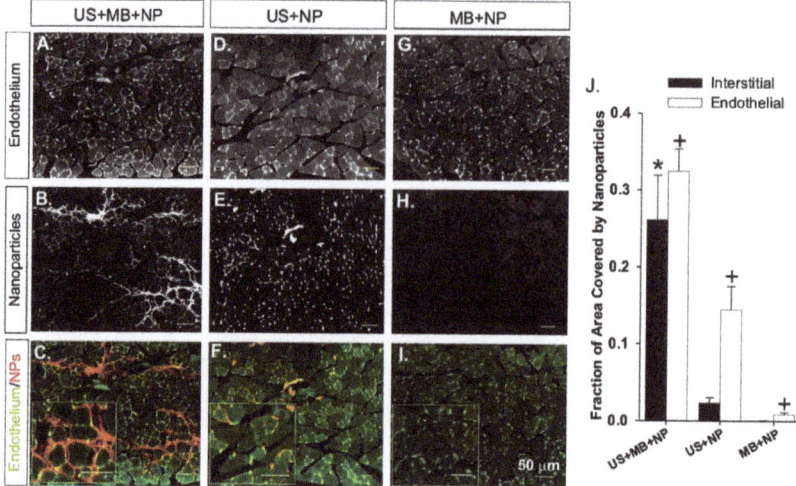

Figure 4. Muscle cross-sections illustrating nanoparticle (NP) delivery. (**A–I**) Representative images of sections taken from gracilis muscles treated with ultrasound (US) + microbubbles (MB) + nanoparticles (NP) (**A–C**), ultrasound + nanoparticles (**D–F**), and microbubbles + nanoparticles (**G–I**) are shown. Note the deposition of nanoparticles (red) in muscle treated with ultrasound + microbubble + nanoparticles. J: Bar graph representing the fraction of interstitial area (regions outside of muscle fibers and vascular structures) or endothelial cell area (cells comprising the walls of blood vessels) occupied by fluorescent polystyrene nanoparticles. Values are means with standard deviations. * Indicates significantly different ($p < 0.05$) to the interstitial area of all other groups. + indicates significantly different ($p < 0.05$) to the endothelial cell area of all other groups. Adapted from Chappell et al. [114].

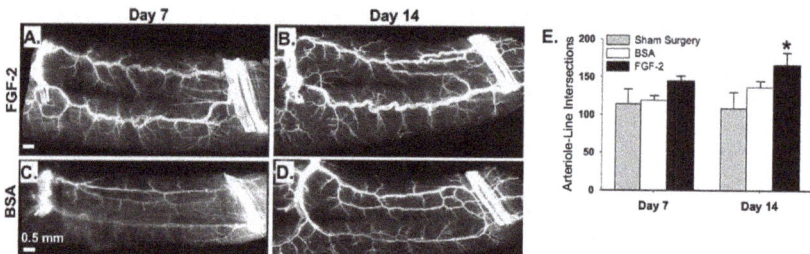

Figure 5. The delivery of FGF-2 bearing nanoparticles by ultrasonic microbubble destruction elicits arteriogenic remodeling in gracilis adductor muscle. (**A–D**) Representative whole-mount images of fluorescently-labeled SM α-actin+ vessels in gracilis adductor muscles seven and 14 days after FGF-2 (**A,B**) and bovine serum albumin (BSA) (**C,D**) treatment. Note the significant increase in arteriolar caliber and density in FGF-2-treated muscles. (**E**) Bar graph of arteriole-line intersections at both time points for FGF-2, BSA, and sham surgery treatment. Values are means with standard errors. * Indicates significantly different ($p < 0.05$) to BSA and sham surgery at day 14. Adapted from Chappell et al. [114].

While US provides a high degree of spatial targeting for treatment, modifications to the MB contrast agents themselves can provide an additional level of specificity. A number of studies have been conducted to modify the shell of the MBs to include targeting ligands, so that the MBs will selectively bind to particular regions of interest. For example, MBs coated with ligands that bind to P-selectin have been developed to target MBs (and thus, their imaging and therapeutic delivery effects) to the endothelium of inflamed blood vessels [115–121]. Other inflammation-related markers that have been used for targeting include E-selectin [122–124], ICAM-1 [125,126], and VCAM-1 [127–130].

A number of ligands against endothelial markers of angiogenesis including $\alpha_v\beta_3$-integrins [131–133], VEGF receptor-2 (VEGFR2) [134–137], and endoglin [138,139] have also been used to target MBs to specific tissues or areas of the vasculature. While the majority of these studies have used the targeted MBs for diagnostic imaging purposes or the delivery of reporter genes or molecules, the method holds great potential for therapeutic applications related to vascular remodeling. Depending on the disease application, this approach allows for enhanced MB accumulation at the desired tissue site, permitting improved delivery of drugs and genes to promote angiogenesis or arteriogenesis.

5. Activation of Implanted Biomaterials with Ultrasound to Elicit Vascular Remodeling

One interesting new therapeutic application of ultrasound has been the advent of acoustically responsive biomaterials. For the past two decades, the principle of acoustic droplet vaporization (ADV) has been utilized to develop phase shift droplet emulsions, sub-micron-sized liquid droplets that vaporize into gas bubbles when exposed to sufficient acoustic pressure [140,141]. The general principle is to stabilize a perfluorocarbon with a relatively low natural boiling point (below body temperature, for example) in a superheated state using a surfactant, trapping the perfluorocarbon within the droplet, and preventing rapid aggregation. The speed of sound in the perfluorocarbon is substantially different than in the plasma surrounding the droplets in the bloodstream, permitting the use of the droplets as both contrast agents in an imaging setting as well as a therapeutic delivery mechanism [142]. Exposure to pressures above a particular threshold can induce the nucleation and growth of gas pockets within the droplets. The droplets then rapidly expand into gas bubbles considerably larger than their initial size [141,143–145], and can release payloads or oscillate like standard microbubbles. Emulsions of such droplets have since been engineered to encapsulate and deliver drugs in a targeted manner for a variety of disease applications [146–150].

Recently, these droplet emulsions have been utilized in a new application, droplet-hydrogel composite materials, where a hydrogel matrix is doped with a perfluorocarbon emulsion containing a therapeutic drug or molecule. This approach allows for both spatial and temporal control of the release of the therapeutic. In a 2013 in vitro study, a fibrin matrix containing perfluorocarbon droplets loaded with bFGF was activated with US, and the releasate from the hydrogel was applied to endothelial cells in culture. The bFGF-containing releasate did indeed stimulate metabolic activity in the cultured endothelial cells, demonstrating that the growth factor maintains functional bioactivity throughout the encapsulation and release processes. Increases in metabolic activity were also observed when endothelial cells were already seeded within the hydrogel at the time of US application [151]. These acoustically-responsive scaffolds (ARS) have also been shown to respond similarly to US in terms of payload release in vivo [152]. A bFGF-loaded ARS was injected subcutaneously into the dorsal region of mice, and later activated with US to release the growth factor. The mice that received the ARS and US demonstrated significantly enhanced perfusion relative to mice that received the ARS without US or a control fibrin hydrogel (with or without free bFGF). Additionally, the ARS + US group showed a significant upregulation in capillary density, indicating the growth factor-loaded ARS approach can be used to stimulate therapeutic angiogenesis [153].

6. Outlook

As reviewed here, over the past 15 years, numerous pre-clinical studies have demonstrated the potential of US to induce revascularization responses through the oscillation and/or destruction of gas-filled MBs, the delivery of therapeutic genes, proteins, or cells, or the activation of acoustically-responsive biomaterials. These approaches present opportunities for novel non-invasive and spatially-targeted treatments for diseases caused or characterized by insufficient or aberrant vasculature, replacing traditional interventions associated with invasive or high-risk procedures (surgery) or off-target effects (systemic delivery). In particular, we believe that US-mediated revascularization has immense potential for treating central nervous system disorders, where the blood–brain barrier poses a significant challenge to many treatment modalities as well as tissue engineering and biomaterials where the ability to non-invasively activate an implanted material would allow for highly tunable and versatile therapies that could be easily adapted to meet the needs of individual patients.

Nonetheless, it is also true that, despite this abundance of pre-clinical investigation, ultrasound-mediated approaches for revascularization have not been successfully translated to the clinic. While this is discouraging, the past few years have seen a handful of ultrasound-mediated drug delivery approaches enter into clinical trials, and we submit that these trials have the potential to open doors for many new applications going forward. This includes the use of ultrasound for stimulating revascularization. Indeed, in combination with i.v. microbubbles, ultrasound has now been used to safely open the blood–brain barrier in Alzheimer's disease patients [154] and to deliver chemotherapy to patients with primary brain tumors [155,156]. Moreover, more trials utilizing focused ultrasound and microbubbles for the blood–brain barrier opening are just now getting underway, signaling an acceleration of clinical activity in this space. Meanwhile, ultrasound-microbubble-mediated drug delivery has also entered clinical trials for an application outside of the CNS, with the targeted delivery of gemcitabine having been performed in patients with pancreatic cancer [157]. With these trials serving as the foundation, we are hopeful that the knowledge gained regarding the safety and relative efficacy of ultrasound-microbubble-mediated treatments will facilitate the adoption of similar approaches for therapeutic revascularization. Overall, we argue that US-based methods of promoting angiogenesis and arteriogenesis still have potential to make an important positive impact on how we treat many vascular pathologies in the future.

Author Contributions: Writing—Original Draft Preparation, C.M.G. and J.C.C.; Writing—Review and Editing, C.M.G., J.C.C., and R.J.P.; Supervision, R.J.P.; Funding Acquisition, R.J.P.

Funding: This study was supported by National Institutes of Health (Grants R01EB020147 and R21EB024323 to R.J.P.). C.M.G. was supported by the American Heart Association Fellowship (18PRE34030022).

Conflicts of Interest: The authors declare no conflict of interest.

References

1. Carmeliet, P. Blood vessels and nerves: Common signals, pathways and diseases. *Nat. Rev. Genet.* **2003**, *4*, 710–720. [CrossRef] [PubMed]
2. Poredos, P.; Poredos, P. Peripheral arterial occlusive disease and perioperative risk. *Int. Angiol.* **2018**, *37*, 93–99. [CrossRef] [PubMed]
3. Lind, B.; Morcos, O.; Ferral, H.; Chen, A.; Aquisto, T.; Lee, S.; Lee, C.J. Endovascular Strategies in the Management of Acute Limb Ischemia. *Vasc. Spec. Int.* **2019**, *35*, 4–9. [CrossRef] [PubMed]
4. Sprengers, R.W.; Teraa, M.; Moll, F.L.; de Wit, G.A.; van der Graaf, Y.; Verhaar, M.C. Quality of life in patients with no-option critical limb ischemia underlines the need for new effective treatment. *J. Vasc. Surg.* **2010**, *52*, 843–849. [CrossRef] [PubMed]
5. Teraa, M.; Conte, M.S.; Moll, F.L.; Verhaar, M.C. Critical Limb Ischemia: Current Trends and Future Directions. *J. Am. Heart Assoc.* **2016**, *5*, e002938. [CrossRef] [PubMed]
6. Henry, T.D.; Satran, D.; Jolicoeur, E.M. Treatment of refractory angina in patients not suitable for revascularization. *Nat. Rev. Cardiol.* **2014**, *11*, 78–95. [CrossRef] [PubMed]
7. Nakagami, H.; Maeda, K.; Morishita, R.; Iguchi, S.; Nishikawa, T.; Takami, Y.; Kikuchi, Y.; Saito, Y.; Tamai, K.; Ogihara, T.; et al. Novel Autologous Cell Therapy in Ischemic Limb Disease Through Growth Factor Secretion by Cultured Adipose Tissue–Derived Stromal Cells. *Arterioscler. Thromb. Vasc. Biol.* **2005**, *25*, 2542–2547. [CrossRef]
8. Biscetti, F.; Bonadia, N.; Nardella, E.; Cecchini, A.L.; Landolfi, R.; Flex, A. The Role of the Stem Cells Therapy in the Peripheral Artery Disease. *Int. J. Mol. Sci.* **2019**, *20*, 2233. [CrossRef]
9. Litwinowicz, R.; Kapelak, B.; Sadowski, J.; Kędziora, A.; Bartus, K. The use of stem cells in ischemic heart disease treatment. *Pol. J. Cardio-Thorac. Surg.* **2018**, *15*, 196–199. [CrossRef]
10. Frangogiannis, N.G. Cell therapy for peripheral artery disease. *Curr. Opin. Pharmacol.* **2018**, *39*, 27–34. [CrossRef]

11. Oduk, Y.; Zhu, W.; Kannappan, R.; Zhao, M.; Borovjagin, A.V.; Oparil, S.; Zhang, J.J. VEGF nanoparticles repair the heart after myocardial infarction. *Am. J. Physiol. Circ. Physiol.* **2018**, *314*, H278–H284. [CrossRef] [PubMed]
12. Marushima, A.; Nieminen, M.; Kremenetskaia, I.; Gianni-Barrera, R.; Woitzik, J.; von Degenfeld, G.; Banfi, A.; Vajkoczy, P.; Hecht, N. Balanced single-vector co-delivery of VEGF/PDGF-BB improves functional collateralization in chronic cerebral ischemia. *J. Cereb. Blood Flow Metab.* **2019**. [CrossRef] [PubMed]
13. Formiga, F.R.; Pelacho, B.; Garbayo, E.; Abizanda, G.; Gavira, J.J.; Simon-Yarza, T.; Mazo, M.; Formiga, F.R.; Tamayo, E.; Jauquicoa, C.; et al. Sustained release of VEGF through PLGA microparticles improves vasculogenesis and tissue remodeling in an acute myocardial ischemia–reperfusion model. *J. Control. Release* **2010**, *147*, 30–37. [CrossRef] [PubMed]
14. Li, X.; Tjwa, M.; Moons, L.; Fons, P.; Noel, A.; Ny, A.; Zhou, J.M.; Lennartsson, J.; Li, H.; Luttun, A.; et al. Revascularization of ischemic tissues by PDGF-CC via effects on endothelial cells and their progenitors. *J. Clin. Investig.* **2005**, *115*, 118–127. [CrossRef] [PubMed]
15. Martins, R.N.; Chleboun, J.O.; Sellers, P.; Sleigh, M.; Muir, J. The Role of PDGF-BB on the Development of the Collateral Circulation after Acute Arterial Occlusion. *Growth Factors* **1994**, *10*, 299–306. [CrossRef]
16. Van Royen, N.; Piek, J.J.; Legemate, D.A.; Schaper, W.; Oskam, J.; Atasever, B.; Voskuil, M.; Ubbink, D.; Schirmer, S.H.; Buschmann, I.; et al. Design of the START-trial: STimulation of ARTeriogenesis using subcutaneous application of GM-CSF as a new treatment for peripheral vascular disease. A randomized, double-blind, placebo-controlled trial. *Vasc. Med.* **2003**, *8*, 191–196. [CrossRef]
17. Marra, S.; Scacciatella, P.; Usmiani, T.; D'Amico, M.; Giorgi, M.; Andriani, M.; Baccega, M.; Boccadoro, M.; Omedè, P.; Sanavio, F.; et al. Concurrent G-CSF and GM-CSF administration for the induction of bone marrow-derived cell mobilization in patients with acute myocardial infarction: A pilot study evaluating feasibility, safety and efficacy. *EuroIntervention* **2006**, *1*, 425–431.
18. JOST, M.M.; Ninci, E.; Meder, B.; Kempf, C.; Van Royen, N.; Hua, J.; Berger, B.; Hoefer, I.; Modolell, M.; Buschmann, I. Divergent effects of GM-CSF and TGFβ$_1$ on bone marrow-derived macrophage arginase-1 activity, MCP-1 expression, and matrix metalloproteinase-12: A potential role during arteriogenesis. *FASEB J.* **2003**, *17*, 2281–2283. [CrossRef]
19. Banfi, A.; von Degenfeld, G.; Gianni-Barrera, R.; Reginato, S.; Merchant, M.J.; McDonald, D.M.; Blau, H.M. Therapeutic angiogenesis due to balanced single-vector delivery of VEGF and PDGF-BB. *FASEB J.* **2012**, *26*, 2486–2497. [CrossRef]
20. Ylä-Herttuala, S.; Bridges, C.; Katz, M.G.; Korpisalo, P. Angiogenic gene therapy in cardiovascular diseases: Dream or vision? *Eur. Heart J.* **2017**, *38*, 1365–1371. [CrossRef]
21. Cooke, J.P.; Losordo, D.W. Modulating the vascular response to limb ischemia: Angiogenic and cell therapies. *Circ. Res.* **2015**, *116*, 1561–1578. [CrossRef] [PubMed]
22. Heuslein, J.L.; Gorick, C.M.; Song, J.; Price, R.J. DNA methyltransferase 1-dependent DNA hypermethylation constrains arteriogenesis by augmenting shear stress set point. *J. Am. Heart Assoc.* **2017**, *6*, e007673. [CrossRef] [PubMed]
23. Heuslein, J.L.; Gorick, C.M.; McDonnell, S.P.; Song, J.; Annex, B.H.; Price, R.J. Exposure of Endothelium to Biomimetic Flow Waveforms Yields Identification of miR-199a-5p as a Potent Regulator of Arteriogenesis. *Mol. Ther. Nucleic Acids* **2018**, *12*, 829–844. [CrossRef] [PubMed]
24. Heuslein, J.L.; McDonnell, S.P.; Song, J.; Annex, B.H.; Price, R.J. MicroRNA-146a Regulates Perfusion Recovery in Response to Arterial Occlusion via Arteriogenesis. *Front. Bioeng. Biotechnol.* **2018**, *6*, 1. [CrossRef] [PubMed]
25. Heuslein, J.L.; Gorick, C.M.; Price, R.J. Epigenetic regulators of the revascularization response to chronic arterial occlusion. *Cardiovasc. Res.* **2019**, *115*, 701–712. [CrossRef] [PubMed]
26. Wei, K.; Skyba, D.M.; Firschke, C.; Jayaweera, A.R.; Lindner, J.R.; Kaul, S. Interactions between microbubbles and ultrasound: In vitro and in vivo observations. *J. Am. Coll. Cardiol.* **1997**, *29*, 1081–1088. [CrossRef]
27. Wei, K.; Jayaweera, A.R.; Firoozan, S.; Linka, A.; Skyba, D.M.; Kaul, S. Quantification of myocardial blood flow with ultrasound-induced destruction of microbubbles administered as a constant venous infusion. *Circulation* **1998**, *97*, 473–483. [CrossRef] [PubMed]
28. Ay, T.; Havaux, X.; van Camp, G.; Campanelli, B.; Gisellu, G.; Pasquet, A.; Denef, J.F.; Melin, J.A.; Vanoverschelde, J.L. Destruction of contrast microbubbles by ultrasound: Effects on myocardial function, coronary perfusion pressure, and microvascular integrity. *Circulation* **2001**, *104*, 461–466. [CrossRef]

29. Li, P.; Cao, L.; Dou, C.-Y.; Armstrong, W.F.; Miller, D. Impact of myocardial contrast echocardiography on vascular permeability: An in vivo dose response study of delivery mode, pressure amplitude and contrast dose. *Ultrasound Med. Biol.* **2003**, *29*, 1341–1349. [CrossRef]
30. Skyba, D.M.; Price, R.J.; Linka, A.Z.; Skalak, T.C.; Kaul, S. Direct in vivo visualization of intravascular destruction of microbubbles by ultrasound and its local effects on tissue. *Circulation* **1998**, *98*, 290–293. [CrossRef]
31. Price, R.J.; Skyba, D.M.; Kaul, S.; Skalak, T.C. Delivery of Colloidal Particles and Red Blood Cells to Tissue Through Microvessel Ruptures Created by Targeted Microbubble Destruction With Ultrasound. *Circulation* **1998**, *98*, 1264–1267. [CrossRef] [PubMed]
32. Song, J.; Qi, M.; Kaul, S.; Price, R.J. Stimulation of arteriogenesis in skeletal muscle by microbubble destruction with ultrasound. *Circulation* **2002**, *106*, 1550–1555. [CrossRef] [PubMed]
33. Miller, D. Overview of experimental studies of biological effects of medical ultrasound caused by gas body activation and inertial cavitation. *Prog. Biophys. Mol. Biol.* **2007**, *93*, 314–330. [CrossRef] [PubMed]
34. Helfield, B.; Chen, X.; Watkins, S.C.; Villanueva, F.S. Biophysical insight into mechanisms of sonoporation. *Proc. Natl. Acad. Sci. USA* **2016**, *113*, 9983–9988. [CrossRef] [PubMed]
35. Chen, W.-S.; Brayman, A.A.; Matula, T.J.; Crum, L.A.; Miller, M.W. The pulse length-dependence of inertial cavitation dose and hemolysis. *Ultrasound Med. Biol.* **2003**, *29*, 739–748. [CrossRef]
36. Chen, W.-S.; Brayman, A.A.; Matula, T.J.; Crum, L.A. Inertial cavitation dose and hemolysis produced in vitro with or without Optison. *Ultrasound Med. Biol.* **2003**, *29*, 725–737. [CrossRef]
37. Dalecki, D.; Raeman, C.H.; Child, S.Z.; Cox, C.; Francis, C.W.; Meltzer, R.S.; Carstensen, E.L. Hemolysis in vivo from exposure to pulsed ultrasound. *Ultrasound Med. Biol.* **1997**, *23*, 307–313. [CrossRef]
38. Poliachik, S.L.; Chandler, W.L.; Mourad, P.D.; Bailey, M.R.; Bloch, S.; Cleveland, R.O.; Kaczkowski, P.; Keilman, G.; Porter, T.; Crum, L.A. Effect of high-intensity focused ultrasound on whole blood with and without microbubble contrast agent. *Ultrasound Med. Biol.* **1999**, *25*, 991–998. [CrossRef]
39. Raymond, S.B.; Skoch, J.; Hynynen, K.; Bacskai, B.J. Multiphoton Imaging of Ultrasound/Optison Mediated Cerebrovascular Effects in vivo. *J. Cereb. Blood Flow Metab.* **2007**, *27*, 393–403. [CrossRef]
40. Basta, G.; Venneri, L.; Lazzerini, G.; Pasanisi, E.; Pianelli, M.; Vesentini, N.; del Turco, S.; Kusmic, C.; Picano, E. In vitro modulation of intracellular oxidative stress of endothelial cells by diagnostic cardiac ultrasound. *Cardiovasc. Res.* **2003**, *58*, 156–161. [CrossRef]
41. Bertuglia, S.; Giusti, A.; Picano, E. Effects of diagnostic cardiac ultrasound on oxygen free radical production and microvascular perfusion during ischemia reperfusion. *Ultrasound Med. Biol.* **2004**, *30*, 549–557. [CrossRef] [PubMed]
42. Kondo, T.; Misík, V.; Riesz, P. Effect of gas-containing microspheres and echo contrast agents on free radical formation by ultrasound. *Free Radic. Biol. Med.* **1998**, *25*, 605–612. [CrossRef]
43. Stride, E.; Saffari, N. The potential for thermal damage posed by microbubble ultrasound contrast agents. *Ultrasonics* **2004**, *42*, 907–913. [CrossRef] [PubMed]
44. Santos, M.A.; Wu, S.-K.; Li, Z.; Goertz, D.E.; Hynynen, K. Microbubble-assisted MRI-guided focused ultrasound for hyperthermia at reduced power levels. *Int. J. Hyperth.* **2018**, *35*, 599–611. [CrossRef] [PubMed]
45. Klotz, A.R.; Lindvere, L.; Stefanovic, B.; Hynynen, K. Temperature change near microbubbles within a capillary network during focused ultrasound. *Phys. Med. Biol.* **2010**, *55*, 1549–1561. [CrossRef] [PubMed]
46. Collis, J.; Manasseh, R.; Liovic, P.; Tho, P.; Ooi, A.; Petkovic-Duran, K.; Zhu, Y. Cavitation microstreaming and stress fields created by microbubbles. *Ultrasonics* **2010**, *50*, 273–279. [CrossRef]
47. Kooiman, K.; Vos, H.J.; Versluis, M.; de Jong, N. Acoustic behavior of microbubbles and implications for drug delivery. *Adv. Drug Deliv. Rev.* **2014**, *72*, 28–48. [CrossRef]
48. Kim, J.; Lindsey, B.D.; Chang, W.-Y.; Dai, X.; Stavas, J.M.; Dayton, P.A.; Jiang, X. Intravascular forward-looking ultrasound transducers for microbubble-mediated sonothrombolysis. *Sci. Rep.* **2017**, *7*, 3454. [CrossRef]
49. Chen, H.; Brayman, A.A.; Kreider, W.; Bailey, M.R.; Matula, T.J. Observations of Translation and Jetting of Ultrasound-Activated Microbubbles in Mesenteric Microvessels. *Ultrasound Med. Biol.* **2011**, *37*, 2139–2148. [CrossRef]
50. Song, J.; Cottler, P.S.; Klibanov, A.L.; Kaul, S.; Price, R.J. Microvascular remodeling and accelerated hyperemia blood flow restoration in arterially occluded skeletal muscle exposed to ultrasonic microbubble destruction. *Am. J. Physiol. Circ. Physiol.* **2004**, *287*, H2754–H2761. [CrossRef]

51. Chappell, J.C.; Klibanov, A.L.; Price, R.J. Ultrasound-microbubble-induced neovascularization in mouse skeletal muscle. *Ultrasound Med. Biol.* **2005**, *31*, 1411–1422. [CrossRef] [PubMed]
52. Chappell, J.C.; Song, J.; Klibanov, A.L.; Price, R.J. Ultrasonic Microbubble Destruction Stimulates Therapeutic Arteriogenesis via the CD18-Dependent Recruitment of Bone Marrow–Derived Cells. *Arterioscler. Thromb. Vasc. Biol.* **2008**, *28*, 1117–1122. [CrossRef] [PubMed]
53. Yoshida, J.; Ohmori, K.; Takeuchi, H.; Shinomiya, K.; Namba, T.; Kondo, I.; Kiyomoto, H.; Kohno, M. Treatment of Ischemic Limbs Based on Local Recruitment of Vascular Endothelial Growth Factor-Producing Inflammatory Cells with Ultrasonic Microbubble Destruction. *J. Am. Coll. Cardiol.* **2005**, *46*, 899–905. [CrossRef] [PubMed]
54. Johnson, C.A.; Sarwate, S.; Miller, R.J.; O'Brien, W.D. A temporal study of ultrasound contrast agent-induced changes in capillary density. *J. Ultrasound Med.* **2010**, *29*, 1267–1275. [CrossRef] [PubMed]
55. Johnson, C.A.; O'Brien, W.D., Jr. The angiogenic response is dependent on ultrasound contrast agent concentration. *Vasc. Cell* **2012**, *4*, 10. [CrossRef] [PubMed]
56. Dörner, J.; Struck, R.; Zimmer, S.; Peigney, C.; Duerr, G.D.; Dewald, O.; Kim, S.C.; Malan, D.; Bettinger, T.; Nickenig, G.; et al. Ultrasound-Mediated Stimulation of Microbubbles after Acute Myocardial Infarction and Reperfusion Ameliorates Left-Ventricular Remodeling in Mice via Improvement of Borderzone Vascularization. *PLoS ONE* **2013**, *8*, e56841. [CrossRef] [PubMed]
57. Hynynen, K.; McDannold, N.; Vykhodtseva, N.; Jolesz, F.A. Non-invasive opening of BBB by focused ultrasound. *Acta Neurochir. Suppl.* **2003**, *86*, 555–558. [PubMed]
58. Hynynen, K.; McDannold, N.; Sheikov, N.A.; Jolesz, F.A.; Vykhodtseva, N. Local and reversible blood–brain barrier disruption by noninvasive focused ultrasound at frequencies suitable for trans-skull sonications. *Neuroimage* **2005**, *24*, 12–20. [CrossRef]
59. Timbie, K.F.; Mead, B.P.; Price, R.J. Drug and gene delivery across the blood-brain barrier with focused ultrasound. *J. Control. Release* **2015**, *219*, 61–75. [CrossRef]
60. Curley, C.T.; Sheybani, N.D.; Bullock, T.N.; Price, R.J. Focused Ultrasound Immunotherapy for Central Nervous System Pathologies: Challenges and Opportunities. *Theranostics* **2017**, *7*, 3608–3623. [CrossRef]
61. McMahon, D.; Hynynen, K. Acute Inflammatory Response Following Increased Blood-Brain Barrier Permeability Induced by Focused Ultrasound is Dependent on Microbubble Dose. *Theranostics* **2017**, *7*, 3989–4000. [CrossRef] [PubMed]
62. McMahon, D.; Mah, E.; Hynynen, K. Angiogenic response of rat hippocampal vasculature to focused ultrasound-mediated increases in blood-brain barrier permeability. *Sci. Rep.* **2018**, *8*, 12178. [CrossRef] [PubMed]
63. Shohet, R.V.; Chen, S.; Zhou, Y.T.; Wang, Z.; Meidell, R.S.; Unger, R.H.; Grayburn, P.A. Echocardiographic destruction of albumin microbubbles directs gene delivery to the myocardium. *Circulation* **2000**, *101*, 2554–2556. [CrossRef] [PubMed]
64. Bekeredjian, R.; Chen, S.; Frenkel, P.A.; Grayburn, P.A.; Shohet, R.V. Ultrasound-Targeted Microbubble Destruction Can Repeatedly Direct Highly Specific Plasmid Expression to the Heart. *Circulation* **2003**, *108*, 1022–1026. [CrossRef] [PubMed]
65. Korpanty, G.; Chen, S.; Shohet, R.V.; Ding, J.; Yang, B.; Frenkel, P.A.; Grayburn, P.A. Targeting of VEGF-mediated angiogenesis to rat myocardium using ultrasonic destruction of microbubbles. *Gene Ther.* **2005**, *12*, 1305–1312. [CrossRef] [PubMed]
66. Sun, L.; Huang, C.-W.; Wu, J.; Chen, K.-J.; Li, S.-H.; Weisel, R.D.; Rakowski, H.; Sung, H.-W.; Li, R.-K. The use of cationic microbubbles to improve ultrasound-targeted gene delivery to the ischemic myocardium. *Biomaterials* **2013**, *34*, 2107–2116. [CrossRef] [PubMed]
67. Yang, L.; Yan, F.; Ma, J.; Zhang, J.; Liu, L.; Guan, L.; Zheng, H.; Li, T.; Liang, D.; Mu, Y. Ultrasound-Targeted Microbubble Destruction-Mediated Co-Delivery of Cxcl12 (Sdf-1alpha) and Bmp2 Genes for Myocardial Repair. *J. Biomed. Nanotechnol.* **2019**, *15*, 1299–1312. [CrossRef] [PubMed]
68. Kondo, I.; Ohmori, K.; Oshita, A.; Takeuchi, H.; Fuke, S.; Shinomiya, K.; Noma, T.; Namba, T.; Kohno, M. Treatment of Acute Myocardial Infarction by Hepatocyte Growth Factor Gene Transfer. *J. Am. Coll. Cardiol.* **2004**, *44*, 644–653. [CrossRef]
69. Christiansen, J.P.; French, B.A.; Klibanov, A.L.; Kaul, S.; Lindner, J.R. Targeted tissue transfection with ultrasound destruction of plasmid-bearing cationic microbubbles. *Ultrasound Med. Biol.* **2003**, *29*, 1759–1767. [CrossRef]

70. Burke, C.W.; Suk, J.S.; Kim, A.J.; Hsiang, Y.-H.J.; Klibanov, A.L.; Hanes, J.; Price, R.J. Markedly enhanced skeletal muscle transfection achieved by the ultrasound-targeted delivery of non-viral gene nanocarriers with microbubbles. *J. Control. Release* **2012**, *162*, 414–421. [CrossRef]
71. Hsiang, Y.-H.; Song, J.; Price, R.J. The partitioning of nanoparticles to endothelium or interstitium during ultrasound-microbubble-targeted delivery depends on peak-negative pressure. *J. Nanopart. Res.* **2015**, *17*, 345. [CrossRef] [PubMed]
72. Song, J.; Chappell, J.C.; Qi, M.; VanGieson, E.J.; Kaul, S.; Price, R.J. Influence of injection site, microvascular pressure and ultrasound variables on microbubble-mediated delivery of microspheres to muscle. *J. Am. Coll. Cardiol.* **2002**, *39*, 726–731. [CrossRef]
73. Leong-Poi, H.; Kuliszewski, M.A.; Lekas, M.; Sibbald, M.; Teichert-Kuliszewska, K.; Klibanov, A.L.; Stewart, D.J.; Lindner, J.R. Therapeutic Arteriogenesis by Ultrasound-Mediated VEGF$_{165}$ Plasmid Gene Delivery to Chronically Ischemic Skeletal Muscle. *Circ. Res.* **2007**, *101*, 295–303. [CrossRef] [PubMed]
74. Taniyama, Y.; Tachibana, K.; Hiraoka, K.; Aoki, M.; Yamamoto, S.; Matsumoto, K.; Nakamura, T.; Ogihara, T.; Kaneda, Y.; Morishita, R. Development of safe and efficient novel nonviral gene transfer using ultrasound: Enhancement of transfection efficiency of naked plasmid DNA in skeletal muscle. *Gene Ther.* **2002**, *9*, 372–380. [CrossRef] [PubMed]
75. Miao, C.H.; Brayman, A.A.; Loeb, K.R.; Ye, P.; Zhou, L.; Mourad, P.; Crum, L.A. Ultrasound Enhances Gene Delivery of Human Factor IX Plasmid. *Hum. Gene Ther.* **2005**, *16*, 893–905. [CrossRef] [PubMed]
76. Shen, Z.P.; Brayman, A.A.; Chen, L.; Miao, C.H. Ultrasound with microbubbles enhances gene expression of plasmid DNA in the liver via intraportal delivery. *Gene Ther.* **2008**, *15*, 1147–1155. [CrossRef] [PubMed]
77. Noble, M.L.; Kuhr, C.S.; Graves, S.S.; Loeb, K.R.; Sun, S.S.; Keilman, G.W.; Morrison, K.P.; Paun, M.; Storb, R.F.; Miao, C.H. Ultrasound-targeted Microbubble Destruction-mediated Gene Delivery Into Canine Livers. *Mol. Ther.* **2013**, *21*, 1687–1694. [CrossRef]
78. Song, S.; Noble, M.; Sun, S.; Chen, L.; Brayman, A.A.; Miao, C.H. Efficient Microbubble- and Ultrasound-Mediated Plasmid DNA Delivery into a Specific Rat Liver Lobe via a Targeted Injection and Acoustic Exposure Using a Novel Ultrasound System. *Mol. Pharm.* **2012**, *9*, 2187–2196. [CrossRef]
79. Song, S.; Shen, Z.; Chen, L.; Brayman, A.A.; Miao, C.H. Explorations of high-intensity therapeutic ultrasound and microbubble-mediated gene delivery in mouse liver. *Gene Ther.* **2011**, *18*, 1006–1014. [CrossRef]
80. Manta, S.; Renault, G.; Delalande, A.; Couture, O.; Lagoutte, I.; Seguin, J.; Lager, F.; Houzé, P.; Midoux, P.; Bessodes, M.; et al. Cationic microbubbles and antibiotic-free miniplasmid for sustained ultrasound–mediated transgene expression in liver. *J. Control. Release* **2017**, *262*, 170–181. [CrossRef]
81. Anderson, C.D.; Moisyadi, S.; Avelar, A.; Walton, C.B.; Shohet, R.V. Ultrasound-targeted hepatic delivery of factor IX in hemophiliac mice. *Gene Ther.* **2016**, *23*, 510–519. [CrossRef] [PubMed]
82. Raju, B.I.; Leyvi, E.; Seip, R.; Sethuraman, S.; Luo, X.; Bird, A.; Li, S.; Koeberl, D. Enhanced gene expression of systemically administered plasmid DNA in the liver with therapeutic ultrasound and microbubbles. *IEEE Trans. Ultrason. Ferroelectr. Freq. Control* **2013**, *60*, 88–96. [CrossRef] [PubMed]
83. Jiang, Z.; Xia, G.; Zhang, Y.; Dong, L.; He, B.; Sun, J. Attenuation of hepatic fibrosis through ultrasound-microbubble-mediated HGF gene transfer in rats. *Clin. Imaging* **2013**, *37*, 104–110. [CrossRef] [PubMed]
84. Tan, J.-K.Y.; Pham, B.; Zong, Y.; Perez, C.; Maris, D.O.; Hemphill, A.; Miao, C.H.; Matula, T.J.; Mourad, P.D.; Wei, H.; et al. Microbubbles and ultrasound increase intraventricular polyplex gene transfer to the brain. *J. Control. Release* **2016**, *231*, 86–93. [CrossRef] [PubMed]
85. Shimamura, M.; Sato, N.; Taniyama, Y.; Yamamoto, S.; Endoh, M.; Kurinami, H.; Aoki, M.; Ogihara, T.; Kaneda, Y.; Morishita, R. Development of efficient plasmid DNA transfer into adult rat central nervous system using microbubble-enhanced ultrasound. *Gene Ther.* **2004**, *11*, 1532–1539. [CrossRef] [PubMed]
86. Lin, C.-Y.; Hsieh, H.-Y.; Pitt, W.G.; Huang, C.-Y.; Tseng, I.-C.; Yeh, C.-K.; Wei, K.-C.; Liu, H.-L. Focused ultrasound-induced blood-brain barrier opening for non-viral, non-invasive, and targeted gene delivery. *J. Control. Release* **2015**, *212*, 1–9. [CrossRef]
87. Fan, C.-H.; Lin, C.-Y.; Liu, H.-L.; Yeh, C.-K. Ultrasound targeted CNS gene delivery for Parkinson's disease treatment. *J. Control. Release* **2017**, *261*, 246–262. [CrossRef]
88. Stavarache, M.A.; Petersen, N.; Jurgens, E.M.; Milstein, E.R.; Rosenfeld, Z.B.; Ballon, D.J.; Kaplitt, M.G. Safe and stable noninvasive focal gene delivery to the mammalian brain following focused ultrasound. *J. Neurosurg.* **2019**, *130*, 989–998. [CrossRef]

89. Huang, Q.; Deng, J.; Xie, Z.; Wang, F.; Chen, S.; Lei, B.; Liao, P.; Huang, N.; Wang, Z.; Wang, Z.; et al. Effective Gene Transfer into Central Nervous System Following Ultrasound-Microbubbles-Induced Opening of the Blood-Brain Barrier. *Ultrasound Med. Biol.* **2012**, *38*, 1234–1243. [CrossRef]
90. Huang, Q.; Deng, J.; Wang, F.; Chen, S.; Liu, Y.; Wang, Z.; Wang, Z.; Cheng, Y. Targeted gene delivery to the mouse brain by MRI-guided focused ultrasound-induced blood–brain barrier disruption. *Exp. Neurol.* **2012**, *233*, 350–356. [CrossRef]
91. Hsu, P.-H.; Wei, K.C.; Huang, C.Y.; Wen, C.J.; Yen, T.C.; Liu, C.L.; Lin, Y.T.; Chen, J.C.; Shen, C.R.; Liu, H.L. Noninvasive and Targeted Gene Delivery into the Brain Using Microbubble-Facilitated Focused Ultrasound. *PLoS ONE* **2013**, *8*, e57682. [CrossRef] [PubMed]
92. Wang, H.-B.; Yang, L.; Wu, J.; Sun, L.; Wu, J.; Tian, H.; Weisel, R.D.; Li, R.-K. Reduced Ischemic Injury After Stroke in Mice by Angiogenic Gene Delivery Via Ultrasound-Targeted Microbubble Destruction. *J. Neuropathol. Exp. Neurol.* **2014**, *73*, 548–558. [CrossRef] [PubMed]
93. Xhima, K.; Nabbouh, F.; Hynynen, K.; Aubert, I.; Tandon, A. Noninvasive delivery of an α-synuclein gene silencing vector with magnetic resonance-guided focused ultrasound. *Mov. Disord.* **2018**, *33*, 1567–1579. [CrossRef] [PubMed]
94. Mead, B.P.; Kim, N.; Miller, G.W.; Hodges, D.; Mastorakos, P.; Klibanov, A.L.; Mandell, J.W.; Hirsh, J.; Suk, J.S.; Hanes, J.; et al. Novel Focused Ultrasound Gene Therapy Approach Noninvasively Restores Dopaminergic Neuron Function in a Rat Parkinson's Disease Model. *Nano Lett.* **2017**, *17*, 3533–3542. [CrossRef] [PubMed]
95. Burgess, A.; Huang, Y.; Querbes, W.; Sah, D.W.; Hynynen, K. Focused ultrasound for targeted delivery of siRNA and efficient knockdown of Htt expression. *J. Control. Release* **2012**, *163*, 125–129. [CrossRef]
96. Thévenot, E.; Jordão, J.F.; O'Reilly, M.A.; Markham, K.; Weng, Y.-Q.; Foust, K.D.; Kaspar, B.K.; Hynynen, K.; Aubert, I. Targeted delivery of self-complementary adeno-associated virus serotype 9 to the brain, using magnetic resonance imaging-guided focused ultrasound. *Hum. Gene Ther.* **2012**, *23*, 1144–1155. [CrossRef] [PubMed]
97. Mead, B.P.; Mastorakos, P.; Suk, J.S.; Klibanov, A.L.; Hanes, J.; Price, R.J. Targeted gene transfer to the brain via the delivery of brain-penetrating DNA nanoparticles with focused ultrasound. *J. Control. Release* **2016**, *223*, 109–117. [CrossRef]
98. Chappell, J.C.; Price, R.J. Targeted Therapeutic Applications of Acoustically Active Microspheres in the Microcirculation. *Microcirculation* **2006**, *13*, 57–70. [CrossRef]
99. Babischkin, J.S.; Aberdeen, G.W.; Lindner, J.R.; Bonagura, T.W.; Pepe, G.J.; Albrecht, E.D. Vascular Endothelial Growth Factor Delivery to Placental Basal Plate Promotes Uterine Artery Remodeling in the Primate. *Endocrinology* **2019**. [CrossRef]
100. Yuan, Q.; Huang, J.; Chu, B.; Li, X.; Li, X.; Si, L. A targeted high-efficiency angiogenesis strategy as therapy for myocardial infarction. *Life Sci.* **2012**, *90*, 695–702. [CrossRef]
101. Sun, Y.; Jin, K.; Xie, L.; Childs, J.; Mao, X.O.; Logvinova, A.; Greenberg, D.A. VEGF-induced neuroprotection, neurogenesis, and angiogenesis after focal cerebral ischemia. *J. Clin. Investig.* **2003**, *111*, 1843–1851. [CrossRef] [PubMed]
102. Zhao, H.; Bao, X.J.; Wang, R.Z.; Li, G.L.; Gao, J.; Ma, S.H.; Wei, J.J.; Feng, M.; Zhao, Y.J.; Ma, W.B.; et al. Postacute Ischemia Vascular Endothelial Growth Factor Transfer by Transferrin-Targeted Liposomes Attenuates Ischemic Brain Injury after Experimental Stroke in Rats. *Hum. Gene Ther.* **2011**, *22*, 207–215. [CrossRef] [PubMed]
103. Li, S.; Sun, Y.; Meng, Q.; Li, S.; Yao, W.; Hu, G.; Li, Z.; Wang, R. Recombinant Adeno-Associated Virus Serotype 1-Vascular Endothelial Growth Factor Promotes Neurogenesis and Neuromigration in the Subventricular Zone and Rescues Neuronal Function in Ischemic Rats. *Neurosurgery* **2009**, *65*, 771–779. [CrossRef] [PubMed]
104. Yoshimura, S.; Morishita, R.; Hayashi, K.; Yamamoto, K.; Nakagami, H.; Kaneda, Y.; Sakai, N.; Ogihara, T. Inhibition of intimal hyperplasia after balloon injury in rat carotid artery model using cis-element 'decoy' of nuclear factor-κB binding site as a novel molecular strategy. *Gene Ther.* **2001**, *8*, 1635–1642. [CrossRef] [PubMed]
105. Inagaki, H.; Suzuki, J.; Ogawa, M.; Taniyama, Y.; Morishita, R.; Isobe, M. Ultrasound-Microbubble-Mediated NF-κB Decoy Transfection Attenuates Neointimal Formation after Arterial Injury in Mice. *J. Vasc. Res.* **2006**, *43*, 12–18. [CrossRef] [PubMed]

106. Yamasaki, K.; Asai, T.; Shimizu, M.; Aoki, M.; Hashiya, N.; Sakonjo, H.; Makino, H.; Kaneda, Y.; Ogihara, T.; Morishita, R. Inhibition of NFκB activation using cis-element 'decoy' of NFκB binding site reduces neointimal formation in porcine balloon-injured coronary artery model. *Gene Ther.* **2003**, *10*, 356–364. [CrossRef]
107. Suzuki, J.; Ogawa, M.; Takayama, K.; Taniyama, Y.; Morishita, R.; Hirata, Y.; Nagai, R.; Isobe, M. Ultrasound-Microbubble–Mediated Intercellular Adhesion Molecule-1 Small Interfering Ribonucleic Acid Transfection Attenuates Neointimal Formation After Arterial Injury in Mice. *J. Am. Coll. Cardiol.* **2010**, *55*, 904–913. [CrossRef] [PubMed]
108. Shintani, S.; Murohara, T.; Ikeda, H.; Ueno, T.; Sasaki, K.; Duan, J.; Imaizumi, T. Augmentation of postnatal neovascularization with autologous bone marrow transplantation. *Circulation* **2001**, *103*, 897–903. [CrossRef]
109. Tateishi-Yuyama, E.; Matsubara, H.; Murohara, T.; Ikeda, U.; Shintani, S.; Masaki, H.; Amano, K.; Kishimoto, Y.; Yoshimoto, K.; Akashi, H.; et al. Therapeutic angiogenesis for patients with limb ischaemia by autologous transplantation of bone-marrow cells: A pilot study and a randomised controlled trial. *Lancet* **2002**, *360*, 427–435. [CrossRef]
110. Imada, T.; Tatsumi, T.; Mori, Y.; Nishiue, T.; Yoshida, M.; Masaki, H.; Okigaki, M.; Kojima, H.; Nozawa, Y.; Nishiwaki, Y.; et al. Targeted Delivery of Bone Marrow Mononuclear Cells by Ultrasound Destruction of Microbubbles Induces Both Angiogenesis and Arteriogenesis Response. *Arterioscler. Thromb. Vasc. Biol.* **2005**, *25*, 2128–2134. [CrossRef]
111. Zen, K.; Okigaki, M.; Hosokawa, Y.; Adachi, Y.; Nozawa, Y.; Takamiya, M.; Tatsumi, T.; Urao, N.; Tateishi, K.; Takahashi, T.; et al. Myocardium-targeted delivery of endothelial progenitor cells by ultrasound-mediated microbubble destruction improves cardiac function via an angiogenic response. *J. Mol. Cell. Cardiol.* **2006**, *40*, 799–809. [CrossRef] [PubMed]
112. Mukherjee, D.; Wong, J.; Griffin, B.; Ellis, S.G.; Porter, T.; Sen, S.; Thomas, J.D. Ten-fold augmentation of endothelial uptake of vascular endothelial growth factor with ultrasound after systemic administration. *J. Am. Coll. Cardiol.* **2000**, *35*, 1678–1686. [CrossRef]
113. Miyake, Y.; Ohmori, K.; Yoshida, J.; Ishizawa, M.; Mizukawa, M.; Yukiiri, K.; Kohno, M. Granulocyte Colony-Stimulating Factor Facilitates the Angiogenesis Induced by Ultrasonic Microbubble Destruction. *Ultrasound Med. Biol.* **2007**, *33*, 1796–1804. [CrossRef] [PubMed]
114. Chappell, J.C.; Song, J.; Burke, C.W.; Klibanov, A.L.; Price, R.J. Targeted delivery of nanoparticles bearing fibroblast growth factor-2 by ultrasonic microbubble destruction for therapeutic arteriogenesis. *Small* **2008**, *4*, 1769–1777. [CrossRef] [PubMed]
115. Rychak, J.J.; Li, B.; Acton, S.T.; Leppänen, A.; Cummings, R.D.; Ley, K.; Klibanov, A.L. Selectin Ligands Promote Ultrasound Contrast Agent Adhesion under Shear Flow. *Mol. Pharm.* **2006**, *3*, 516–524. [CrossRef]
116. Rychak, J.J.; Klibanov, A.L.; Ley, K.F.; Hossack, J.A. Enhanced Targeting of Ultrasound Contrast Agents Using Acoustic Radiation Force. *Ultrasound Med. Biol.* **2007**, *33*, 1132–1139. [CrossRef] [PubMed]
117. Takalkar, A.M.; Klibanov, A.L.; Rychak, J.J.; Lindner, J.R.; Ley, K. Binding and detachment dynamics of microbubbles targeted to P-selectin under controlled shear flow. *J. Control. Release* **2004**, *96*, 473–482. [CrossRef]
118. Rychak, J.J.; Lindner, J.R.; Ley, K.; Klibanov, A.L. Deformable gas-filled microbubbles targeted to P-selectin. *J. Control. Release* **2006**, *114*, 288–299. [CrossRef]
119. Klibanov, A.L.; Rychak, J.J.; Yang, W.C.; Alikhani, S.; Li, B.; Acton, S.; Lindner, J.R.; Ley, K.; Kaul, S. Targeted ultrasound contrast agent for molecular imaging of inflammation in high-shear flow. *Contrast Media Mol. Imaging* **2006**, *1*, 259–266. [CrossRef]
120. Lindner, J.R.; Song, J.; Christiansen, J.; Klibanov, A.L.; Xu, F.; Ley, K. Ultrasound assessment of inflammation and renal tissue injury with microbubbles targeted to P-selectin. *Circulation* **2001**, *104*, 2107–2112. [CrossRef]
121. Shentu, W.; Yan, C.; Liu, C.; Qi, R.; Wang, Y.; Huang, Z.; Zhou, L.; You, X. Use of cationic microbubbles targeted to P-selectin to improve ultrasound-mediated gene transfection of hVEGF165 to the ischemic myocardium. *J. Zhejiang Univ. B* **2018**, *19*, 699–707. [CrossRef] [PubMed]
122. Fokong, S.; Fragoso, A.; Rix, A.; Curaj, A.; Wu, Z.; Lederle, W.; Iranzo, O.; Gätjens, J.; Kiessling, F.; Palmowski, M. Ultrasound Molecular Imaging of E-Selectin in Tumor Vessels Using Poly n-Butyl Cyanoacrylate Microbubbles Covalently Coupled to a Short Targeting Peptide. *Investig. Radiol.* **2013**, *48*, 843–850. [CrossRef] [PubMed]

123. Spivak, I.; Rix, A.; Schmitz, G.; Fokong, S.; Iranzo, O.; Lederle, W.; Kiessling, F. Low-Dose Molecular Ultrasound Imaging with E-Selectin-Targeted PBCA Microbubbles. *Mol. Imaging Biol.* **2016**, *18*, 180–190. [CrossRef] [PubMed]
124. Leng, X.; Wang, J.; Carson, A.; Chen, X.; Fu, H.; Ottoboni, S.; Wagner, W.R.; Villanueva, F.S. Ultrasound detection of myocardial ischemic memory using an E-selectin targeting peptide amenable to human application. *Mol. Imaging* **2014**, *13*, 1–9. [CrossRef] [PubMed]
125. Weller, G.E.R.; Villanueva, F.S.; Tom, E.M.; Wagner, W.R. Targeted ultrasound contrast agents: In vitro assessment of endothelial dysfunction and multi-targeting to ICAM-1 and sialyl Lewisx. *Biotechnol. Bioeng.* **2005**, *92*, 780–788. [CrossRef] [PubMed]
126. Wang, B.-P.; Luo, L.-H.; Wu, F.-L. Evaluation of renal tissue ischemia-reperfusion injury with ultrasound radiation force and targeted microbubbles. *Nan Fang Yi Ke Da Xue Xue Bao* **2017**, *37*, 402–406. [PubMed]
127. Moccetti, F.; Weinkauf, C.C.; Davidson, B.P.; Belcik, J.T.; Marinelli, E.R.; Unger, E.; Lindner, J.R. Ultrasound Molecular Imaging of Atherosclerosis Using Small-Peptide Targeting Ligands Against Endothelial Markers of Inflammation and Oxidative Stress. *Ultrasound Med. Biol.* **2018**, *44*, 1155–1163. [CrossRef] [PubMed]
128. Samiotaki, G.; Acosta, C.; Wang, S.; Konofagou, E.E. Enhanced delivery and bioactivity of the neurturin neurotrophic factor through focused ultrasound-mediated blood-brain barrier opening in vivo. *J. Cereb. Blood Flow Metab.* **2015**, *35*, 611–622. [CrossRef] [PubMed]
129. Wang, S.; Unnikrishnan, S.; Herbst, E.B.; Klibanov, A.L.; Mauldin, F.W.; Hossack, J.A. Ultrasound Molecular Imaging of Inflammation in Mouse Abdominal Aorta. *Investig. Radiol.* **2017**, *52*, 499–506. [CrossRef]
130. Phillips, L.C.; Klibanov, A.L.; Wamhoff, B.R.; Hossack, J.A. Intravascular ultrasound detection and delivery of molecularly targeted microbubbles for gene delivery. *IEEE Trans. Ultrason. Ferroelectr. Freq. Control* **2012**, *59*, 1596–1601. [CrossRef] [PubMed]
131. Daeichin, V.; Kooiman, K.; Skachkov, I.; Bosch, J.G.; Theelen, T.L.; Steiger, K.; Needles, A.; Janssen, B.J.; Daemen, M.J.; van der Steen, A.F.; et al. Quantification of Endothelial $\alpha_v\beta_3$ Expression with High-Frequency Ultrasound and Targeted Microbubbles: In Vitro and In Vivo Studies. *Ultrasound Med. Biol.* **2016**, *42*, 2283–2293. [CrossRef] [PubMed]
132. Yuan, H.; Wang, W.; Wen, J.; Lin, L.; Exner, A.A.; Guan, P.; Chen, X. Dual-Targeted Microbubbles Specific to Integrin $\alpha_v\beta_3$ and Vascular Endothelial Growth Factor Receptor 2 for Ultrasonography Evaluation of Tumor Angiogenesis. *Ultrasound Med. Biol.* **2018**, *44*, 1460–1467. [CrossRef] [PubMed]
133. Yan, F.; Xu, X.; Chen, Y.; Deng, Z.; Liu, H.; Xu, J.; Zhou, J.; Tan, G.; Wu, J.; Zheng, H. A Lipopeptide-Based $\alpha_v\beta_3$ Integrin-Targeted Ultrasound Contrast Agent for Molecular Imaging of Tumor Angiogenesis. *Ultrasound Med. Biol.* **2015**, *41*, 2765–2773. [CrossRef] [PubMed]
134. Pochon, S.; Tardy, I.; Bussat, P.; Bettinger, T.; Brochot, J.; von Wronski, M.; Passantino, L.; Schneider, M. BR55: A Lipopeptide-Based VEGFR2-Targeted Ultrasound Contrast Agent for Molecular Imaging of Angiogenesis. *Investig. Radiol.* **2010**, *45*, 89–95. [CrossRef] [PubMed]
135. Eschbach, R.S.; Clevert, D.A.; Hirner-Eppeneder, H.; Ingrisch, M.; Moser, M.; Schuster, J.; Tadros, D.; Schneider, M.; Kazmierczak, P.M.; Reiser, M.; et al. Contrast-Enhanced Ultrasound with VEGFR2-Targeted Microbubbles for Monitoring Regorafenib Therapy Effects in Experimental Colorectal Adenocarcinomas in Rats with DCE-MRI and Immunohistochemical Validation. *PLoS ONE* **2017**, *12*, e0169323. [CrossRef]
136. Baetke, S.C.; Rix, A.; Tranquart, F.; Schneider, R.; Lammers, T.; Kiessling, F.; Lederle, W. Squamous Cell Carcinoma Xenografts: Use of VEGFR2-targeted Microbubbles for Combined Functional and Molecular US to Monitor Antiangiogenic Therapy Effects. *Radiology* **2016**, *278*, 430–440. [CrossRef]
137. Chang, E.-L.; Ting, C.Y.; Hsu, P.H.; Lin, Y.C.; Liao, E.C.; Huang, C.Y.; Chang, Y.C.; Chan, H.L.; Chiang, C.S.; Liu, H.L.; et al. Angiogenesis-targeting microbubbles combined with ultrasound-mediated gene therapy in brain tumors. *J. Control. Release* **2017**, *255*, 164–175. [CrossRef]
138. Liu, C.; Yan, F.; Xu, Y.; Zheng, H.; Sun, L. In Vivo Molecular Ultrasound Assessment of Glioblastoma Neovasculature with Endoglin-Targeted Microbubbles. *Contrast Media Mol. Imaging* **2018**, *2018*, 1–10. [CrossRef]
139. Zhou, Y.; Gu, H.; Xu, Y.; Li, F.; Kuang, S.; Wang, Z.; Zhou, X.; Ma, H.; Li, P.; Zheng, Y.; et al. Targeted Antiangiogenesis Gene Therapy Using Targeted Cationic Microbubbles Conjugated with CD105 Antibody Compared with Untargeted Cationic and Neutral Microbubbles. *Theranostics* **2015**, *5*, 399–417. [CrossRef]
140. Kripfgans, O.D.; Fowlkes, J.B.; Miller, D.L.; Eldevik, O.P.; Carson, P.L. Acoustic droplet vaporization for therapeutic and diagnostic applications. *Ultrasound Med. Biol.* **2000**, *26*, 1177–1189. [CrossRef]

141. Kripfgans, O.D.; Fabiilli, M.L.; Carson, P.L.; Fowlkes, J.B. On the acoustic vaporization of micrometer-sized droplets. *J. Acoust. Soc. Am.* **2004**, *116*, 272–281. [CrossRef]
142. Dayton, P.A.; Zhao, S.; Bloch, S.H.; Schumann, P.; Penrose, K.; Matsunaga, T.O.; Zutshi, R.; Doinikov, A.; Ferrara, K.W. Application of ultrasound to selectively localize nanodroplets for targeted imaging and therapy. *Mol. Imaging* **2006**, *5*, 160–174. [CrossRef] [PubMed]
143. Shpak, O.; Stricker, L.; Versluis, M.; Lohse, D. The role of gas in ultrasonically driven vapor bubble growth. *Phys. Med. Biol.* **2013**, *58*, 2523–2535. [CrossRef] [PubMed]
144. Sheeran, P.S.; Wong, V.P.; Luois, S.; McFarland, R.J.; Ross, W.D.; Feingold, S.; Matsunaga, T.O.; Dayton, P.A. Decafluorobutane as a Phase-Change Contrast Agent for Low-Energy Extravascular Ultrasonic Imaging. *Ultrasound Med. Biol.* **2011**, *37*, 1518–1530. [CrossRef] [PubMed]
145. Kang, S.-T.; Lin, Y.-C.; Yeh, C.-K. Mechanical bioeffects of acoustic droplet vaporization in vessel-mimicking phantoms. *Ultrason. Sonochem.* **2014**, *21*, 1866–1874. [CrossRef] [PubMed]
146. Hwang, T.-L.; Lin, Y.-K.; Chi, C.-H.; Huang, T.-H.; Fang, J.-Y. Development and Evaluation of Perfluorocarbon Nanobubbles for Apomorphine Delivery. *J. Pharm. Sci.* **2009**, *98*, 3735–3747. [CrossRef] [PubMed]
147. Fang, J.-Y.; Hung, C.-F.; Hua, S.-C.; Hwang, T.-L. Acoustically active perfluorocarbon nanoemulsions as drug delivery carriers for camptothecin: Drug release and cytotoxicity against cancer cells. *Ultrasonics* **2009**, *49*, 39–46. [CrossRef]
148. Fabiilli, M.L.; Lee, J.A.; Kripfgans, O.D.; Carson, P.L.; Fowlkes, J.B. Delivery of Water-Soluble Drugs Using Acoustically Triggered Perfluorocarbon Double Emulsions. *Pharm. Res.* **2010**, *27*, 2753–2765. [CrossRef]
149. Fabiilli, M.L.; Haworth, K.J.; Sebastian, I.E.; Kripfgans, O.D.; Carson, P.L.; Fowlkes, J.B. Delivery of Chlorambucil Using an Acoustically-Triggered Perfluoropentane Emulsion. *Ultrasound Med. Biol.* **2010**, *36*, 1364–1375. [CrossRef]
150. Wang, C.-H.; Kang, S.-T.; Lee, Y.-H.; Luo, Y.-L.; Huang, Y.-F.; Yeh, C.-K. Aptamer-conjugated and drug-loaded acoustic droplets for ultrasound theranosis. *Biomaterials* **2012**, *33*, 1939–1947. [CrossRef]
151. Fabiilli, M.L.; Wilson, C.G.; Padilla, F.; Martín-Saavedra, F.M.; Fowlkes, J.B.; Franceschi, R.T. Acoustic droplet–hydrogel composites for spatial and temporal control of growth factor delivery and scaffold stiffness. *Acta Biomater.* **2013**, *9*, 7399–7409. [CrossRef] [PubMed]
152. Moncion, A.; Arlotta, K.J.; O'Neill, E.G.; Lin, M.; Mohr, L.A.; Franceschi, R.T.; Kripfgans, O.D.; Putnam, A.J.; Fabiilli, M.L. In vitro and in vivo assessment of controlled release and degradation of acoustically responsive scaffolds. *Acta Biomater.* **2016**, *46*, 221–233. [CrossRef] [PubMed]
153. Moncion, A.; Lin, M.; O'Neill, E.G.; Franceschi, R.T.; Kripfgans, O.D.; Putnam, A.J.; Fabiilli, M.L. Controlled release of basic fibroblast growth factor for angiogenesis using acoustically-responsive scaffolds. *Biomaterials* **2017**, *140*, 26–36. [CrossRef] [PubMed]
154. Lipsman, N.; Meng, Y.; Bethune, A.J.; Huang, Y.; Lam, B.; Masellis, M.; Herrmann, N.; Heyn, C.; Aubert, I.; Boutet, A.; et al. Blood–brain barrier opening in Alzheimer's disease using MR-guided focused ultrasound. *Nat. Commun.* **2018**, *9*, 2336. [CrossRef] [PubMed]
155. Carpentier, A.; Canney, M.; Vignot, A.; Reina, V.; Beccaria, K.; Horodyckid, C.; Karachi, C.; Leclercq, D.; Lafon, C.; Chapelon, J.Y.; et al. Clinical trial of blood-brain barrier disruption by pulsed ultrasound. *Sci. Transl. Med.* **2016**, *8*, 343. [CrossRef] [PubMed]
156. Mainprize, T.; Lipsman, N.; Huang, Y.; Meng, Y.; Bethune, A.; Ironside, S.; Heyn, C.; Alkins, R.; Trudeau, M.; Sahgal, A.; et al. Blood-Brain Barrier Opening in Primary Brain Tumors with Non-invasive MR-Guided Focused Ultrasound: A Clinical Safety and Feasibility Study. *Sci. Rep.* **2019**, *9*, 321. [CrossRef] [PubMed]
157. Dimcevski, G.; Kotopoulis, S.; Bjånes, T.; Hoem, D.; Schjøtt, J.; Gjertsen, B.T.; Biermann, M.; Molven, A.; Sorbye, H.; McCormack, E.; et al. A human clinical trial using ultrasound and microbubbles to enhance gemcitabine treatment of inoperable pancreatic cancer. *J. Control. Release* **2016**, *243*, 172–181. [CrossRef]

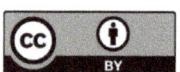

© 2019 by the authors. Licensee MDPI, Basel, Switzerland. This article is an open access article distributed under the terms and conditions of the Creative Commons Attribution (CC BY) license (http://creativecommons.org/licenses/by/4.0/).

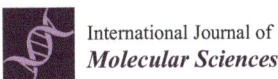

Article

Development of an Exercise Training Protocol to Investigate Arteriogenesis in a Murine Model of Peripheral Artery Disease

Ayko Bresler [1], Johanna Vogel [2], Daniel Niederer [2], Daphne Gray [1], Thomas Schmitz-Rixen [1] and Kerstin Troidl [1,3,*]

[1] Department of Vascular and Endovascular Surgery, University Hospital Frankfurt, Theodor-Stern-Kai 7, 60590 Frankfurt, Germany
[2] Department of Sports Medicine, Institute of Sport Sciences, Goethe University, Ginnheimer Landstraße 39, 60487 Frankfurt, Germany
[3] Department of Pharmacology, Max-Planck-Institute for Heart and Lung Research, Ludwigstr. 43, 61231 Bad Nauheim, Germany
* Correspondence: Kerstin.troidl@mpi-bn.mpg.de; Tel.: +49-6032-705-1205

Received: 27 July 2019; Accepted: 13 August 2019; Published: 14 August 2019

Abstract: Exercise is a treatment option in peripheral artery disease (PAD) patients to improve their clinical trajectory, at least in part induced by collateral growth. The ligation of the femoral artery (FAL) in mice is an established model to induce arteriogenesis. We intended to develop an animal model to stimulate collateral growth in mice through exercise. The training intensity assessment consisted of comparing two different training regimens in C57BL/6 mice, a treadmill implementing forced exercise and a free-to-access voluntary running wheel. The mice in the latter group covered a much greater distance than the former pre- and postoperatively. C57BL/6 mice and hypercholesterolemic ApoE-deficient (ApoE$^{-/-}$) mice were subjected to FAL and had either access to a running wheel or were kept in motion-restricting cages (control) and hind limb perfusion was measured pre- and postoperatively at various times. Perfusion recovery in C57BL/6 mice was similar between the groups. In contrast, ApoE$^{-/-}$ mice showed significant differences between training and control 7 d postoperatively with a significant increase in pericollateral macrophages while the collateral diameter did not differ between training and control groups 21 d after surgery. ApoE$^{-/-}$ mice with running wheel training is a suitable model to simulate exercise induced collateral growth in PAD. This experimental set-up may provide a model for investigating molecular training effects.

Keywords: arteriogenesis; exercise training; mouse model; femoral artery ligation; running wheel; voluntary training; peripheral artery disease

---

1. Introduction

Patients with peripheral arterial disease (PAD) often suffer from intermittent claudication, leading to a significant walking impairment. According to the 2017 guidelines of the European Society of Vascular Surgery (ESVS), supervised exercise training is a Class I, Level A recommendation in patients presenting intermittent claudication, whereas unsupervised training is a Class I, Level C recommendation. Walking has thus been shown to be a safe and effective treatment for patients with PAD [1,2]. In particular, walking performance, cardiovascular parameters, and quality of life can be improved by exercise.

Some potential exercise effects and scheduling modifiers are still unclear, in particular, risk factors such as smoking, dyslipidemia, diabetes mellitus, obesity, and arterial hypertension as major comorbidities of PAD are only considered infrequently [3–6]. Physical activity has suppressive effects on inflammation [7] and proinflammatory immune cells [8,9], as well as beneficial effects on endothelial function [10]. Additionally, physical training has the potential to promote an additional vascularization in hypoxic/ischemic tissues, such as the myocardium or peripheral limb [11]. Arteriogenesis, can be induced by exercise in human [12–14] and in animal studies [15]. The driving force of arteriogenesis is altered fluid shear stress (FSS) in the preformed collateral arteries due to increased blood flow [16]. The increased blood flow initiates vascular remodeling and diameter growth [17] and alters the miRNA profile [18].

Nevertheless, the physiological pathways of how exercise affects collateral growth at the molecular level are still not finally delineated.

Arteriogenesis is the process that results in growth of pre-existing collateral arterioles into functional collateral arteries, triggered by a hemodynamically relevant stenosis of supplying blood vessels. These bypassing vessels can sometimes be remarkably efficient and nearly completely replace the occluded arteries [19]. This formation is stimulated by an increase of shear stress on the endothelium [20]. An increase of blood flow can be achieved by a high demand and walking exercise gives the best possibility to maximize the flow physiologically [6].

In past decades various models have been developed that help in understanding the mechanisms of arteriogenesis. The ligation of the femoral artery (FAL) in mammals, especially the mouse, has become a well-established model for the induction of arteriogenesis [3,21,22]. Exercise stress tests are widely used for a variety of training protocols [23–25]. In most of the mice models, the training is voluntary (treadmill or running wheel), only a minor share of the protocols is forced. As exercise characteristics like frequency, intensity, type, and time cannot be controlled, a forced protocol may be appropriate. On the other hand, forced exercise is, unlike voluntary exercise, affected by distress [25–27].

The aim of this study was to find a suitable mouse model for simulating PAD as well as to establish a training protocol that would be accepted by cardiovascular-diseased animals and stimulate arteriogenesis. Such a protocol could provide the basis to methodically investigate effects of training on PAD at the molecular level in an experimental setup.

2. Results

2.1. Evaluation of a Training Regime in C57BL/6

In order to maximize training intensity, we compared two training regimens: A treadmill to implement forced exercise and a free-to-access voluntary running wheel. During the treadmill protocol the mice were trained using an incremental protocol: initial running speed was 0.2 m/s, increased daily to the maximal speed of 0.3 m/s at day 7. The training frequency was twice per day, and each training lasted 30 min. A maximum distance of 1.08 km was covered each day. Distances traveled and running wheel speeds were recorded continuously. After an adaptation period a running distance of 4.36 ± 0.41 km/d with an average speed of 0.5 m/s of was recorded. We observed increased speed and distance values for the voluntary exercise mice when compared to those forced to exercise in a treadmill throughout the observation period (Figure 1a,b).

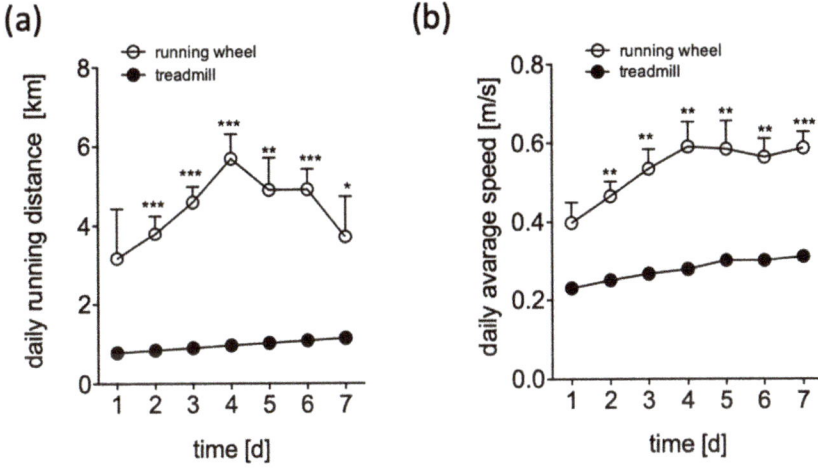

Figure 1. Daily running distance (**a**) and daily average speed (**b**) of C57BL/6 mice over time, during 7 days of adaptation in a treadmill receiving forced exercise (filled circles) or in a voluntary running wheel (open circles). Data are displayed as mean ± SEM. * $p < 0.05$; ** $p < 0.01$; *** $p < 0.005$.

2.2. Acceptance of Voluntary Training in ApoE$^{-/-}$ Mice after HFD and Post-Surgery

To further increase a similarity to patients presenting PAD we included ApoE$^{-/-}$ mice fed with a high fat diet (HFD; 21% butter fat, 1.5% cholesterol) to the exercise study. These mice showed numerous plaques throughout the whole arterial system including the femoral artery and the aortic root as well as fat deposition in the collateral arterioles (Figure 2a–c).

Given the health constraints of ApoE$^{-/-}$ mice following 12 weeks of HFD, we intended to evaluate whether they were able to cover the same distance as healthy C57BL/6 mice pre- and post-FAL. During the adaptation the mean distance covered was 3.93 ± 0.28 km/d which was not significantly different to C57BL/6 mice ($p = 0.36$). Post-FAL the re-adjustment period was similar to C57BL/6 mice, with no significant difference, as visualized in the equal progression of running performance (Figure 2d). Both strains, before and after surgery, recovered quickly to their initial distance when they had access to a voluntary running wheel.

2.3. Reperfusion Recovery after FAL in C57BL/6 and ApoE$^{-/-}$ Mice with and without Training

In order to evaluate training effects on reperfusion recovery, 18-week-old ApoE$^{-/-}$ mice that had been fed with an HFD for 12 weeks and 12-week-old healthy C57BL/6 mice were subjected to the experimental protocols shown in Figure 3a,b. Both mouse strains were randomly subdivided into training or control groups. The control group was housed in motion-restricting cages. The training group was held in single cages containing a free-to-access running wheel starting 7 days prior surgery. FAL was performed on day 0 and perfusion of the hind-limb was measured by LDPI pre- and postoperatively and on postoperative days, d3, d7, and d14. Adductor muscle tissue was harvested from ApoE$^{-/-}$ mice at different time points following FAL. The ratio of hind-limb perfusion in the operated leg to that in the non-operated leg dropped to 10% on average in C57BL/6 mice (training: 11 ± 4%, $n = 12$, control: mean 8 ± 1%, $n = 16$; $p > 0.05$), whereas perfusion recovery increased similarly within 14 days in the control (69 ± 10%) and training group (69 ± 4%) (Figure 3c).

In contrast, exercising ApoE$^{-/-}$ mice showed a significantly faster approximation of perfusion with training ($n = 19$). A maximum of 78 ± 8% perfusion of the hind limbs could be reached within 7 days postoperatively, compared with the control group ($n = 21$) averaging 53 ± 3% ($p = 0.012$) (Figure 3d,e). Interestingly, immediately postoperatively ApoE$^{-/-}$ mice showed a baseline perfusion of 25% independent of a training adaptation that was significantly higher than that of C57BL/6 mice ($p = 0.001$) (Figure 3f).

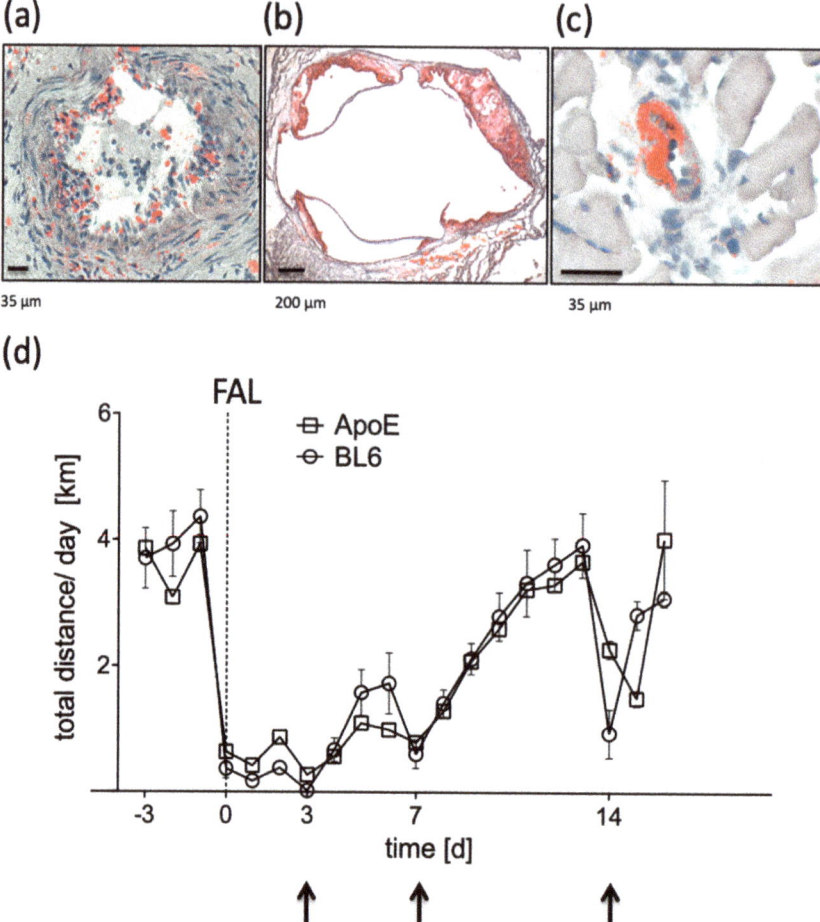

Figure 2. Plaque development in (**a**) the femoral artery, (**b**) the aortic root, and (**c**) the collateral artery of ApoE$^{-/-}$ mice following 12 weeks of high fat diet, as visualized by Oil-red-O staining. (**d**) Daily running distances of C57BL/6 mice (BL6, circles) compared to ApoE$^{-/-}$ mice (ApoE, squares) over time, pre- and post-ligation of the femoral artery (FAL). Arrows indicate short term running breaks due to anesthesia during perfusion measurements.

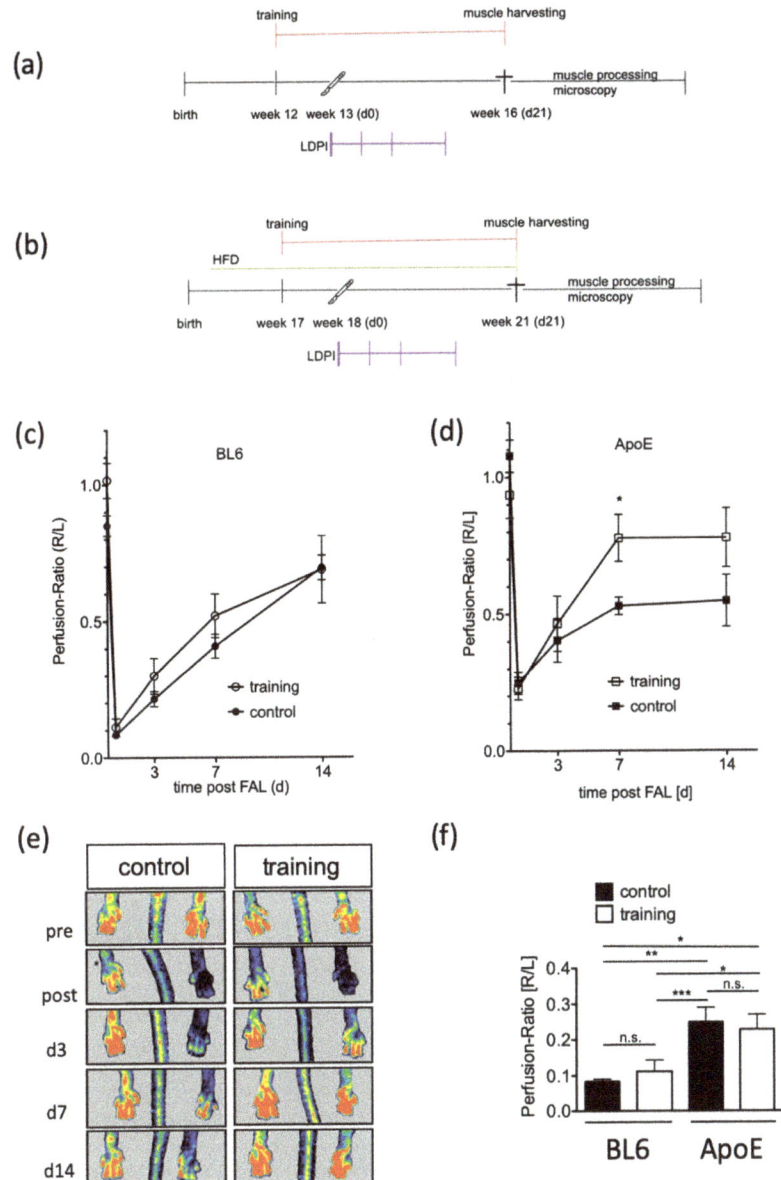

Figure 3. Functional effects on hind limb perfusion in response to training. (**a**) Schematic of experimental setup in C57BL/6, (**b**) schematic of experimental setup in ApoE$^{-/-}$, and (**c**,**d**) laser Doppler perfusion imaging in C57BL/6 and ApoE$^{-/-}$ as indicated. Data are expressed as ratio of the operated leg to the non-operated leg and represent mean ± SEM. Open symbols show the data of the training group whereas filled symbols represent the control group. As a statistical test, the unpaired t-test was used; * $p < 0.05$. (**e**) Representative laser Doppler perfusion images indicate the effect of training in the operated hind limb when compared to the control group. (**f**) Postoperative perfusion ratio (R/L). Open symbols show the data of the training group whereas filled symbols represent the control group. As a statistical test, the one-way ANOVA was used; * $p < 0.05$; ** $p < 0.01$; *** $p < 0.005$; n.s. not significant.

2.4. Increased Accumulation of Macrophages after Training in ApoE$^{-/-}$ Mice

In order to investigate the beneficial influence of exercise training on the vascular remodeling process in ApoE$^{-/-}$ mice, adductor muscle tissue was harvested from these mice 21 days following FAL. Early perfusion benefits were not reflected by morphometric examination at the end of the experimental period. There was no difference of the size of the wall area between training and control groups on day 21 post-surgery (2.15 ± 0.53 mm^2 and 2.46 ± 0.53 mm^2, respectively; $p > 0.05$; Figure 4a,b).

In the initial phase, collateral growth is critically driven by pericollateral macrophage assembly. Therefore, adductor muscle tissue was harvested from ApoE$^{-/-}$ mice 3 or 7 days following FAL and the macrophage number was quantified in the vascular nerve sheath of the collateral vessels. Seven days after FAL the number of macrophages in close proximity of growing collaterals was significantly higher in the training group with an average of 3.9 ± 0.8 compared to the control group with an average of 2.3 ± 0.4 ($p = 0.042$; Figure 4c,d).

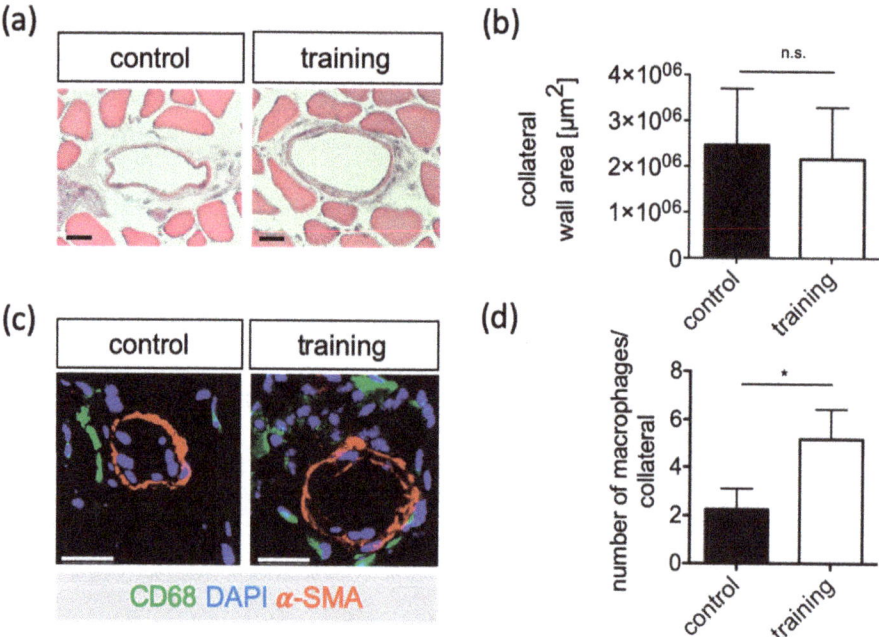

Figure 4. Histological evaluation of collateral growth in cross sections of the adductor muscles of ApoE$^{-/-}$ mice in response to training. (**a**) Representative micrographs of collateral arteries for morphometry. Scale bar: 200μm. (**b**) Quantification of wall area 21 days after FAL of the training and control group. (**c**) Immunostaining to determine macrophage accumulation around collaterals 7 d after FAL of the training and control groups. Representative images of CD68 (green) and αSMA (red) immunostaining. Blue staining indicates nuclei and scale bars are 25 μm. (**d**) Quantification of macrophage number. Data are expressed as mean ± SEM of three collateral cross-sections per mouse of at least three mice per group ($n \geq 3$). As a statistical test, the unpaired t-test was used; * $p < 0.05$.

3. Discussion

Arteriogenesis is the natural compensation mechanism through which collateral circulation develops. This formation is stimulated by an increase of shear stress on the endothelium [20]. An increase of blood flow can be achieved by a high demand and walking exercise is the best possibility to maximize the flow physiologically [6]. Therefore, the aim of the study was to establish a training protocol in a murine model of PAD that increases arteriogenesis through exercise. Our results suggest that a FAL surgery in ApoE$^{-/-}$ mice having free access to a voluntary running wheel serves best for future studies of exercise-induced arteriogenesis.

To increase physiologic shear stress on the arterioles it is preferable to develop an exercise program that maximizes intensity.

Initially we compared activity of healthy young C57BL/6 mice trained either with forced exercise by treadmill twice daily or with a 24 h accessible running wheel. Forced exercise is controlled and reproducible, but usually depends on a negative impulse. In models with forced exercise regimens, increased distress values, depressive behavior, inflammation reactions, and elevated corticosterone levels have been shown [26,28–30]. Distress, for example, may limit physiological remodeling normally associated with exercise training in humans [31,32]. The transferability of forced exercise models into humans may thus be limited. In contrast, similar structural and functional cardiac changes occurred in forced and voluntary exercise regimens [33]. The pros and cons of a forced versus a voluntary exercise model are thus not finally delineated.

We further showed that voluntary training leads to a much greater distance covered than forced exercise. Furthermore, voluntary running resulted in a higher running speed. Resulting from this higher exercise dose, a higher training effect response of voluntary running than of forced treadmill walking would be expected. Free-to-access running wheels are an easy way to record and store activity data without disturbing the habitual behavior. Likewise, voluntary access to running wheels permits reasonable adaptation to exercise after surgery and provides an excellent tool to monitor the behavior of mice. We could show that mice do tolerate this voluntary training much better with an increase of the distance travelled compared to forced exercise. For the reasons given above we continued our studies with voluntary training knowing well that this cannot be directly translated to the human situation. There is a discrepancy in intrinsic exercise capacity and response to exercise training between mice and humans. Mice do have a natural drive for running. Humans with sedentary behavior do not push their maximum limit. The focus of our study was to establish a protocol in mice which was adapted to their natural behavior and allowed for future investigations on collateral growth.

Since in PAD a stenosis is progressing over time and involves the whole arterial system, there is an uncertainty if healthy animals can be used to simulate the human patient's illness [3,23,34,35]. An acute occlusion in healthy participants by e.g., arterial emboli or trauma demands an instant intervention. The sudden tissue hypoxia can lead to an acute inflammatory–angiogenic–myogenic response which could result in massive loss of tissue. Patients suffering from PAD usually better tolerate an acute occlusion [36].

In order to increase the similarity to patients presenting PAD we used ApoE$^{-/-}$ mice fed with a HFD, that show numerous plaques throughout the whole arterial system [21,23,24,37] including fat deposition in collaterals.

It was expected that different mouse strains don't have similar responses to voluntary training [27,38]. Our findings showed that C57BL/6 and ApoE$^{-/-}$ animals accepted the voluntary training without a notable difference between the two strains. In this study we showed that there was just a short postoperative readjustment period of 10 days needed to get mice back to the initial distance. Whether this delay was due to the surgical intervention alone (opening and closing of the skin) cannot be fully excluded, because a sham treatment group without FAL was not investigated.

Next, the voluntary training protocol (running wheel) was tested in both strains to evaluate the reperfusion recovery after FAL.

The LDPI data acquired showed a significant higher perfusion immediately after the occlusion in ApoE$^{-/-}$ mice. This could be explained due to an increased collateral growth as a result of arteriosclerotic plaques in the major arteries [21]. C57BL/6 as well as ApoE$^{-/-}$ mice presented a maximum re-perfusion up to 69% and 77% with no significant difference in between the two strains.

It could be shown that having training possibility allowed ApoE$^{-/-}$ mice to reach the maximum reperfusion alignment one week post-FAL.

In order to correlate the increased perfusion to arteriogenesis we performed histological analyses of collateral tissue of ApoE$^{-/-}$ mice with and without exercise training. It is well accepted that mechanical, cellular, and molecular factors influence collateral growth [39]. Macrophages accumulate around the growing collaterals and cytokine secretion improves that process [40,41]. After training, ApoE$^{-/-}$ mice show a higher accumulation of CD68$^+$ macrophages in the vascular nerve sheath of the collateral vessels than without training.

The presented experimental setup involves atherosclerotic ApoE$^{-/-}$ mice subjected to an acute FAL. Functional as well as histological findings implicate an improvement of arteriogenesis after exercise training in the proposed model.

4. Materials and Methods

4.1. Ethics Statement

Animal handling and all experimental procedures carried out were in full compliance with the Directive 2010/63/EU of the European Parliament on protection of animals used for scientific purposes. Approval was given by the responsible local authority, the Darmstadt governmental council for animal protection and handling (permit reference numbers V54-19c20/15-B2/360, permit date: 30 October 2013). Throughout this study all mice had access to water and food ad libitum.

4.2. Femoral Artery Ligation (FAL)

Twenty-eight male C57BL/6 mice (Charles River, Sulzfeld, Germany) and 40 male ApoE$^{-/-}$ mice were subjected to FAL as described [22]. The contralateral leg served as the reference. During the surgical procedure mice were kept on a heating plate with a temperature of 38 °C. Anesthesia was applied using ketamine (120 mg/kg BW) and xylazine (16 mg/kg BW) i.p.. For postoperative analgesia carprofen (5 mg/kg BW) was injected s.c.. After termination of experiments the mice were euthanized by an anesthetic overdose.

4.3. Forced Exercise on Treadmill

Mice were first accustomed by using a treadmill (Exer 3/6, Columbus Instruments, Columbus, OH, USA) with a motivation grid for 15 min/day. This applied small amounts of electric shock for conditioning when the mice stopped running.

After being conditioned, the mice started training at a light intensity with a preset speed of 0.2 m/s leading up to a maximum of 0.3 m/s with no further resistance. Training frequency was 2 times per day. Training was terminated at exhaustions. Exhaustion was defined as pause of more than 5 s at a time, or three times for two or more seconds on the shock pad without trying to get back on the treadmill.

4.4. Voluntary Running Wheels

To evaluate voluntary training each animal was individually housed in a cage equipped with a free-to-access running wheel. The running wheels were connected to a computer equipped with TSE PhenoMaster V5.1.6 (2014-4115) (TSE Systems GmbH, Bad Homburg, Germany). This setup gave accurate data on each animal, recording time and traveled distances and it allowed evaluation of activity patterns during an adaptation period as well as identifing post-surgery effects.

4.5. Restraining Cages

For simulating inactivity, mice were kept as a reference (control) group in smaller cages without the possibility to climb in order to minimize movement.

4.6. Laser Doppler Perfusion Imaging (LDPI)

Perfusion of the paws was recorded using the laser Doppler imaging device PIM3 (Perimed Instruments, Järfälla, Sweden; Software: LDPIwin for PIM3 3.1.3), on a heating plate at 38 °C, before FAL (d0 pre), immediately after FAL (d0 post), as well as at d3, d7, and d14 after FAL.

The mean perfusion was shown as the ratio of the ligated hind limb to the contralateral, non-ischemic hind limb.

4.7. Histology

Mice were perfused with 10 mL vasodilation buffer (100 µg adenosine, 1 µg sodium nitroprusside, 0.05% BSA in PBS, pH7.4) followed by 10 mL 4% PFA post mortem. Adductor muscles from ligated or sham-operated mice were harvested and placed in 15% sucrose in PBS for 4 h and overnight at 4 °C in 30% sucrose in PBS. Tissue was cryopreserved in Tissue-Tek O.C.T. (Sakura, Alphen aan den Rijn, The Netherlands) and cut in 8 µm cryosections. Morphometric analyses were performed using a hematoxylin-eosin stain to evaluate the dimensions of collateral arteries.

4.8. Immunohistochemistry

Cryosections were stained with blue-fluorescent DNA stain DAPI (4′,6-Diaminidino-2-phenyllindole-dilactate; Thermo Fisher Scientific, Waltham, MA, USA) and counterstained for αSMA-Cy3 (C6198, Sigma-Aldrich GmbH, Taufkirchen, Germany) or αSMA-FITC (F3777, Sigma-Aldrich GmbH, Taufkirchen, Germany) and CD68 (MCA1957A448T, AbD Serotec, BioRad, Feldkirchen, Germany).

4.9. Statistical Analysis

All statistical analyses were supported by GraphPad software PRISM5 for Mac (GraphPad Software, La Jolla, CA, USA), JMP for Mac (Version 9.0.12010 SAS Institute Inc., Heidelberg, Germany), Image J (National Institutes of Health, Bethesda, Maryland, USA) and Microsoft Excel for Mac (Version16.15, Microsoft, Redmond, Washington, USA). Comparisons between groups were based on unpaired student's t-test. One-way or two-way ANOVA were used to determine differences between the means of three or more independent groups as indicated. Data were reported as standard error of mean (SEM). Data deviations were considered to be statistically significant differences at $p < 0.05$.

5. Conclusions

Femoral artery ligated ApoE$^{-/-}$ mice on HFD with running wheel training is a suitable model to simulate exercise induced collateral growth. This experimental set-up may provide a model for investigating molecular training effects on arteriogenesis.

Author Contributions: A.B., K.T., and T.S.-R. designed the experiments. A.B., J.V., D.N. and K.T. interpreted the findings. A.B. and K.T. wrote the first draft of the manuscript. A.B and K.T. analyzed and performed experiments, A.B. performed statistical analyses; D.G., J.V., D.N., and T.S.-R. discussed the results and revised the manuscript. All authors edited and approved the manuscript.

Funding: This research was funded by the Anna-Maria and Uwe-Karsten Kühl Foundation (T0188/28514/2016, Bad Nauheim, Germany to K.T.).

Acknowledgments: The authors thank Christina Reschke and Brigitte Matzke for excellent technical assistance and Amir Kauveh Panah for proofreading the manuscript.

Conflicts of Interest: The authors declare no conflict of interest.

Abbreviations

PAD	Peripheral artery disease
CVD	Cardiovascular disease
ApoE$^{-/-}$	Apolipoprotein E knockout
FAL	Femoral artery ligation
HFD	High fat diet

References

1. Naci, H.; Ioannidis, J.P. Comparative effectiveness of exercise and drug interventions on mortality outcomes: Metaepidemiological study. *Br. J. Sports Med.* **2015**, *49*, 1414–1422. [CrossRef] [PubMed]
2. Lyu, X.; Li, S.; Peng, S.; Cai, H.; Liu, G.; Ran, X. Intensive walking exercise for lower extremity peripheral arterial disease: A systematic review and meta-analysis. *J. Diabetes* **2016**, *8*, 363–377. [CrossRef] [PubMed]
3. Gardner, A.W.; Montgomery, P.S.; Parker, D.E. Physical activity is a predictor of all-cause mortality in patients with intermittent claudication. *J. Vasc. Surg.* **2008**, *47*, 117–122. [CrossRef] [PubMed]
4. Aherne, T.; McHugh, S.; Kheirelseid, E.A.; Lee, M.J.; McCaffrey, N.; Moneley, D.; Leahy, A.L.; Naughton, P. Comparing Supervised Exercise Therapy to Invasive Measures in the Management of Symptomatic Peripheral Arterial Disease. *Surg. Res. Pract.* **2015**, *2015*, 960402. [CrossRef] [PubMed]
5. Larsen, O.A.; Lassen, N.A. Effect of daily muscular exercise in patients with intermittent claudication. *Lancet* **1966**, *2*, 1093–1096. [CrossRef]
6. Haas, T.L.L.P.; Yang, H.-T.; Terjung, R.L. Exercise Training and Peripheral Arterial Disease. *Compr. Physiol.* **2012**, *2*, 2933–3017. [CrossRef] [PubMed]
7. Niessner, A.; Richter, B.; Penka, M.; Steiner, S.; Strasser, B.; Ziegler, S.; Heeb-Elze, E.; Zorn, G.; Leitner-Heinschink, A.; Niessner, C.; et al. Endurance training reduces circulating inflammatory markers in persons at risk of coronary events: Impact on plaque stabilization? *Atherosclerosis* **2006**, *186*, 160–165. [CrossRef] [PubMed]
8. Timmerman, K.L.; Flynn, M.G.; Coen, P.M.; Markofski, M.M.; Pence, B.D. Exercise training-induced lowering of inflammatory (CD14+CD16+) monocytes: A role in the anti-inflammatory influence of exercise? *J. Leukoc. Biol.* **2008**, *84*, 1271–1278. [CrossRef] [PubMed]
9. Michishita, R.; Shono, N.; Inoue, T.; Tsuruta, T.; Node, K. Effect of exercise therapy on monocyte and neutrophil counts in overweight women. *Am. J. Med. Sci.* **2010**, *339*, 152–156. [PubMed]
10. Higashi, Y.; Sasaki, S.; Kurisu, S.; Yoshimizu, A.; Sasaki, N.; Matsuura, H.; Kajiyama, G.; Oshima, T. Regular aerobic exercise augments endothelium-dependent vascular relaxation in normotensive as well as hypertensive subjects: Role of endothelium-derived nitric oxide. *Circulation* **1999**, *100*, 1194–1202. [CrossRef]
11. Guerreiro, L.F.; Rocha, A.M.; Martins, C.N.; Ribeiro, J.P.; Wally, C.; Strieder, D.L.; Carissimi, C.G.; Oliveira, M.G.; Pereira, A.A.; Biondi, H.S.; et al. Oxidative status of the myocardium in response to different intensities of physical training. *Physiol. Res.* **2016**, *65*, 737–749. [PubMed]
12. Huonker, M.; Halle, M.; Keul, J. Structural and functional adaptations of the cardiovascular system by training. *Int. J. Sports Med.* **1996**, *17* (Suppl. 3), S164–S172. [CrossRef]
13. Nash, M.S.; Montalvo, B.M.; Applegate, B. Lower extremity blood flow and responses to occlusion ischemia differ in exercise-trained and sedentary tetraplegic persons. *Arch. Phys. Med. Rehabil.* **1996**, *77*, 1260–1265. [CrossRef]
14. Dopheide, J.F.; Rubrech, J.; Trumpp, A.; Geissler, P.; Zeller, G.C.; Schnorbus, B.; Schmidt, F.; Gori, T.; Münzel, T.; Espinola-Klein, C. Supervised exercise training in peripheral arterial disease increases vascular shear stress and profunda femoral artery diameter. *Eur. J. Prev. Cardiol.* **2017**, *24*, 178–191. [CrossRef] [PubMed]
15. Sayed, A.; Schierling, W.; Troidl, K.; Ruding, I.; Nelson, K.; Apfelbeck, H.; Benli, I.; Schaper, W.; Schmitz-Rixen, T. Exercise linked to transient increase in expression and activity of cation channels in newly formed hind-limb collaterals. European journal of vascular and endovascular surgery. *Eur. J. Soc. Vasc. Endovasc. Surg.* **2010**, *40*, 81–87. [CrossRef] [PubMed]
16. Heil, M.; Eitenmüller, I.; Schmitz-Rixen, T.; Schaper, W. Arteriogenesis versus angiogenesis: Similarities and differences. *J. Cell. Mol. Med.* **2006**, *10*, 45–55. [CrossRef] [PubMed]
17. Ben Driss, A.; Benessiano, J.; Poitevin, P.; Levy, B.I.; Michel, J.B. Arterial expansive remodeling induced by high flow rates. *Am. J. Physiol.* **1997**, *272*, H851–H858. [CrossRef]

18. Vogel, J.; Niederer, D.; Engeroff, T.; Vogt, L.; Troidl, C.; Schmitz-Rixen, T.; Banzer, W.; Troidl, K. Effects on the Profile of Circulating miRNAs after Single Bouts of Resistance Training with and without Blood Flow Restriction-A Three-Arm, Randomized Crossover Trial. *Int. J. Mol. Sci.* **2019**, *20*, 3249. [CrossRef]
19. Hendrikx, G.; Voo, S.; Bauwens, M.; Post, M.J.; Mottaghy, F.M. SPECT and PET imaging of angiogenesis and arteriogenesis in pre-clinical models of myocardial ischemia and peripheral vascular disease. *Eur. J. Nucl. Med. Mol. Imaging* **2016**, *43*, 2433–2447. [CrossRef]
20. Eitenmuller, I.; Volger, O.; Kluge, A.; Troidl, K.; Barancik, M.; Cai, W.J.; Heil, M.; Pipp, F.; Fischer, S.; Horrevoets, A.J.; et al. The range of adaptation by collateral vessels after femoral artery occlusion. *Circ. Res.* **2006**, *99*, 656–662. [CrossRef]
21. Lee-Young, R.S.; Griffee, S.R.; Lynes, S.E.; Bracy, D.P.; Ayala, J.E.; McGuinness, O.P.; Wasserman, D.H. Skeletal muscle AMP-activated protein kinase is essential for the metabolic response to exercise in vivo. *J. Biol. Chem.* **2009**, *284*, 23925–23934. [CrossRef] [PubMed]
22. Limbourg, A.; Korff, T.; Napp, L.C.; Schaper, W.; Drexler, H.; Limbourg, F.P. Evaluation of postnatal arteriogenesis and angiogenesis in a mouse model of hind-limb ischemia. *Nat. Protoc.* **2009**, *4*, 1737–1746. [CrossRef] [PubMed]
23. Baltgalvis, K.A.; White, K.; Li, W.; Claypool, M.D.; Lang, W.; Alcantara, R.; Singh, B.K.; Friera, A.M.; McLaughlin, J.; Hansen, D.; et al. Exercise performance and peripheral vascular insufficiency improve with AMPK activation in high-fat diet-fed mice. *Am. J. Physiol. Heart Circ. Physiol.* **2014**, *306*, H1128–H1145. [CrossRef] [PubMed]
24. Lo Sasso, G.; Schlage, W.K.; Boue, S.; Veljkovic, E.; Peitsch, M.C.; Hoeng, J. The Apoe(-/-) mouse model: A suitable model to study cardiovascular and respiratory diseases in the context of cigarette smoke exposure and harm reduction. *J. Trans. Med.* **2016**, *14*, 146. [CrossRef] [PubMed]
25. Schirmer, S.H.; Millenaar, D.N.; Werner, C.; Schuh, L.; Degen, A.; Bettink, S.I.; Lipp, P.; van Rooijen, N.; Meyer, T.; Böhm, M.; et al. Exercise promotes collateral artery growth mediated by monocytic nitric oxide. *Arterioscler. Thromb. Vasc. Biol.* **2015**, *35*, 1862–1871. [CrossRef] [PubMed]
26. Morgan, J.A.; Corrigan, F.; Baune, B.T. Effects of physical exercise on central nervous system functions: A review of brain region specific adaptations. *J. Mol. Psychiatry* **2015**, *3*, 3. [CrossRef] [PubMed]
27. Manzanares, G.; Brito-da-Silva, G.; Gandra, P.G. Voluntary wheel running: Patterns and physiological effects in mice. *Braz. J. Med. Biol. Res.* **2019**, *52*, e7830. [CrossRef] [PubMed]
28. Slattery, D.A.; Cryan, J.F. Using the rat forced swim test to assess antidepressant-like activity in rodents. *Nat. Protoc.* **2012**, *7*, 1009. [CrossRef]
29. Cook, M.D.; Martin, S.A.; Williams, C.; Whitlock, K.; Wallig, M.A.; Pence, B.D.; Woods, J.A. Forced treadmill exercise training exacerbates inflammation and causes mortality while voluntary wheel training is protective in a mouse model of colitis. *Brain Behav. Immun.* **2013**, *33*, 46–56. [CrossRef]
30. Gong, S.; Miao, Y.L.; Jiao, G.Z.; Sun, M.J.; Li, H.; Lin, J.; Luo, M.J.; Tan, J.H. Dynamics and correlation of serum cortisol and corticosterone under different physiological or stressful conditions in mice. *PLoS ONE* **2015**, *10*, e0117503. [CrossRef]
31. Billman, G.E.; Cagnoli, K.L.; Csepe, T.; Li, N.; Wright, P.; Mohler, P.J.; Fedorov, V.V. Exercise training-induced bradycardia: Evidence for enhanced parasympathetic regulation without changes in intrinsic sinoatrial node function. *J. Appl. Physiol. (1985)* **2015**, *118*, 1344–1355. [CrossRef] [PubMed]
32. Bartolomucci, A.; Palanza, P.; Costoli, T.; Savani, E.; Laviola, G.; Parmigiani, S.; Sgoifo, A. Chronic psychosocial stress persistently alters autonomic function and physical activity in mice. *Physiol. Behav.* **2003**, *80*, 57–67. [CrossRef]
33. Lakin, R.; Guzman, C.; Izaddoustdar, F.; Polidovitch, N.; Goodman, J.M.; Backx, P.H. Changes in Heart Rate and Its Regulation by the Autonomic Nervous System Do Not Differ Between Forced and Voluntary Exercise in Mice. *Front. Physiol.* **2018**, *9*, 841. [CrossRef] [PubMed]
34. Ziegler, M.A.; Distasi, M.R.; Bills, R.G.; Miller, S.J.; Alloosh, M.; Murphy, M.P.; Akingba, A.G.; Sturek, M.; Dalsing, M.C.; Unthank, J.L. Marvels, mysteries, and misconceptions of vascular compensation to peripheral artery occlusion. *Microcirculation* **2010**, *17*, 3–20. [CrossRef] [PubMed]
35. Leeper, N.J.; Myers, J.; Zhou, M.; Nead, K.T.; Syed, A.; Kojima, Y.; Caceres, R.D.; Cooke, J.P. Exercise capacity is the strongest predictor of mortality in patients with peripheral arterial disease. *J. Vasc. Surg.* **2013**, *57*, 728–733. [CrossRef] [PubMed]

36. Dragneva, G.; Korpisalo, P.; Yla-Herttuala, S. Promoting blood vessel growth in ischemic diseases: Challenges in translating preclinical potential into clinical success. *Dis. Model. Mech.* **2013**, *6*, 312–322. [CrossRef] [PubMed]
37. Berger, J.S.; Hochman, J.; Lobach, I.; Adelman, M.A.; Riles, T.S.; Rockman, C.B. Modifiable risk factor burden and the prevalence of peripheral artery disease in different vascular territories. *J. Vasc. Surg.* **2013**, *58*, 673.e1–681.e1. [CrossRef] [PubMed]
38. Goh, J.; Ladiges, W. Voluntary Wheel Running in Mice. *Curr. Protoc. Mouse Biol.* **2015**, *5*, 283–290. [CrossRef] [PubMed]
39. Heil, M.; Schaper, W. Influence of mechanical, cellular, and molecular factors on collateral artery growth (arteriogenesis). *Circ. Res.* **2004**, *95*, 449–458. [CrossRef] [PubMed]
40. Troidl, C.; Jung, G.; Troidl, K.; Hoffmann, J.; Mollmann, H.; Nef, H.; Schaper, W.; Hamm, C.W.; Schmitz-Rixen, T. The temporal and spatial distribution of macrophage subpopulations during arteriogenesis. *Curr. Vasc. Pharmacol.* **2013**, *11*, 5–12. [CrossRef]
41. van Royen, N.; Piek, J.J.; Buschmann, I.; Hoefer, I.; Voskuil, M.; Schaper, W. Stimulation of arteriogenesis; a new concept for the treatment of arterial occlusive disease. *Cardiovasc. Res.* **2001**, *49*, 543–553. [CrossRef]

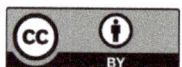

© 2019 by the authors. Licensee MDPI, Basel, Switzerland. This article is an open access article distributed under the terms and conditions of the Creative Commons Attribution (CC BY) license (http://creativecommons.org/licenses/by/4.0/).

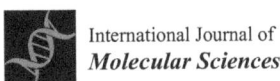

Article

Effects on the Profile of Circulating miRNAs after Single Bouts of Resistance Training with and without Blood Flow Restriction—A Three-Arm, Randomized Crossover Trial

Johanna Vogel [1,*], Daniel Niederer [1], Tobias Engeroff [1], Lutz Vogt [1], Christian Troidl [2,3,4], Thomas Schmitz-Rixen [5], Winfried Banzer [6] and Kerstin Troidl [5,7,*]

[1] Department of Sports Medicine, Institute of Sport Sciences, Goethe University, Ginnheimer Landstraße 39, 60487 Frankfurt, Germany
[2] Department of Experimental Cardiology, Medical Faculty, Justus-Liebig-University, 35392 Giessen, Germany
[3] Department of Cardiology, Kerckhoff Heart and Thorax Center, 61231 Bad Nauheim, Germany
[4] German Center for Cardiovascular Research (DZHK), Partner Site RheinMain, Frankfurt am Main, Germany
[5] Department of Vascular and Endovascular Surgery, University Hospital Frankfurt, Theodor-Stern-Kai 7, 60590 Frankfurt, Germany
[6] Institute for Occupational Medicine, Social Medicine and Environmental Medicine, University Hospital Frankfurt, Theodor-Stern-Kai 7, 60590 Frankfurt, Germany
[7] Department of Pharmacology, Max-Planck-Institute for Heart and Lung Research, Ludwigstrasse 43, 61231 Bad Nauheim, Germany
* Correspondence: johvogel@em.uni-frankfurt.de (J.V.); kerstin.troidl@mpi-bn.mpg.de (K.T.); Tel.: +49-69-798-24426 (J.V.); +49-6032-7051205 (K.T.); Fax: +49-69-798-24592 (J.V.); +49-6032-7051204 (K.T.)

Received: 31 May 2019; Accepted: 28 June 2019; Published: 2 July 2019

Abstract: Background: The effects of blood flow restriction (training) may serve as a model of peripheral artery disease. In both conditions, circulating micro RNAs (miRNAs) are suggested to play a crucial role during exercise-induced arteriogenesis. We aimed to determine whether the profile of circulating miRNAs is altered after acute resistance training during blood flow restriction (BFR) as compared with unrestricted low- and high-volume training, and we hypothesized that miRNA that are relevant for arteriogenesis are affected after resistance training. Methods: Eighteen healthy volunteers (aged 25 ± 2 years) were enrolled in this three-arm, randomized-balanced crossover study. The arms were single bouts of leg flexion/extension resistance training at (1) 70% of the individual single-repetition maximum (1RM), (2) at 30% of the 1RM, and (3) at 30% of the 1RM with BFR (artificially applied by a cuff at 300 mm Hg). Before the first exercise intervention, the individual 1RM (N) and the blood flow velocity (m/s) used to validate the BFR application were determined. During each training intervention, load-associated outcomes (fatigue, heart rate, and exhaustion) were monitored. Acute effects (circulating miRNAs, lactate) were determined using pre-and post-intervention measurements. Results: All training interventions increased lactate concentration and heart rate ($p < 0.001$). The high-intensity intervention (HI) resulted in a higher lactate concentration than both lower-intensity training protocols with BFR (LI-BFR) and without (LI) (LI, $p = 0.003$; 30% LI-BFR, $p = 0.008$). The level of miR-143-3p was down-regulated by LI-BFR, and miR-139-5p, miR-143-3p, miR-195-5p, miR-197-3p, miR-30a-5p, and miR-10b-5p were up-regulated after HI. The lactate concentration and miR-143-3p expression showed a significant positive linear correlation ($p = 0.009$, $r = 0.52$). A partial correlation (intervention partialized) showed a systematic impact of the type of training (LI-BFR vs. HI) on the association ($r = 0.35$ remaining after partialization of training type). Conclusions: The strong effects of LI-BFR and HI on lactate- and arteriogenesis-associated miRNA-143-3p in young and healthy athletes are consistent with an important role of this particular miRNA in metabolic processes during (here) artificial blood flow restriction. BFR may be able to mimic the occlusion of a larger artery which leads to increased collateral flow, and it may therefore serve as an external stimulus of arteriogenesis.

Keywords: circulating miRNA; miR-143-3p; blood flow restriction; peripheral artery disease; arteriogenesis; strength training

1. Introduction

Arteriogenesis is defined as the growth of functional collateral arteries from pre-existing arterio-arteriolar anastomoses [1,2]. An initial trigger is the occlusion of a main artery, which occurs during peripheral artery disease (PAD). Such an occlusion redirects the blood flow to the pre-formed collateral arteries and thereby alters the fluid shear stress (FSS) [3]. The increased blood flow initiates vascular remodeling and diameter growth [4]. Several mechano-sensors and transducers that convey the FSS message during collateral remodeling have been proposed, including ion channels [5], the glycocalyx layer of endothelial cells (ECs) [6], nitric oxide (NO) [7], and microRNAs (miRNAs) [8].

These small, non-coding ribonucleic acids have been shown to play a decisive role in processes such as heart development, vascular regeneration, and tissue repair [9–12]. miRNAs are involved in post-transcriptional gene regulation by binding to mRNAs, causing the repression of translation and mRNA degradation, thus fine-tuning protein expression. Several miRNAs have been shown to control the response of vascular cells to hemodynamic stress [8]. In addition, miRNAs can be secreted and can thereby contribute to intercellular communication [13] or serve as circulating biomarkers [14].

Arteriogenesis can be amplified by exercise, as documented in human trials [15–17] and animal studies [18]. Therefore, according to international guidelines, PAD patients in Fontaine stage I or IIA/B (Rutherford 1–3) should be recommended for exercise training [19,20]. Mechanisms involved in the exercise-mediated benefits of treating PAD are thought to be the suppression of inflammation [1], expression of pro-inflammatory immune cells [21,22], and the improvement of endothelial function [23]. Beyond that, physical training has the potential to promote additional vascularization [24,25].

Comparable mechanisms have been discussed for the training effects of blood flow restriction exercises: Blood flow restriction training (BFR) is a resistance training method in which blood flow is reduced artificially. The decreased blood flow is usually caused by applying a blood pressure cuff at the origin of the extremity (arms or legs) to be trained. The mechanisms of BFR are thought to involve ischemic hypoxia and the increased expression of vascular endothelial growth factors [26]. The hemodynamic stimuli amplified by BFR (e.g., shear stress at the endothelium) lead to an increased release of the endothelial NO synthase, among other responses [27].

To achieve systematic effects during BFR, a lower resistance load is used than in classic resistance training without BFR: An intensity of 20% of the single repetition maximum (1RM) and a reduced training time of about 4–8 weeks have been demonstrated to have effects on muscle hypertrophy and muscular strength [28–30]. BFR training with a lower load in a shorter time can lead to the same results as resistance training with significantly higher loads (at 65% 1RM). In particular, increases in muscle thickness and strength are comparable between these strategies [31,32]. Due to the comparable effects and lower loads, BFR is of great relevance for training persons with physical limitations (e.g., patients with injuries, patients with cardiovascular diseases, or elderly persons) [33,34].

Despite the promising results derived from BFR as a method to mimic exercise effects under different occlusion conditions like PAD and the potential role of miRNAs as effectors after hemodynamic stress or FSS, nothing is known about the acute effects of strength training during BFR on miRNA levels. Therefore, this study was designed to determine whether the profile of circulating miRNAs is altered after resistance training during BFR, as compared with low- and high-volume training protocols with no BFR. Our hypotheses were: (1) Blood flow restriction leads to a reduced blood flow velocity; (2) low-intensity blood flow restriction training leads to metabolic responses that are similar to those of high-intensity strength training without blood flow restriction; (3) low-intensity blood flow restriction training and training without blood flow restriction lead to different expression characteristics of miRNAs.

2. Results

2.1. Sample

None of the participants withdrew their consent, and none had to be excluded. Eighteen healthy adults (females = 11; mean age 25 ± standard deviation (SD) 2 years; body mass index 22.1 ± 1.8 kg/m^2) were included.

2.2. Blood Flow Velocity

The blood flow velocity in the A. poplitea was significantly reduced by wearing the BFR cuff (compared to unrestricted, $p = 0.002$; mean intraindividual difference: −7.6 cm/s, −14%, Figure 1).

a
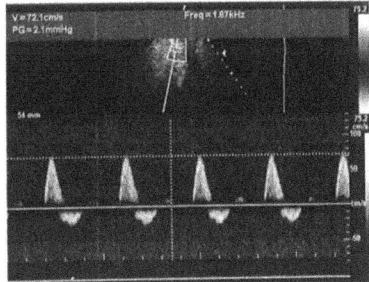

b
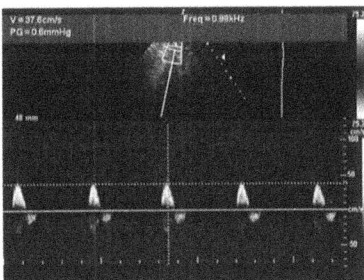

c
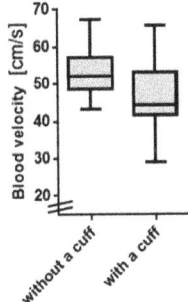

Figure 1. Blood flow velocity in the A. poplitea: (**a,b**) Representative original Doppler sonography blood flow profiles at rest: The upper images show the region of interest of the A.poplitea; the lower diagrams show the time course on the x-axis and the blood flow velocity heartbeat by heartbeat on the y-axis. (**a**) Blood flow velocity without wearing a cuff. (**b**) Blood flow velocity while wearing the cuff (occlusion pressure 300 mm Hg). (**c**) Boxplots of the grouped pre-post differences in blood flow velocity with and without cuff. Data are displayed as median and inter-quartile ranges plus range (whisker bars).

2.3. Basic Resistance Training Outcomes

2.3.1. Objective Outcomes of the Training Interventions

Lactate concentration and heart rate were increased after all training interventions ($p < 0.001$) (Figure 2a,b). The lactate concentration was different between the groups: The high-intensity (HI) intervention resulted in a higher lactate concentration than both lower-intensity (LI) training protocols

(LI, $p = 0.003$; LI-BFR, $p = 0.008$). In the HI group, the mechanical pain threshold increased from before to after training ($p < 0.05$) (Figure 2c).

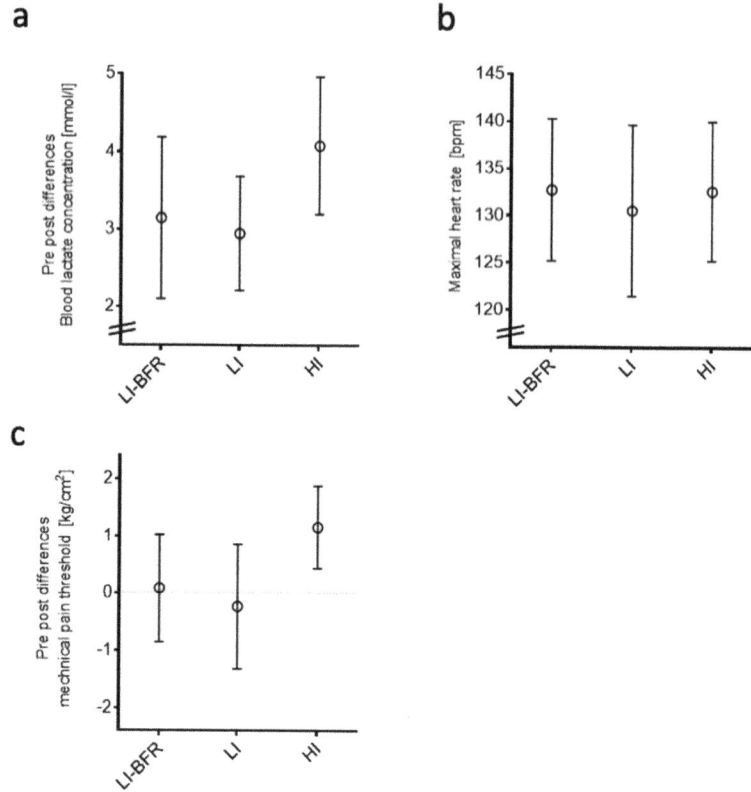

Figure 2. Objective outcomes of training interventions. Data are displayed as mean and 95% confidence intervals. Bpm, beats per minute; LI-BFR, low-intensity training with blood flow restriction; LI, low-intensity training; HI, high-intensity training. (**a**) Differences in blood lactate concentration pre- and post-training, (**b**) maximal heart rate, and (**c**) differences in mechanical pain threshold pre- and post-training.

2.3.2. Participant-Reported Outcomes

The perceived exertion was greater during the HI intervention than in the LI interventions (LI, $p = 0.005$; LI-BFR, $p = 0.028$). The HI group scored a lower value than the LI group in the feeling scale ($p < 0.05$). Participants in the LI group reported lower values on the fatigue scale than the LI-BFR group ($p = 0.028$) and the HI group ($p = 0.004$). The corresponding values are displayed in Figure 3.

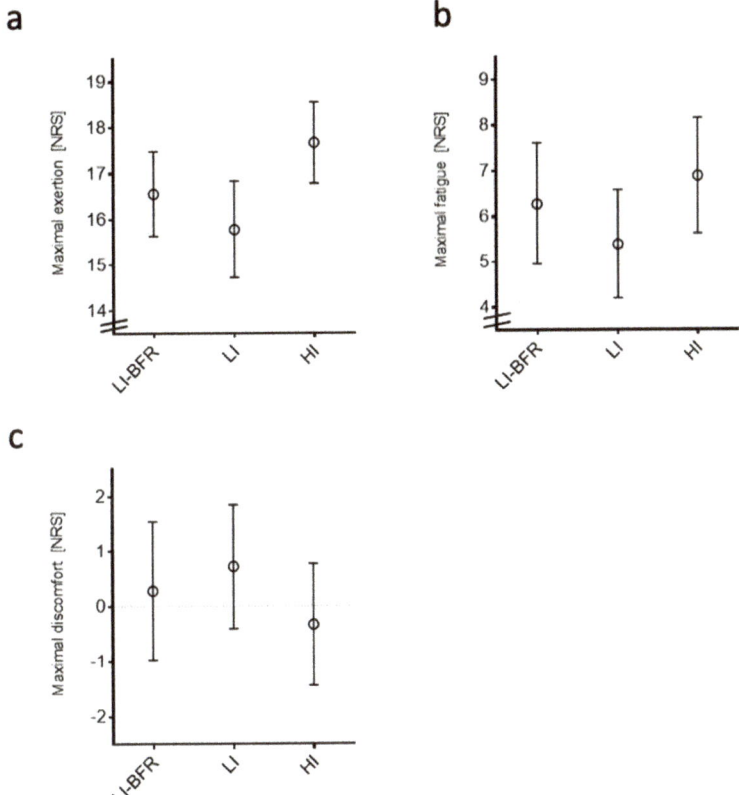

Figure 3. Participant-reported outcomes of training interventions. Data are displayed as mean and 95% confidence intervals. (**a**) Maximal exertion. (**b**) Maximal fatigue. (**c**) Maximal discomfort. NRS, numeric rating scale; LI-BFR, low-intensity training with blood flow restriction; LI, low-intensity training; HI, high-intensity training.

2.4. Profiling of Circulating miRNAs

2.4.1. Capillary Blood for miRNA Isolation, Expression Analysis, and Quantification

A single capillary blood draw resulted in ≥50 µL plasma, and, in comparison to venous blood sampling, the average degree of hemolysis differed significantly ($p < 0.05$) as determined by OD_{414} in a pilot study (Figure 4a,b). Only 50 µL of plasma were sufficient to isolate total RNA and to reverse-transcribe miRNAs for real-time PCR-based quantification. In order to identify stably expressed reference genes for normalization, five candidate miRNAs (hsa-miR-30e-5p, hsa-miR-148b-3p, hsa-miR-222-3p, hsa-miR-425-5p, hsa-miR-484) were tested for stable expression over the entire range of samples being investigated. Except for hsa-miR-222-3p, all miRNAs were suitable for normalization (Figure 4c).

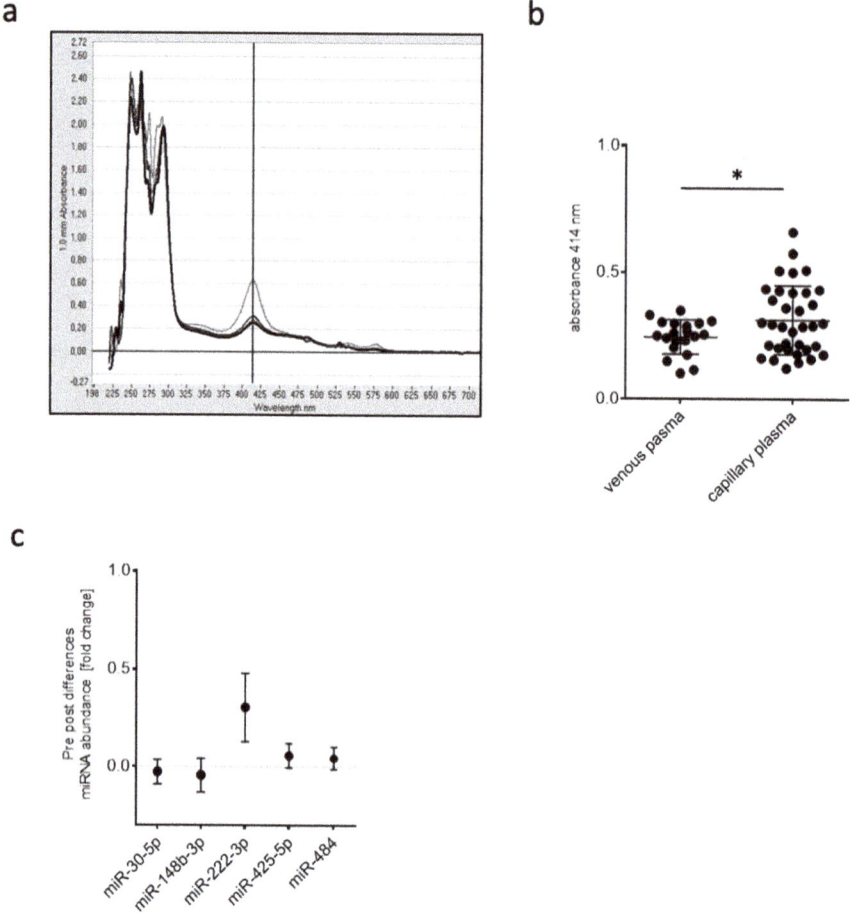

Figure 4. (a) Example of an OD scan from 200 to 700 nm with a distinct absorbance peak at 414 nm to assess hemolysis. Different lines depict different plasma samples. (b) OD_{414} values in plasma samples after venous or capillary blood draw (* $p < 0.05$). (c) Differences in miRNA abundance of typically detected miRNAs in plasma to determine stable expression pre- and post-training intervention.

2.4.2. Screening of Expression Changes in Circulating miRNAs before and after BFR Training

Based on the assumption that the LI-BFR reduces blood flow to the periphery in a way that is comparable to that of a PAD, eight plasma samples of four participants pre- (control) and post-training were selected and subjected to the human serum/plasma focus panel consisting of 179 miRNA assays targeting human plasma-relevant miRNAs, reference miRNAs, and spike-in controls. A global C_T mean of expressed miRNAs was used for normalization, and cel-miR-39-3p was included as an internal amplification control. In each sample, more than 80% of miRNAs surpassed the lower limit of detection of a $C_t < 35$ (Figure 5a). Significant miRNA expression changes were visualized in the volcano plot (Figure 5b). A total of 11 miRNAs were selected for further validation due to their markedly altered expression or previous association with collateral growth (Table 1). Interestingly, among the differentially expressed miRNAs identified, three arteriogenesis-associated, previously detected miRNAs were recovered: miR-143-3p, miR-195-5p, and miR-126-5p.

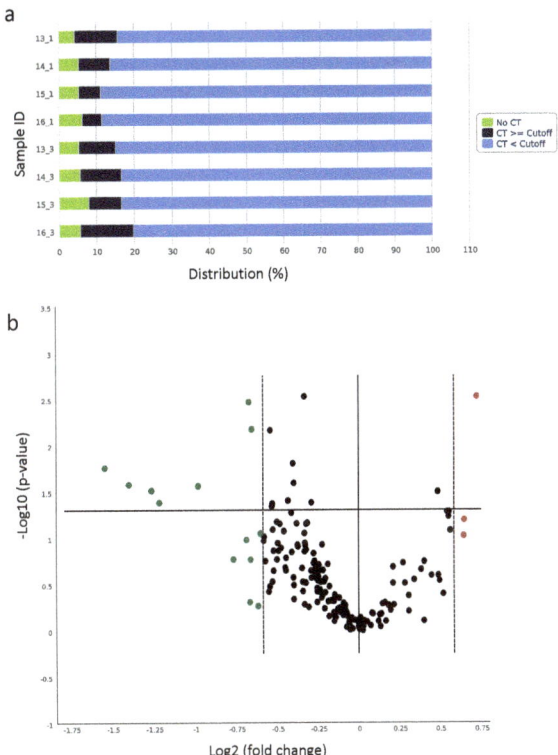

Figure 5. qPCR-based serum/plasma focus panel of circulating miRNAs (**a**) Distribution of C_t values for the processed data of each plasma sample. (**b**) Volcano plot of differentially expressed miRNAs pre- and post-LI-BFR training. Data points outside the two dashed lines are up-regulated (red) or down-regulated (green) more than x-fold. Data points above the solid horizontal line have *p*-values less than 0.05.

Table 1. Over-expressed miRNAs (fold regulation values greater than 1.5) and under-expressed miRNAs (fold regulation values less than −1.5) detected in the screen and analyzed in the three different training groups.

miRNA ID	Fold Change Screen	*p*-Value	HI	LI-BFR	LI
hsa-miR-197-3p	1.56	0.094			
hsa-miR-326	1.65	0.002 **			
hsa-miR-136-3p	1.57	0.063			
hsa-miR-143-3p	−1.7	0.170	up *		down *
hsa-miR-30a-5p	−1.59	0.003 **	up **		
hsa-miR-139-5p	−1.97	0.027 *	up *		
hsa-miR-125a-5p	−2.63	0.026 *			
hsa-miR-375	−1.59	0.492			
hsa-miR-99a-5p	−1.58	0.171			
hsa-miR-126-5p	−1.57	0.006 **			
hsa-miR-10b-5p	−2.4	0.030 *	up **		
hsa-miR-195-5p	−2.92	0.017 *	up *		
hsa-miR-125b-5p	−2.32	0.041 *			
hsa-miR-100-5p	−1.61	0.104			
hsa-miR-362-3p	−1.52	0.088			
hsa-miR-376c-3p	−1.53	0.540			

* *p*-value < 0.05, ** *p*-value < 0.01, HI: High intensity training, LI-BFR: Low intensity training with blood flow restriction, LI: Low intensity training. Bold text shows the miRNAs that have been previously associated with collateral growth.

2.4.3. Analysis of miRNAs in Different Training Intervention Groups

The abundance of these 11 differentially expressed miRNAs was analyzed in each training group in individual assays in a larger cohort of 12 participants. Only miR-143-3p was confirmed to be down-regulated after LI-BFR. In contrast to the initial screening results, miR-139-5p, miR-143-3p, miR-195-5p, miR-197-3p, miR-30a-5p, and miR-10b-5p were up-regulated after HI. There was no differential expression after LI. (Figure 6, Table 1)

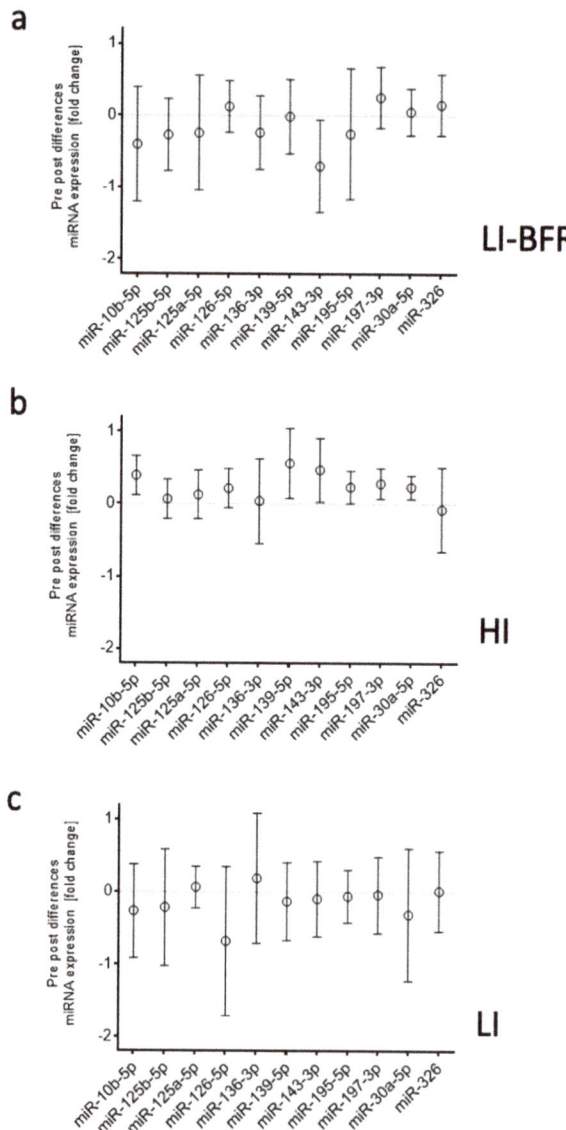

Figure 6. Differences in miRNA expression pre- and post-training. Data are displayed as mean and 95% confidence intervals. (**a**) LI-BFR, low-intensity training with blood flow restriction. (**b**) HI; high-intensity training. (**c**) LI, low-intensity training.

2.5. Associations between Training Outcomes and Circulating miRNAs

The pre-to-post changes in lactate concentration and miR-143-3p expression showed a significant linear positive correlation (intervention partialized) of $r = 0.34$ ($p = 0.048$). This correlation is visualized in Figure 7. Without considering the group as a partializing co-variate, lactate and miRNA-143-3p differences were associated with a coefficient of $r = 0.305$; however, this correlation lacks statistical significance ($p = 0.075$). No other systematic correlation between lactate concentration and miRNA expressions occurred.

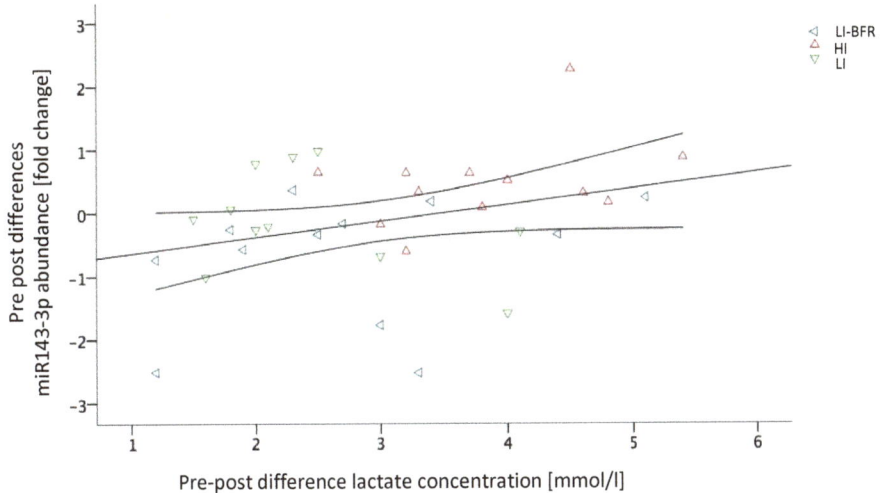

Figure 7. Scatterplot diagram of miR-143-3p and lactate concentration with a correlation line (including confidence intervals); LI-BFR, low-intensity training with blood flow restriction; HI, high-intensity training, LI, low-intensity training.

3. Discussion

In this three-armed crossover study, we investigated the miRNA profiles in young, healthy athletes before and after various resistance training interventions (HI and LI). In addition, we employed peripheral blood flow restriction (LI-BFR) that was achieved by applying an external cuff during the resistance training at LI. We assumed that BFR can mimic the occlusion of a larger artery, leading to an increased collateral flow, and would therefore serve as an external stimulus of arteriogenesis.

The BFR application led to a decreased blood flow velocity in the popliteal artery, confirming our first hypothesis. The HI intervention showed the largest effects on lactate, and all interventions led to a comparable heart rate response. The LI intervention resulted in the smallest pre to post differences. Hypothesis 2 was thus partially verified (depending on the outcome). Our results further suggest that miRNA profiles were acutely affected by HI training and LI-BFR training but not by LI training alone. In particular, miR-143-3p expression correlated with training intensity, which verifies Hypothesis 3.

The fact that BFR application led to a decrease in the blood flow velocity (Hypothesis 1) confirms the validity of BFR. The reduction of 7.6 cm/s is far beyond the standard error of measurement found in inter-rater reliability analyses [35] and can thus be considered as clinically relevant. The mean blood flow velocity in the popliteal artery in PAD patients was recently found to be 41 ± 17 (SD) cm/s [36], which is considerably lower than the velocity we found in the no-cuff condition and is comparable to the one we found in the blood flow-restricted condition. Consequently, one may consider our model valid in terms of blood flow restriction and velocity, although the study population does not fully mimic the PAD caused by atherosclerosis.

All interventions induced increases in lactate and heart rate; the largest effects on lactate occurred after the HI intervention, whereas all interventions led to a comparable heart rate response. The LI intervention resulted in the smallest differences in pre- and post-intervention values in objective and participant-reported outcomes. The finding of a BFR-induced increase in lactate concentration is in accordance with previous reports [23]. The metabolic response thus varies with varying training intensity. If BFR training effects comparable to those of 70% 1RM sessions without BFR are to be reached, the current literature recommends BFR training at 30% of the individual 1RM [18]. Though we followed this recommendation, BFR elicited lower values/effects in some of the outcomes than during/after HI training; this is in contrast to our second hypothesis, which was only partially verified. One possible reason may be due to our sample. The majority of current studies adopting BFR training or interventions at 30% of the 1RM refer to an elderly or untrained population [18]. For a trained study population, a minority of studies in the literature suggest that 50% of the 1RM should be used to achieve a sufficient metabolic response [24].

We further analyzed the profiles of circulating miRNAs before and after resistance training. Our results of the quantification in each intervention group suggest that the profile of circulating miRNAs is altered as an acute effect of resistance training. In particular, we identified six miRNAs (miR-139-5p, miR-143-3p, miR-195-5p, miR-197-3p, miR-30a-5p, and miR-10b-5p) that are up-regulated after HI training. Only miR-143 was found to be down-regulated after LI-BFR training. The LI training, in contrast, had no systematic effect of either miRNA. Other studies also demonstrated both acute effects of intensive stimuli (miRNA-21, miRNA-146a, miRNA-221, and miRNA-222) and training effects (miRNA-146a, miRNA-222, and miRNA-20a) [37]. Consequently, we conclude that increased training intensity leads to increased miR-143-3p. The correlation of the lactate difference (BFR-LI, LI, and HI) and miR-143-3p abundance further indicates a decisive role depending on training intensity. In detail, 3.5 mmol/L of pre-to-post lactate difference was determined as a potential threshold from miR-143-3p down-regulation to its up-regulation. Consequently, a major share, but not only the lactate concentration (or the intensity of the training), is decisive for miRNA expression—as is (to a minor share) the type of training. More concretely, BFR seems not only to lead to lower lactate increases but also tendentiously leads to a down-regulation of miRNA-143-3p, whereas LI seems to be able to increase lactate concentration but does not affect miRNA-143-3p expression. The HI, in contrast, seemed to be able to both up-regulate lactate and miRNA-143-3p. Whether the differences between the conditions are due to the lower intensity or the type of training may be finally delineated by using the intensity increase up to 50% during BFR, as described above.

We have previously shown an association of miR-195-5p and miR-143-3p with collateral growth [38]. Both of these species were found to be highly up-regulated in the vascular tissue itself, and miR-143-3p was identified as an essential factor for proper collateral formation following femoral artery ligation in mice. The acute and local blockade of miR-143-3p in these mice completely abrogated arteriogenesis. In blood vessels, miR-143 is one of the most-studied miRNAs expressed by vascular smooth muscle cells, and, together with miR-145, this miRNA is thought to play a pivotal role in smooth muscle cell differentiation and vascular disease [8,13,39]. Furthermore, circulating miR-143-3p has been associated with cardiovascular disease [40] and is considered to be a predictor of aging and the acute adaptive response to resistance exercise [41].

Small volumes of capillary blood are routinely used for lactate diagnostics. We aimed to establish this routinely used, less invasive method of fingertip blood drawing for obtaining cell-free, non-hemolytic plasma samples suitable for the isolation and quantification of circulating miRNAs. Indeed, this method was successful in yielding plasma samples reproducible in quality and volume. All miRNAs identified, with the exception of miR-10b-5p, were validated in terms of independency of hemolytic score. For miRNA profiling, we included plasma samples of four participants with an $OD_{414} < 0.3$ and an increased lactate concentration after training intervention, a maximal heart rate during training of at least 60% of maximal calculated heart rate, and a participant-reported "very hard" intensity on the Borg scale of at least 16 points (data not shown).

Our results are in line with the proposed epigenetic potential of lifestyle interventions that may alter gene expression [42,43]. Therefore, we postulate that in order to maximize the beneficial role of miR-143-3p in collateral growth, training intensity will have to be adjusted. For symptomatic PAD patients, controlled training is an efficient, conservative therapy that is a good alternative to invasive therapies. The formation of collaterals and compensatory blood flow is the goal of conservative treatment. However, since the success of training varies, responders and non-responders must be identified. Thus, future studies are needed to (1) confirm our findings in PAD patients, (2) delineate the mechanisms of how miRNA-143-3p may be decisive in response or non-response to resistance training, and (3) determine how a pre-intervention screening of miRNA-143-3p or other microRNAs can be used to stratify responders and non-responders for the individualization of intervention/training goals.

4. Materials and Methods

4.1. Ethical Standard and Study Design

The study had a randomized-balanced crossover design. Ethical approval was obtained from the local institutional review board (protocol number 2018-16, 17.06.2018, Ethics Committee Department 5 Psychology and Sports Sciences Goethe-University Frankfurt). The trial was conducted in accordance with the ethical standards set down by the declaration of Helsinki (World medical Association) Declaration of Helsinki–Ethical Principles for Medical Research Involving Human Subjects) with its recent modification of 2013 (Fortaleza). All participants gave written informed consent prior to study enrollment.

4.2. Sample

Participants were considered eligible if they fulfilled the following criteria: (1) Healthy and (2) aged 18 to 30 years. Exclusion criteria comprised (1) severe psychiatric, neurological, or cardiovascular diseases; (2) acute orthopedic disorders; (3) pregnancy; (4) muscle soreness; and (5) intake of painkillers, analgesics, or muscle relaxants within the previous 48 hours.

4.3. Experimental Design

The experimental design incorporated three arms. Each participant performed each of the three conditions once (on three different days with a washout of at least 7 days in between) in a randomized, balanced sequence. Before the first exercise intervention, blood flow velocity to validate the BFR application and the individual 1RM from the knee extensor and knee flexor were determined. During each training intervention, loading-associated outcomes were monitored. Acute effects were determined using pre- and post-intervention measurements.

4.4. Blood Flow Velocity Measurement

The arterial blood flow velocity in the popliteal artery was measured in one leg (side randomly chosen, in the prone position) with and without external blood flow restriction caused/provoked by the BFR cuff (7 cm wide; nylon pneumatic cuff) at 300 mm Hg. Doppler sonography (Siemens Acuson X300, Munich, Germany) was used with spectral analysis, and data were gathered about components of the flow profile. The procedure is reliable [35].

4.5. RM Determination

Prior to the 1RM determination, participants warmed up by cycling for 5 min on a stationary bicycle. After a one-minute rest, an individualized starting load (~80% of estimated the 1RM, estimation based on sex, weight, and strength training experience) was moved through the full range of motion in sagittal plane (knee extension and flexion). After each successful performance, the weight increased until an attempt failed. One-minute rests were given between each attempt, and the 1RM was attained within a maximum of 5 attempts.

4.6. Intervention

The three training conditions were (1) resistance training during BFR at 30% of the 1RM, (2) resistance training without BFR at 30% of the 1RM, and (3) resistance training without BFR at 70% of the 1RM. The possible sequences of the conditions to be performed were randomly assigned to the participants in a balanced frequency. Resistance training comprised knee extensors and flexors on a combination training device (Schnell M3 Diagnosis, Peutenhausen, Germany). In conditions (1) and (2), resistance training with 30% of 1RM was adopted, and each exercise period consisted of 75 repetitions divided into 4 sets with a rest period of 90 s. In contrast, in condition (3), the resistance training was performed at 70% of the 1RM; here, 30 repetitions divided into 3 sets with a break of 90 seconds between sets. During condition (1), blood pressure cuffs inflated to 300 mm Hg were applied to both legs. The exercise protocols have been used previously in other studies and have been classified as low risk [44]. The washout phase between test days was at least 7 days. On each test day, a standardized control condition ("do-nothing" phase) was performed for 20 min before the test condition.

4.7. Assessments

4.7.1. Laboratory Analytic Outcomes

Blood Lactate Concentration

Before and directly after each intervention, capillary blood was taken by pricking the earlobe with a safety lancet. The sample was applied directly to a test strip to determine lactate concentration (mmol/l) by means of a portable, hand-held unit (Lactate Scout, SensLab GmbH, Leipzig, Germany).

Heart Rate

During the intervention, a chest belt (Polar H7) and heart rate receiver (Polar M 430) continuously measured heart rate (beats/min). The maximum heart rate was selected for further analyses.

Mechanical Pain Threshold

Before and directly after each intervention, the mechanical pain threshold (N/cm^2) was determined. Participants reclined supine on a bench with their legs extended. With an algometer (FPK, Wagner Instruments, Greenwich, CT, USA) pressure was applied on the skin (1 cm^2). Three measurements were taken in the middle of both mm. recti femoris. The average of the three measurements was selected for further analyses.

Blood Sampling and Plasma Preparation for miRNA Profiling

In order to minimize pre-analytical variables that might influence the miRNA expression profile, care was taken in the collection of blood and the preparation of plasma to prevent blood cell contamination and hemolysis. Before and after each intervention, fingertip capillary blood samples (≥200 µL) were collected in microvettes (system for capillary blood collection) containing Ethylenediaminetetraacetic acid (EDTA). Blood samples were centrifuged for 10 min at 3000 rpm and 4 °C. After the first centrifugation step, the upper plasma phase was transferred to a new tube without disturbing the intermediate buffy coat layer. The plasma samples were centrifuged a second time for 10 min at 15,000 rpm and 4 °C. The cleared supernatant was carefully transferred to a new tube and frozen at −80 °C.

Determination of Hemolysis

To assess hemolysis, oxyhemoglobin absorbance was measured at 414 nm in plasma samples using NanoDrop (peqlab Biotechnologie GmbH; Erlangen, Germany).

miRNA Isolation

Sample amounts were standardized by volume: The same volume of plasma was used for each RNA isolation, and the same volume of purified RNA was used for all further analyses. The miRNAs were isolated from 50 µL (qRT-PCR) or 200 µL (PANEL screen) of plasma using a column-based protocol (miRNeasy Serum/Plasma Advanced Kit, (Qiagen, Hilden, Germany) according to the manufacturer's protocol. cel-miR-39 from *Caenorhabditis elegans* (1 nM) was spiked in. In the final step, total RNA (>18 nucleotides) was eluted using 20 µL of RNase-free water.

Reverse Transcription and miRNA Profiling

For reverse transcription, the miRCURY LNA RT Kit (Qiagen, Hilden, Germany) was used. Undiluted complementary DNA (cDNA, 20 µL) was used for miRCURY LNA miRNA Focus Panel Human Serum/Plasma (YAHS-106Y) in the 2 × 96-well plate format. The Human Serum/Plasma Focus Panel includes 179 miRNA assays targeting relevant miRNAs, reference miRNAs, and spike-in controls.

Reverse Transcription and qRT-PCR

Following reverse transcription as described above, quantitative real-time PCR was performed using miRCURY LNA miRNA PCR assays (Appendix A) in a 10-µL reaction containing 3 µL of cDNA (1:30) and a CFX real-time PCR detection system (BioRad, Munich, Germany). Assays were performed in triplicate. The amount of the respective miRNA was normalized to miR-425-3p and cel-miR-39.

For the miRCURY miRNA PCR analysis, v1.0 raw C_t data from real-time PCR were up-loaded at (https://www.qiagen.com/us/shop/genes-and-pathways/data-analysis-center-overview-page). Cel-miR-39-3p was used as an internal spike-in amplification control. A C_t cut-off of 35 was set as the lower limit of detection. A global C_t mean of expressed miRNAs was used for normalization, and the fold change was calculated as ($2^{-\Delta\Delta Ct}$), which represents the average normalized miRNA expression ($2^{-\Delta\Delta Ct}$) of the samples in the test group divided by the average normalized miRNA expression ($2^{-\Delta\Delta Ct}$) of the samples in the control group.

4.7.2. Self-Reported Outcomes

Self-reported outcomes consisted of rates of perceived exertion (RPE-Borg; Likert 6 to 20 point scale) [45], current well-being assessments (feeling scale: (+5 to −5, 10 point Likert scale)), and fatigue reporting (numeric rating scale NRS: 0 to 10 points). All self-reported parameters were assessed once after each intervention. The participants were asked to refer to the highest intensity during (RPE and feeling scale) or at the end (fatigue) of each intervention.

4.8. Data Analyses and Statistics

For all outcomes assessed before and after each intervention, real values and absolute pre-to-post differences were used for further analysis. Continuously assessed variables were processed in their real values.

After the following plausibility control, all analyses were performed based on the results of the initial checking for relevant underlying assumptions to test for parametric or nonparametric characteristics (data, distribution of the variances and variance homogeneity). Between-group differences and pre-to-post changes were assessed using omnibus and follow-up post-hoc testing. SPSS 23 (SPSS Inc., Chicago, IL, USA) and GraphPad software PRISM5 for Mac (GraphPad Software, La Jolla, CA, USA) were used to conduct all statistical calculations and create figures. An alpha-error level of 5% was considered to be a relevant cut-off value for significance testing, with p-values below 0.05 indicating significant differences.

Friedman tests were performed for omnibus between-group comparisons for all resistance training outcomes (or the a priori calculated differences). For significant omnibus testing, post-hoc comparisons using post-hoc Bonferroni–Holm tests and alpha-error-adjusted Mann–Whitney-U-tests were performed. For pre-to-post significance testing, Wilcoxon tests were performed.

To identify significant miRNA expression changes between conditions, a fold regulation was calculated, and a fold-change threshold of 1.5 was defined. Significant miRNA expression changes were visualized using the volcano plot. For each miRNA showing a significant expression change, a pairwise group comparison (Student's t-test) was made based on the $2^{-\Delta\Delta Ct}$ value of the replicate samples. The p-value calculation was based on a parametric, two-sample, equal variance, unpaired, and two-tailed distribution.

The potential associations between the kinematic (treatment) effects of the miRNA and lactate were analyzed using partial linear regression with the covariate group allocation.

Author Contributions: J.V., K.T., T.E. and L.V. designed the experiments. J.V., K.T., T.E., D.N. and L.V. interpreted the findings. J.V. and K.T. wrote the first draft of the manuscript. J.V., K.T., C.T. and D.N. analyzed and performed the experiments. D.N. performed statistical analyses. C.T., T.S.-R. and W.B. discussed the results and revised the manuscript. All authors edited and approved the manuscript.

Funding: This research was funded by the German Research Foundation (Bonn, Germany, TR 1137/2-1 to K.T) and the Anna-Maria and Uwe-Karsten Kühl Foundation (T188/30462/2017, Bad Nauheim, Germany to K.T.).

Acknowledgments: The authors thank Monika Rieschel for excellent technical assistance, Jan Wilke for excellent support in the preparation of the study design, Andres Rosenhagen for excellent technical support in the ultrasonography. Elizabeth Martinson of the KHFI Editorial Office provided editorial assistance during preparation of this manuscript.

Conflicts of Interest: The authors declare no conflict of interest.

Abbreviations

miRNA	microRNA
PAD	Peripheral artery disease
BFR	Blood flow restriction
FSS	Fluid shear stress
HI	High intensity
LI	Low intensity
LI-BFR	Low intensity with blood flow restriction

Appendix A

Table A1. miRCURY LNA miRNA PCR assays for normalization.

hsa-miR-30e-5p	YP00204714	5'UGUAAACAUCCUUGACUGGAAG
hsa-miR-148b-3p	YP00204047	5'UCAGUGCAUCACAGAACUUUGU
hsa-miR-222-3p	YP00204551	5'AGCUACAUCUGGCUACUGGGU
hsa-miR-425-5p	YP00204337	5'AAUGACACGAUCACUCCCGUUGA
hsa-miR-484	YP00205636	5'UCAGGCUCAGUCCCCUCCCGAU

Table A2. miRCURY LNA miRNA PCR assays for screening hits.

hsa-miR-197-3p	YP00204380	5'UUCACCACCUUCUCCACCCAGC
hsa miR-326	YP00204512	5'CCUCUGGGCCCUUCCUCCAG
hsa-miR-136-3p	YP00205503	5'CAUCAUCGUCUCAAAUGAGUCU
hsa-miR-143-3p	YP00205992	5'UGAGAUGAAGCACUGUAGCUC
hsa-miR-30a-5p	YP00205695	5'UGUAAACAUCCUCGACUGGAAG
hsa-miR-139-5p	YP00205874	5'UCUACAGUGCACGUGUCUCCAGU
hsa-miR-125a-5p	YP00204339	5'UCCCUGAGACCCUUUAACCUGUGA
hsa-miR-125b-5p	YP00205713	5'UCCCUGAGACCCUAACUUGUGA
hsa-miR-126-5p	YP00206010	5'CAUUAUUACUUUUGGUACGCG
hsa-miR-10b-5p	YP00205637	5'UACCCUGUAGAACCGAAUUUGUG
hsa-miR-195-5p	YP00205869	5'UAGCAGCACAGAAAUAUUGGC

References

1. Schaper, W. On arteriogenesis—A reply. *Basic Res. Cardiol.* **2003**, *98*, 183–184. [PubMed]
2. Heil, M.; Eitenmüller, I.; Schmitz-Rixen, T.; Schaper, W. Arteriogenesis versus angiogenesis: Similarities and differences. *J. Cell. Mol. Med.* **2006**, *10*, 45–55. [CrossRef]
3. Ben Driss, A.; Benessiano, J.; Poitevin, P.; Levy, B.I.; Michel, J.B. Arterial expansive remodeling induced by high flow rates. *Am. J. Physiol.* **1997**, *272*, H851–H858. [CrossRef] [PubMed]
4. Gerhold, K.A.; Schwartz, M.A. Ion Channels in Endothelial Responses to Fluid Shear Stress. *Physiology* **2016**, *31*, 359–369. [CrossRef] [PubMed]
5. Shi, Z.-D.; Tarbell, J.M. Fluid Flow Mechanotransduction in Vascular Smooth Muscle Cells and Fibroblasts. *Ann. Biomed. Eng.* **2011**, *39*, 1608–1619. [CrossRef] [PubMed]
6. Tronc, F.; Mallat, Z.; Lehoux, S.; Wassef, M.; Esposito, B.; Tedgui, A. Role of matrix metalloproteinases in blood flow-induced arterial enlargement: Interaction with NO. *Arterioscler. Thromb. Vasc. Biol.* **2000**, *20*, E120–E126. [CrossRef]
7. Neth, P.; Nazari-Jahantigh, M.; Schober, A.; Weber, C. MicroRNAs in flow-dependent vascular remodelling. *Cardiovasc. Res.* **2013**, *99*, 294–303. [CrossRef]
8. Wang, G.-K.; Zhu, J.-Q.; Zhang, J.-T.; Li, Q.; Li, Y.; He, J.; Qin, Y.-W.; Jing, Q. Circulating microRNA: A novel potential biomarker for early diagnosis of acute myocardial infarction in humans. *Eur. Heart J.* **2010**, *31*, 659–666. [CrossRef]
9. Zhang, C. MicroRNAs in Vascular Biology and Vascular Disease. *J. Cardiovasc. Trans. Res.* **2010**, *3*, 235–240. [CrossRef]
10. Chan, S.Y.; Zhang, Y.-Y.; Hemann, C.; Mahoney, C.E.; Zweier, J.L.; Loscalzo, J. MicroRNA-210 Controls Mitochondrial Metabolism during Hypoxia by Repressing the Iron-Sulfur Cluster Assembly Proteins ISCU1/2. *Cell Metab.* **2009**, *10*, 273–284. [CrossRef]
11. Williams, A.H.; Liu, N.; van Rooij, E.; Olson, E.N. MicroRNA control of muscle development and disease. *Curr. Opin. Cell Biol.* **2009**, *21*, 461–469. [CrossRef] [PubMed]
12. Hergenreider, E.; Heydt, S.; Tréguer, K.; Boettger, T.; Horrevoets, A.J.G.; Zeiher, A.M.; Scheffer, M.P.; Frangakis, A.S.; Yin, X.; Mayr, M.; et al. Atheroprotective communication between endothelial cells and smooth muscle cells through miRNAs. *Nat. Cell Biol.* **2012**, *14*, 249–256. [CrossRef] [PubMed]
13. Chen, L.-J.; Wei, S.-Y.; Chiu, J.-J. Mechanical regulation of epigenetics in vascular biology and pathobiology. *J. Cell. Mol. Med.* **2013**, *17*, 437–448. [CrossRef] [PubMed]
14. Huonker, M.; Halle, M.; Keul, J. Structural and functional adaptations of the cardiovascular system by training. *Int. J. Sports Med.* **1996**, *17*, S164–S172. [CrossRef] [PubMed]
15. Nash, M.S.; Montalvo, B.M.; Applegate, B. Lower extremity blood flow and responses to occlusion ischemia differ in exercise-trained and sedentary tetraplegic persons. *Arch. Phys. Med. Rehab.* **1996**, *77*, 1260–1265. [CrossRef]
16. Dopheide, J.F.; Rubrech, J.; Trumpp, A.; Geissler, P.; Zeller, G.C.; Schnorbus, B.; Schmidt, F.; Gori, T.; Münzel, T.; Espinola-Klein, C. Supervised exercise training in peripheral arterial disease increases vascular shear stress and profunda femoral artery diameter. *Eur. J. Prev. Cardiol.* **2017**, *24*, 178–191. [CrossRef]
17. Sayed, A.; Schierling, W.; Troidl, K.; Rüding, I.; Nelson, K.; Apfelbeck, H.; Benli, I.; Schaper, W.; Schmitz-Rixen, T. Exercise Linked to Transient Increase in Expression and Activity of Cation Channels in Newly Formed Hind-limb Collaterals. *Eur. J. Vasc. Endovasc. Surg.* **2010**, *40*, 81–87. [CrossRef]
18. Anderson, J.L.; Halperin, J.L.; Albert, N.M.; Bozkurt, B.; Brindis, R.G.; Curtis, L.H.; DeMets, D.; Guyton, R.A.; Hochman, J.S.; Kovacs, R.J.; et al. Management of patients with peripheral artery disease (compilation of 2005 and 2011 ACCF/AHA guideline recommendations): A report of the American College of Cardiology Foundation/American Heart Association Task Force on Practice Guidelines. *Circulation* **2013**, *127*, 1425–1443. [CrossRef]
19. Tendera, M.; Aboyans, V.; Bartelink, M.-L.; Baumgartner, I.; Clément, D.; Collet, J.-P.; Cremonesi, A.; de Carlo, M.; Erbel, R.; Fowkes, F.G.R.; et al. ESC Guidelines on the diagnosis and treatment of peripheral artery diseases: Document covering atherosclerotic disease of extracranial carotid and vertebral, mesenteric, renal, upper and lower extremity arteries: The Task Force on the Diagnosis and Treatment of Peripheral Artery Diseases of the European Society of Cardiology (ESC). *Eur. Heart J.* **2011**, *32*, 2851–2906.

20. Niessner, A.; Richter, B.; Penka, M.; Steiner, S.; Strasser, B.; Ziegler, S.; Heeb-Elze, E.; Zorn, G.; Leitner-Heinschink, A.; Niessner, C.; et al. Endurance training reduces circulating inflammatory markers in persons at risk of coronary events: Impact on plaque stabilization? *Atherosclerosis* **2006**, *186*, 160–165. [CrossRef]
21. Michishita, R.; Shono, N.; Inoue, T.; Tsuruta, T.; Node, K. Effect of exercise therapy on monocyte and neutrophil counts in overweight women. *Am. J. Med. Sci.* **2010**, *339*, 152–156. [PubMed]
22. Timmerman, K.L.; Flynn, M.G.; Coen, P.M.; Markofski, M.M.; Pence, B.D. Exercise training-induced lowering of inflammatory ($CD14^+CD16^+$) monocytes: A role in the anti-inflammatory influence of exercise? *J. Leuk. Biol.* **2008**, *84*, 1271–1278. [CrossRef] [PubMed]
23. Higashi, Y.; Sasaki, S.; Kurisu, S.; Yoshimizu, A.; Sasaki, N.; Matsuura, H.; Kajiyama, G.; Oshima, T. Regular aerobic exercise augments endothelium-dependent vascular relaxation in normotensive as well as hypertensive subjects: Role of endothelium-derived nitric oxide. *Circulation* **1999**, *100*, 1194–1202. [CrossRef] [PubMed]
24. Guerreiro, L.F.; Rocha, A.M.; Martins, C.N.; Ribeiro, J.P.; Wally, C.; Strieder, D.L.; Carissimi, C.G.; Oliveira, M.G.; Pereira, A.A.; Biondi, H.S.; et al. Oxidative status of the myocardium in response to different intensities of physical training. *Physiol. Res.* **2016**, *65*, 737–749. [PubMed]
25. Menêses, A.L.; Ritti-Dias, R.M.; Parmenter, B.; Golledge, J.; Askew, C.D. Combined Lower Limb Revascularisation and Supervised Exercise Training for Patients with Peripheral Arterial Disease: A Systematic Review of Randomised Controlled Trials. *Sports Med.* **2017**, *47*, 987–1002. [CrossRef] [PubMed]
26. Takano, H.; Morita, T.; Iida, H.; Asada, K.; Kato, M.; Uno, K.; Hirose, K.; Matsumoto, A.; Takenaka, K.; Hirata, Y.; et al. Hemodynamic and hormonal responses to a short-term low-intensity resistance exercise with the reduction of muscle blood flow. *Eur. J. Appl. Physiol.* **2005**, *95*, 65–73. [CrossRef] [PubMed]
27. Green, D.J.; Hopman, M.T.E.; Padilla, J.; Laughlin, M.H.; Thijssen, D.H.J. Vascular Adaptation to Exercise in Humans: Role of Hemodynamic Stimuli. *Physiol. Rev.* **2017**, *97*, 495–528. [CrossRef]
28. Loenneke, J.P.; Abe, T.; Wilson, J.M.; Thiebaud, R.S.; Fahs, C.A.; Rossow, L.M.; Bemben, M.G. Blood flow restriction: An evidence based progressive model. *Acta Physiol. Hung.* **2012**, *99*, 235–250. [CrossRef]
29. Alberti, G.; Cavaggioni, L.; Silvaggi, N.; Caumo, A.; Garufi, M. Resistance Training with Blood Flow Restriction Using the Modulation of the Muscle's Contraction Velocity. *Strength Cond. J.* **2013**, *35*, 42–47.
30. Formenti, D.; Perpetuini, D.; Iodice, P.; Cardone, D.; Michielon, G.; Scurati, R.; Alberti, G.; Merla, A. Effects of knee extension with different speeds of movement on muscle and cerebral oxygenation. *PeerJ* **2018**, *6*, e5704. [CrossRef]
31. Bagley, J.R.; Rosengarten, J.J.; Galpin, A.J. Is Blood Flow Restriction Training Beneficial for Athletes? *Strength Cond. J.* **2015**, *37*, 48–53. [CrossRef]
32. Loenneke, J.P.; Pujol, T.J. The Use of Occlusion Training to Produce Muscle Hypertrophy. *Strength Cond. J.* **2009**, *31*, 77–84. [CrossRef]
33. Cook, S.B.; Brown, K.A.; Deruisseau, K.; Kanaley, J.A.; Ploutz-Snyder, L.L. Skeletal muscle adaptations following blood flow-restricted training during 30 days of muscular unloading. *J. Appl. Physiol.* **2010**, *109*, 341–349. [CrossRef] [PubMed]
34. Gualano, B.; Neves, M.; Lima, F.R.; Pinto, A.L.D.S.; Laurentino, G.; Borges, C.; Baptista, L.; Artioli, G.G.; Aoki, M.S.; Moriscot, A.; et al. Resistance training with vascular occlusion in inclusion body myositis: A case study. *Med. Sci. Sports Exerc.* **2010**, *42*, 250–254. [CrossRef] [PubMed]
35. Guirro, E.C.O.; Leite, G.P.M.F.; Dibai-Filho, A.V.; Borges, N.C.S.; Guirro, R.R.J. Intra- and Inter-rater Reliability of Peripheral Arterial Blood Flow Velocity by Means of Doppler Ultrasound. *J. Manipul. Physiol. Therap.* **2017**, *40*, 236–240. [CrossRef] [PubMed]
36. Venous flow volume measured by duplex ultrasound can be used as an indicator of impaired tissue perfusion in patients with peripheral arterial disease. *Med. Ultrason* **2015**, *17*.
37. Baggish, A.L.; Hale, A.; Weiner, R.B.; Lewis, G.D.; Systrom, D.; Wang, F.; Wang, T.J.; Chan, S.Y. Dynamic regulation of circulating microRNA during acute exhaustive exercise and sustained aerobic exercise training: Circulating microRNA in exercise. *J. Physiol.* **2011**, *589*, 3983–3994. [CrossRef]
38. Troidl, K.; Hammerschick, T.; Albarran-Juarez, J.; Jung, G.; Schierling, W.; Krüger, M.; Matuschke, B.; Triodl, C.; Schaper, W.; Schmitz-Rixen, T.; et al. Shear stress-induced miR-143-3p in collateral arteries contributes to outward vessel growth by targeting collagenV-α2. "Manuscript submitted for publication".

39. Lagos-Quintana, M. Identification of Novel Genes Coding for Small Expressed RNAs. *Science* **2001**, *294*, 853–858. [CrossRef]
40. Tiedt, S.; Prestel, M.; Malik, R.; Schieferdecker, N.; Duering, M.; Kautzky, V.; Stoycheva, I.; Böck, J.; Northoff, B.H.; Klein, M.; et al. RNA-Seq Identifies Circulating miR-125a-5p, miR-125b-5p, and miR-143-3p as Potential Biomarkers for Acute Ischemic Stroke. *Circ. Res.* **2017**, *121*, 970–980. [CrossRef]
41. Margolis, L.M.; Lessard, S.J.; Ezzyat, Y.; Fielding, R.A.; Rivas, D.A. Circulating MicroRNA Are Predictive of Aging and Acute Adaptive Response to Resistance Exercise in Men. *GERONA* **2016**, glw243. [CrossRef]
42. Barber, J.L.; Zellars, K.N.; Barringhaus, K.G.; Bouchard, C.; Spinale, F.G.; Sarzynski, M.A. The Effects of Regular Exercise on Circulating Cardiovascular-related MicroRNAs. *Sci. Rep.* **2019**, *9*, 7527. [CrossRef] [PubMed]
43. Domańska-Senderowska, D.; Laguette, M.-J.; Jegier, A.; Cięszczyk, P.; September, A.; Brzeziańska-Lasota, E. MicroRNA Profile and Adaptive Response to Exercise Training: A Review. *Int. J. Sports Med.* **2019**, *40*, 227–235. [CrossRef] [PubMed]
44. Karabulut, M.; Abe, T.; Sato, Y.; Bemben, M.G. The effects of low-intensity resistance training with vascular restriction on leg muscle strength in older men. *Eur. J. Appl. Physiol.* **2010**, *108*, 147–155. [CrossRef] [PubMed]
45. Borg, G.A. Psychophysical bases of perceived exertion. *Med. Sci. Sports Exerc.* **1982**, *14*, 377–381. [CrossRef]

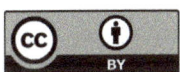

© 2019 by the authors. Licensee MDPI, Basel, Switzerland. This article is an open access article distributed under the terms and conditions of the Creative Commons Attribution (CC BY) license (http://creativecommons.org/licenses/by/4.0/).

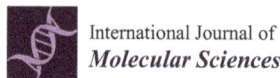

Review

The Human Coronary Collateral Circulation, Its Extracardiac Anastomoses and Their Therapeutic Promotion

Bigler Marius Reto and Christian Seiler *

Department of Cardiology, Inselspital, Bern University Hospital, University of Bern, 3010 Bern, Switzerland
* Correspondence: christian.seiler@insel.ch; Tel.: +41-31-632-36-93

Received: 30 May 2019; Accepted: 12 July 2019; Published: 30 July 2019

Abstract: Cardiovascular disease remains the leading global cause of death, and the number of patients with coronary artery disease (CAD) and exhausted therapeutic options (i.e., percutaneous coronary intervention (PCI), coronary artery bypass grafting (CABG) and medical treatment) is on the rise. Therefore, the evaluation of new therapeutic approaches to offer an alternative treatment strategy for these patients is necessary. A promising research field is the promotion of the coronary collateral circulation, an arterio-arterial network able to prevent or reduce myocardial ischemia in CAD. This review summarizes the basic principles of the human coronary collateral circulation, its extracardiac anastomoses as well as the different therapeutic approaches, especially that of stimulating the extracardiac collateral circulation via permanent occlusion of the internal mammary arteries.

Keywords: human coronary collateral circulation; extracardiac anastomoses; collateral flow index; collateral artery growth in man; permanent internal mammary artery occlusion

1. Introduction

According to the American Heart Association, "cardiovascular disease is the leading global cause of death", accounting for more than 17.6 million deaths in 2016, a number that is expected to grow to more than 23.6 million by 2030 [1] In the event of acute coronary syndrome, percutaneous coronary intervention (PCI) has been shown to be beneficial on outcome [2]. The beneficial effect of PCI on the course of chronic stable coronary artery disease (CAD) has, so far, not been proven yet [3]. A recently published randomized controlled trial among patients with stable, single-vessel CAD, the so called ORBITA trial (e.g., Objective Randomised Blinded Investigation With Optimal Medical Therapy of Angioplasty in Stable Angina) [4], found that PCI of the stenotic lesion did not prolong exercise time by more than the effect of a sham procedure during the short observation period of six weeks. The new aspect of the ORBITA trial was a methodological one, that is, the use of a sham control group of patients undergoing the invasive coronary procedure, but not the actual PCI. The importance of a sham control group in interventional procedures is pivotal, especially in a population with a high level of suffering [5,6]. After all, it is known that the placebo effect can cause significant clinical improvements (e.g., an increased exercise duration of >90 s [7]). Coronary artery bypass grafting (CABG), on the other hand, has been found superior to PCI with respect to all-cause or cardiovascular mortality [8].

The number of patients with incomplete revascularization as well as so-called "no-option"-patients (i.e., patients without options for PCI or CABG still suffering from symptoms of CAD despite optimal medical therapy) is on the rise. It is estimated, that 30,000–50,000 new patients are affected in continental Europe per year [9] and Williams et al. reported a prevalence of 25.8% of incomplete revascularization in patients with CAD [10]. Apart from the limited quality of life, these patients also have a higher mortality at three years than patients with complete revascularization [10].

Accordingly, new therapeutic approaches are required. Because of the known survival benefit of patients with a well-developed coronary collateral circulation [11,12], interventions aiming at the promotion of coronary collaterals are a promising strategy. Coronary collaterals represent pre-existing inter-arterial anastomoses and as such are the natural counterpart of surgically created bypasses. To this end, biochemical (e.g., intracoronary vascular-endothelial growth factor or intravenous granulocyte-macrophage colony-stimulating factor) as well as biophysical (e.g., external counterpulsation) approaches have been evaluated for the promotion of those collaterals.

The aim of this review is to describe basic principles of the coronary collateral circulation, its extracardiac anastomoses as well as different therapeutic approaches, especially that of stimulating extracardiac coronary supply via permanent occlusion of the internal mammary arteries.

2. Basic Principles of the Human Coronary Collateral Circulation

2.1. Coronary Collateral Circulation

The development of the cardiovascular system during embryogenesis occurs by vasculogenesis, a process defined as "the de novo formation of blood vessels from endothelial precursor cells" [13]. Directed by the concentration of local messenger substance, endothelial precursor cells sprout out and start forming a dense vascular network with multiple anastomoses. The density of this network is at its peak in neonates and declines subsequently by physiological regression, a process called pruning [14–16].

Nevertheless, it has been hypothesized early on and tested that the coronary anastomoses of the neonate do not vanish completely but some collaterals rather recede in calibre. This concept has been decisively advanced by the findings of the Scottish pathologist W.F. Fulton, who found "numerous anastomoses in all normal hearts" by using a vascular overlay detecting technique with radiographic contrast medium containing uniform particles sized 0.5–2.0 µm to visualize even small arteries [17].

Interestingly, with changing vascular pressure- and resistance conditions, it is possible to recruit these receded arterial anastomoses. This process is often seen during the course of CAD with development of a pressure gradient across a stenotic lesion, which itself induces augmented flow in preformed arterial anastomoses and finally, structural augmentation of these collateral arteries (arteriogenesis). Accordingly, the prevalence of functional coronary anastomoses depends on the presence of CAD and is highest in chronic total coronary occlusions [16].

Coronary collaterals in patients without coronary atherosclerosis range in calibre between 10–200 µm; collateral arteries of patients with CAD are approximately four times bigger (100–800 µm) [17]. This observation is in accordance with an experimental rabbit model, where occlusion of the femoral artery increased the lumen diameter of pre-existent arterioles four- to fivefold [18]. "At the same time, the growth in structural size goes along with a decreasing number of collateral arteries, a process called pruning. Pathophysiologically and in the sense of the Hagen Poiseuille law, pruning may be interpreted as a way of effectively reducing vascular resistance to collateral flow" [13].

2.2. Extracardiac Coronary Supply

Apart from inter-coronary arterial anastomoses, the human coronary arterial circulation is supplied by several extracardiac anastomoses, also called the non-coronary collateral myocardial blood flow (NCCMBF) [19]. Hence, the heart receives additional blood from the arteries of surrounding structures [20–24]. Most of the extracardiac anastomoses originate from arteries, which supply the pericardium [21] and these arteries are typically located at the sites of pericardial reflections (e.g., the entry of the caval veins or the exit of the great arteries) [22]. Thus, a well-known extracardiac anastomosis connects the right internal mammary artery (IMA, also called internal thoracic artery) to the right coronary artery via the pericardiacophrenic branch and the sinus node artery [25] (Figure 1). This extracardiac coronary supply can also develop after coronary bypass surgery as shown exemplary in Figure 2 [22].

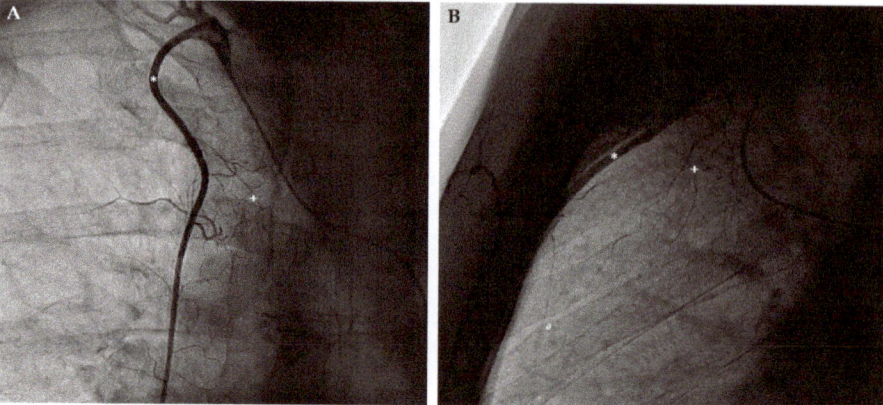

Figure 1. Angiographic demonstration of extracardiac coronary supply. (**A**) Posterior-anterior projection of the right internal mammary artery (IMA, marked by *) and its connection to the right coronary artery via the pericardiacophrenic branch (marked by +). (**B**) Lateral projection using the same markers. Noteworthy, additional branches of the IMA (marked by #) heading towards the heart.

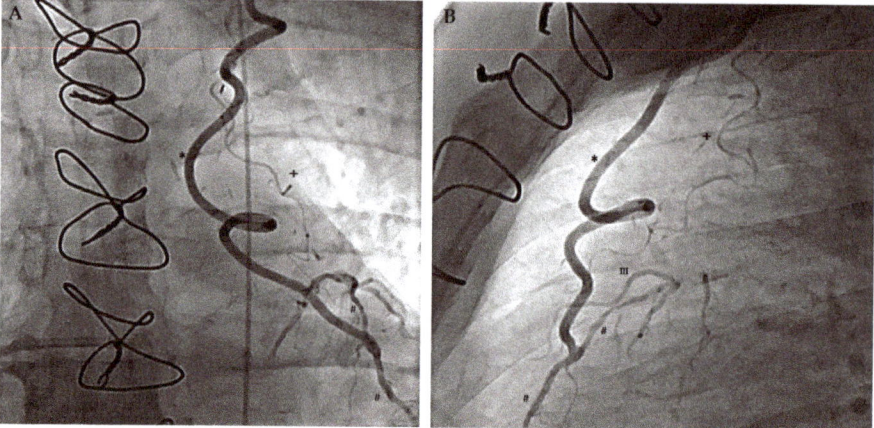

Figure 2. Angiographic demonstration of extracardiac coronary supply after coronary artery bypass surgery. (**A**) Posterior-anterior projection of the left internal mammary artery bypass (marked by a *) on the left anterior descending coronary artery (LAD, marked by a #). Upstream of the bypass anastomosis, retrograde filling of the LAD is incomplete revealing coronary occlusion, which triggered the arteriogenesis of the pericardiacophrenic branch (marked by a +) (**B**) Lateral projection using the same markers revealing the connection of the pericardiacophrenic branch with the third diagonal branch (marked by III).

Most commonly, NCCMBF originates from the bronchial or the internal mammary arteries [22]. Bjork et al. showed a prevalence for bronchial-coronary-anastomoses of more than 20% by reviewing 200 coronary angiographies [26]. According to this observation, most of the anastomoses connect to the left circumflex artery (LCX) and demonstrate poor blood flow. However, blood flow within an anastomosis between two arterial beds depends on the respective vascular resistances. Thus, a constant decrease of vascular resistance in one arterial bed causes an increased blood flow to it with associated arteriogenesis. Consequently and depending on the underlying pathology, bronchial-to-coronary (e.g., in the case of a chronic occluded coronary artery [27]) as well as coronary-to-bronchial anastomoses (e.g., during chronic pulmonary diseases [28]) have been described.

Additional evidence for extracardiac anastomoses comes from the work of Hudson et al., who, by injecting ink into the coronary arteries, demonstrated anastomoses with anterior mediastinal, phrenic and intercostal arteries as well as with esophageal arterial branches of the aorta [21].

NCCMBF has also been increasingly recognized by cardiac surgeons as they discovered that anastomotic blood flow can dilute, and thus, be a potential hazard to cardioplegia [23]. To quantify this phenomenon, several studies have been conducted with reported values of anastomotic perfusion ranging between 3.4 to 14 mL/100 g/min [29,30] during cardiopulmonary bypass with cross-clamping of the aorta.

2.3. Quantitative Evaluation of the Coronary Collateral Circulation

The first in vivo functional coronary collateral measurements were conducted in the 1970s, showing a direct relation between "angiographic appearance and functional performance of coronary collaterals during bypass surgery" [31]. Rentrop et al. proposed a transluminal coronary angioplasty approach, which divided the appearance of coronary collaterals in four groups (0 = no collateral filling from the contralateral vessel to 3 = "complete filling of the epicardial segment of the artery") [32]. Unfortunately, the method is only qualitative and evaluation of extracardiac collaterals is not feasible.

Thereafter a method for quantitative coronary collateral function assessment based on coronary occlusive pressure measurements was introduced. The so called collateral flow index (CFI) [33,34] "is the ratio between mean coronary occlusive and aortic pressure both subtracted by central venous pressure as obtained during a 1-min proximal coronary balloon occlusion" [33] (Figure 3). The method is accepted as the reference method for functional collateral assessment in patients with chronic stable CAD [35,36]. In terms of sufficient collateral blood supply, it has been demonstrated that a CFI of >0.20–0.25 is related to absent signs of ischemia on the intracoronary electrocardiogram (i.c.ECG) during this 1-min coronary artery balloon occlusion [37,38].

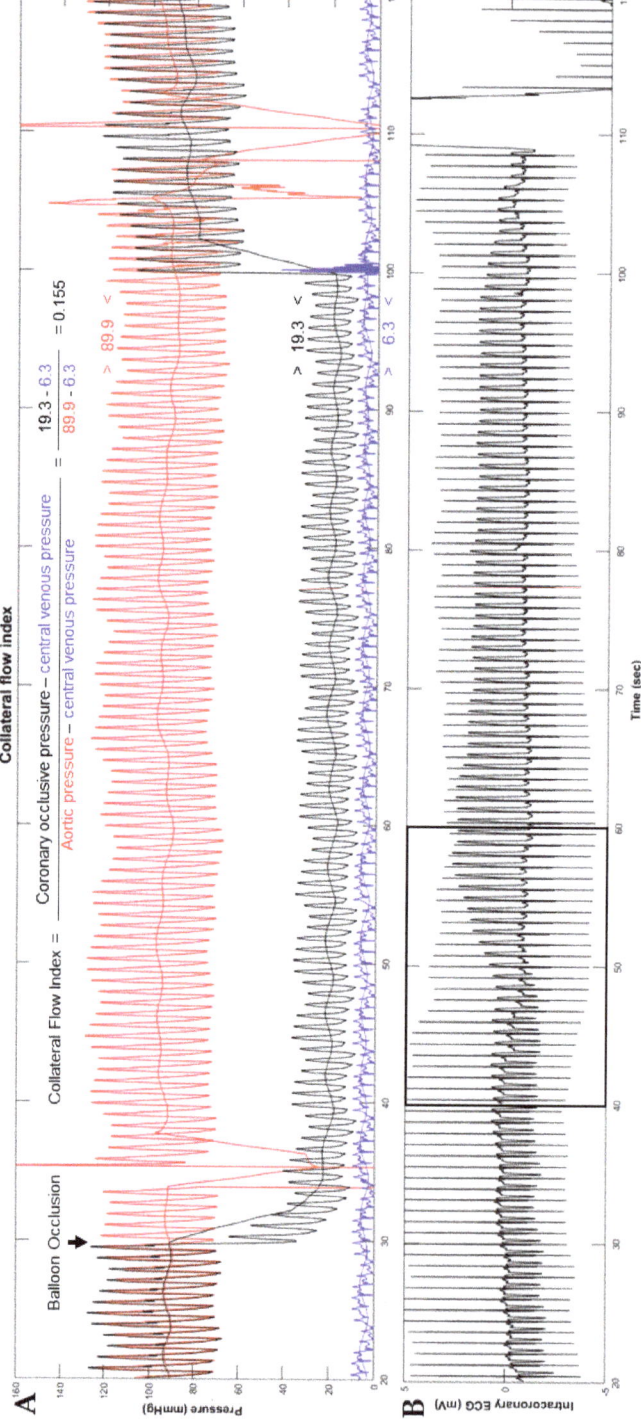

Figure 3. Collateral flow index (CFI) measurement. (**A**) Simultaneous recordings of mean and phasic aortic (red signals, Pao), coronary occlusive (black signals, Poccl) and central venous pressure (blue signals, CVP) immediately before (left side) and during coronary artery occlusion in a patient with poorly functional collaterals. (**B**) Detection of myocardial ischemia during the coronary artery occlusion by the intracoronary electrocardiogram (i.c.ECG). Immediately after balloon occlusion, the i.c.ECG shows marked electrical alternations with flipped T-waves and ST-segment elevation (marked by the black square). Generally, a CFI of >0.20–0.25 is related to absent signs of ischemia on i.c.ECG during a 1-min proximal coronary occlusion.

CFI has also been determined in patients with angiographically normal coronary arteries, revealing functional collateral arteries "to the extent, that one fifth to one quarter of them (i.e., the patients without coronary stenoses) do not show signs of myocardial ischemia during the brief vascular occlusions" [39]. Those findings of functional sufficient collaterals even in the absence of CAD support the above mentioned pathoanatomic observations [17], that coronary anastomoses calibre remain functional to a considerable degree.

3. Angiogenesis and Arteriogenesis

To understand the different therapeutic approaches for promoting the coronary collateral circulation, it is crucial to differentiate between two basic physiologic principles, that is, angiogenesis and arteriogenesis.

3.1. Angiogenesis

The formation of capillaries from pre-existing vessels to expand the microvascular system by increasing the capillary density is called angiogenesis. Driven by several growth factors such as hypoxia-inducible factor 1α, vascular endothelial growth factor (VEGF) [40] and inflammatory mediators as well as inflammatory cells (mainly monocytes [41]), a local milieu is formed [42] which promotes the proliferation and migration of endothelial cells, pericytes and smooth muscle cells. Thereby, "the amplification of the vascular network occurs within a short time due to either abluminal outgrowth (sprouting) or intraluminal division (intussusceptive growth) of capillaries" [43]. In contrast to arteriogenesis, angiogenesis is mostly driven by metabolic demands (i.e., hypoxemia) [44]

3.2. Arteriogenesis

"Although capillary sprouting may deliver some relief to the underperfused territory, only true collateral arteries are principally capable of providing large enough amounts of blood flow to the ischemic area at risk for necrosis or loss of function." [41] Hence, arteriogenesis is the process of outward remodelling [44] (i.e., growth in diameter and length) of pre-existing anastomoses [45], resulting in an increased flow capacity of the artery.

Fluid shear stress, "the product of spatial flow velocity changes during the cardiac cycle and blood viscosity" [46] "is the primary and strongest arteriogenic stimulus" [47]. It leads to the expression of nitric oxide (NO), VEGF and monocyte chemoattractant protein-1 (MCP-1), resulting in the attraction and activation of monocytes [41,44,48–51]. Those inflammatory cells conduct the process of arteriogenesis with induction of cell proliferation as well as preparation of the extracellular matrix to enable cell migration [48].

Arteriogenesis is a common phenomenon that interventional cardiologists encounter on a daily basis as it appears (e.g., in the course of hypertensive heart disease with concentric left ventricular hypertrophy and augmented myocardial mass). Due to the direct and curvilinear relationship between myocardial mass and coronary arterial cross-sectional area [52], structural remodelling (i.e., arteriogenesis of the epicardial coronary arteries) occurs, resulting in large vascular calibres and, because of undirected growth, also affecting vascular length. Thus, this leads to the typical corkscrew pattern that is seen in this condition (Figure 4A).

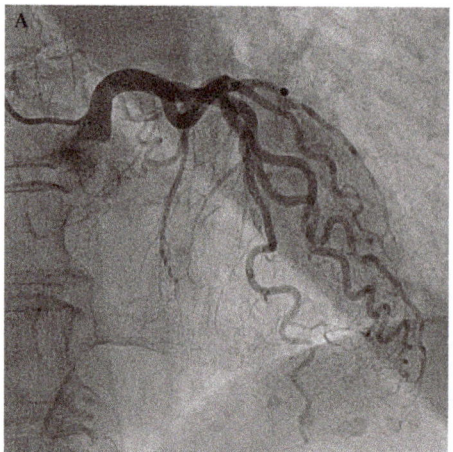 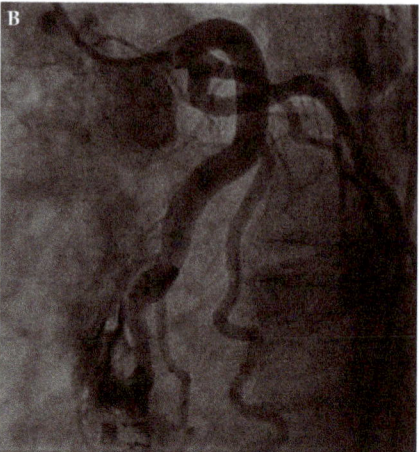

Figure 4. Angiographic presentation of two different pathophysiological etiologies of arteriogenesis. (**A**) Arteriogenesis in the course of hypertensive heart disease with concentric left ventricular hypertrophy. Enlarged myocardial mass is the driving force behind this arterial growth. (**B**) Arteriogenesis solely initiated by constant elevation of fluid shear stress. Iatrogenic drainage of the left anterior descending artery (LAD) into the right ventricular cavity after myocardial biopsy significantly increased coronary blood flow and consequently vascular size.

Importantly and in contrast to the previously outlined process of angiogenesis, myocardial ischemia is unrelated to this process [53,54]. Arteriogenesis depends solely on physical pressure gradients across pre-formed anastomoses between different arterial territories with consequent augmentation of endothelial fluid shear stress [47,53,55]. Figure 4B illustrates this concept: After myocardial biopsy with perforation of the LAD and consecutive drainage into the (low resistance) right ventricular cavity, blood flow in the LAD increased due to the abrupt decrease in "vascular" resistance. As a consequence, abundant growth of the LAD, both in cross-sectional area and length, could be observed [56].

4. Therapeutic Promotion of the Coronary Collateral Circulation

The following chapter summarizes the most promising therapeutic approaches of coronary collateral promotion divided according to the basic concept of biochemical or biophysical methods.

4.1. Biochemical Concepts

In general, biochemical concepts are "prone to potentially harmful effects, since arteriogenesis shares many common mechanisms with inflammatory diseases, such as atherosclerosis" [44]. Accordingly, Epstein et al. coined (biochemical) collateral promotion a "Janus Phenomenon", that is, "whatever intervention enhances collaterals increases atherogenesis and vice versa" [57].

With the rapid development of angiogenic growth factors and the growing understanding of their mechanisms of action, multiple trials testing collateral growth promotion have been initiated. Because of the known pivotal role of monocytes in orchestrating the different processes of angio- and arteriogenesis [50], most of the projects focused on the activation or the recruitment of this cell line. Growth factors most extensively studied have been granulocyte-macrophage colony-stimulating factor (GM-CSF) [58–62], granulocyte colony-stimulating factor (G-CSF) [63–66] or monocyte chemoattractant protein-1 (MCP-1) [41]. Besides, also different fibroblast growth factors (FGF) [67–69] and VEGF [70] have been clinically tested. Altogether, this study showed that angiogenesis is less efficient than arteriogenesis [71] for promoting bulk collateral blood flow, since it only promotes microvascular density. Consequently, clinical trials evaluating the effect of angiogenetic factors such as FGF or VEGF have failed to demonstrate a therapeutic effect that exceeds the effect of placebo treatment [67,68,70].

Colony-stimulating factors, on the other hand, have been found to promote the formation of large interconnecting arterioles (arteriogenesis), which are required for the salvage of myocardium in the presence of occlusive CAD [58]. Buschmann et al. [61] found that a continuous infusion of GM-CSF into the stump of the acutely occluded femoral artery of rabbits enhanced blood flow to the hind limb five-fold. The mechanism of action in that study has been found to be the prolonged survival of monocytes, "known to play a decisive role in arteriogenesis" [61]. In two small but randomized and placebo-controlled clinical trials with 35 patients in total, GM-CSF has been shown to be efficacious in a short-term subcutaneous administration protocol of two weeks [58,59]. Both studies have demonstrated a significant increase in CFI (from 0.116 to 0.159; $p = 0.028$ respectively from 0.21 to 0.31; $p < 0.05$). Of note, this beneficial effect of GM-CSF in the promotion of coronary collateral growth could not be transferred to the clinical setting of peripheral vascular disease, where it failed to improve the walking time [60]. Further, one of the clinical trials using GM-CSF for arteriogenesis had to be stopped prematurely for safety concerns in the context of two patients with acute coronary syndrome in the treatment group [59].

G-CSF has been reported in meta-analyses to be safe in terms of major adverse cardiovascular events (cardiovascular death, recurrent myocardial infarction and in-stent restenosis) and toleration of the treatment injections [72–74]. These findings and promising animal test results [75] have led to a randomized, placebo-controlled clinical trial in humans, in which subcutaneous G-CSF was shown to increase CFI from 0.121 to 0.166 ($p < 0.0001$) when administered every other day for two weeks [63]. Despite the above meta-analyses, one study assessing the outcomes and risks of G-CSF in patients with CAD has reported an increased frequency of adverse outcomes (i.e., acute coronary syndrome) [64].

In conclusion, despite the promising results of small clinical trials or animal models using biochemical concepts to therapeutically promote the coronary collateral circulation, none of the approaches evaluated so far could be successfully translated into clinical practice. Besides the above mentioned limitations such as inefficient collateral formation (i.e., angiogenesis) or potentially harmful propagation of atherogenesis (i.e., the "Janus Phenomenon" [57]), a number of additional unresolved issues remains. These include questions relating to the dosage, the application route and the timing of administration of growth factors [44]. Importantly, considering that "no-option" patients with extensive CAD are the most likely candidates for coronary arteriogenesis, safety of any collateral-promoting substance is crucial [59].

4.2. Biophysical Concepts

The biophysical concept of arteriogenesis is to increase tangential vascular shear stress in preformed coronary anastomoses. One of the natural ways of increasing vascular shear stress is physical exercise [76]. However, because of different comorbidities it is often not feasible for patients with CAD to perform physical exercise training sufficiently. Thus, several other biophysical approaches have been introduced and will be described subsequently.

4.2.1. Physical Exercise

The positive effects of physical exercise on the cardiovascular system have been known for a long time [77]. For instance, it was concluded in 1958 by Morris and Crawford that physically active people are less prone to develop stable CAD in comparison with sedentary people [78]. Physical exercise has a positive effect on several cardiovascular aspects such as vascular remodelling, increase of the maximal coronary blood flow (i.e., coronary flow reserve; CFR) as well as a decrease of coronary artherogenesis [79,80].

Concerning the effect of training on coronary collateral function, Scheel et al. observed an arteriogenetic effect of physical exercise in dogs with a constricted coronary artery whereas this effect was not observed in dogs without coronary stenosis [81]. In the groups with artificial coronary occlusion, exercise stress doubled the collateral growth and hence, the coronary flow reserve when compared to none exercised dogs. In humans, Zbinden et al. documented an increase of the quantitative parameter CFI in a proof-of-concept study [82]. They evaluated CFI, CFR and other cardiac parameters before and immediately after exercise training of a healthy marathon runner and demonstrated an increase of CFI from 0.23 to 0.37. Two small, non-randomized clinical trials have supported the positive effect of physical exercise on coronary collateral function, the increase in coronary cross-sectional area [83] as well as dose-dependent relation between training and increase in CFI [84]. Those results are in agreement with several other studies [80,85–89], which showed augmented perfusion by collateral vessels in response to exercise training. Besides, there have been other clinical trials failing to show a beneficial effect on the collateral circulation by exercise as assessed by angiographic imaging, but not by functional measurements [90]. However, the authors mention the limited validity of the angiographic approach and despite the negative outcome on coronary collateral formation, the exercise group had a significant better clinical outcome concerning the frequency of cardiac symptoms and the physical performance.

Recently, the first randomized clinical trial on the effect of physical exercise on coronary collateral function has been published [91]. Möbius-Winkler et al. randomly assigned 60 patients to two training groups (moderate- and high-intensity exercise with 10 h of training per week in each group) and one control group (usual care with encouragement to perform regular physical activity according to current recommendations). After four weeks, both exercise groups showed a significant increase in CFI (from 0.142 to 0.198, $p = 0.005$ respectively from 0.143 to 0.202, $p = 0.004$) without a statistically relevant difference between the training modalities whereas CFI in the control group remained unchanged (from 0.149 to 0.150, $p =$ n.s.).

In conclusion, the positive effect of physical exercise on the human coronary collateral circulation has been repeatedly demonstrated. However, there remain important questions concerning the type and extent of physical exercise for optimal promotion as well as the implementation for patients with limited physical possibilities.

4.2.2. External Counterpulsation (ECP)

"External counterpulsation therapy was first developed as a resuscitative tool to support the failing heart and was based on the hemodynamic principles of the intra-aortic balloon pump", which is the augmentation of diastolic blood flow with consecutive improvement of coronary perfusion as well as ventricular afterload reduction [92]. ECP uses three pairs of pneumatic cuffs wrapped around each of the lower extremities. Those cuffs are sequentially inflated from distal to proximal triggered by the ECG. Besides augmenting diastolic blood flow and reducing ventricular afterload, ECP increases tangential endothelial shear stress triggering arteriogenesis. Used as a safe, effective and low-cost second line treatment in refractory angina pectoris, ECP has been shown to be efficacious in reducing CAD symptoms as well as improving exercise time [92–96]. Of note, the positive effect appears to outlast the actual, conventional seven week period of treatment [97].

The effects of ECP on the coronary collateral circulation have been evaluated in two invasive clinical trials. Buschmann et al. demonstrated in a non-randomized study a significant increase in CFI. Other invasive parameters obtained in that study as the index of microvascular resistance (IMR) or quantitative coronary angiography (QCA) remained unchanged and hence, the increase of CFI reflected a "true" improvement of the myocardial blood flow [98]. These results have been confirmed in a randomized, sham-controlled clinical trial with an increase in CFI from 0.125 to 0.174 at a four-week follow-up exam ($p = 0.006$) in the experimental, but not in the placebo group (CFI changed from 0.129 to 0.111, $p = 0.14$) [46].

Recently, the principle of external counterpulsation has been individualized in order to alleviate the side effects of ECP (i.e., the cumbersome procedure with high pressure levels), thus increasing its acceptance. The so called individual shear rate therapy (ISRT) adjusts the used treatment pressures of the pneumatic cuffs according to individually adapted intra-arterial shear rates to achieve the same effect with reduced pressure values [99]. The calculation is based on Doppler-flow parameters in the common carotid artery at different treatment pressure values. Due to this procedure, the individually calculated treatment pressure ranged between 160 to 220 mmHg instead of the regular treatment pressure of 250 to 300 mmHg.

4.2.3. Coronary Sinus Reducer

The biophysical concept of the coronary sinus reducer is based on a perioperative approach during heart surgery with artificially narrowed coronary sinus for augmented retro-perfusion [100]. The exact pathophysiologic principle for a beneficial effect remains unclear [101]. One proposed mechanism assumes that the venous back pressure as applied in the coronary sinus is regionally balanced in the venous, but not in the vascular bed upstream of the microcirculation [102]. Based on the two regionally counteracting responses of the microcirculation during myocardial ischemia, that is maximal vasodilatation and increased myocardial compressive forces (i.e., augmented ventricular wall stress due to diminished myocardial thickness), regional imbalance in microvascular resistance with higher resistance in the ischemic area arises. Thus, augmented venous back pressure is able to reach the non-ischaemic microcirculation more easily than the ischaemic one, thereby increasing the microcirculatory resistance in the non-ischaemic zone. This leads to a flow diversion of arterialised blood to the ischaemic area at risk under the necessary condition of functional collateral connections originating from the non-ischaemic area [102].

Due to advances in percutaneous coronary intervention, and at the same time, increasing number of patients with refractory angina pectoris, several investigators have picked up this approach by using balloon-expandable, hourglass-shaped devices to physically narrow the coronary sinus [103–105]. In a first-in-man study, this device has demonstrated relief of angina pectoris in 12 out of 14 patients without options for coronary revascularization [103]. Subsequently, Verheye et al. performed a randomized, sham-controlled clinical trial in 104 patients, which confirmed the results of the first study [101]. They showed an improvement in Canadian Cardiovascular Society (CCS) score as well as quality of life. Nevertheless, exercise time and mean change in the wall motion index as assessed by means of dobutamine stress echocardiography remained unchanged [101]. Subsequently and to evaluate the role of this device in future clinical practice, a post marketing study is currently enrolling selected patients without revascularization options (called Reducer-I-study; NCT02710435). They plan to recruit over 400 patients and assess the clinical efficacy as well as the long-term outcome with follow-ups up to five years after implantation [104].

4.2.4. Pharmacologic Biophysical Arteriogenesis

Ivabradine, a specific inhibitor of the I_f-channel mainly expressed in sinoatrial nodal cells [106], specifically decreases the heart rate without affecting cardiac contractility, afterload or vasomotion as it occurs with beta-blockers [107,108]. Based on the biophysical rationale of diastolic prolongation by ivabradine with extension of diastolic vascular shear stress, a small randomized placebo-controlled trial has demonstrated a significant increase in CFI by ivabradine (from 0.107 to 0.152, $p = 0.0461$) [109]. This result is in accordance with several other trials, which have shown an arteriogenic effect on coronary arteries by initiating bradycardia [110–112]). However, despite the promotion of coronary collateral supply, ivabradine has not been shown to be efficacious with respect to cardiovascular outcomes (composite of death from cardiovascular causes or nonfatal myocardial infarction) in patients with stable CAD [106] in bigger randomized trials such as the BEAUTIFUL [113] and SIGNIFY trials [114].

5. Therapeutic Promotion of Extracardiac Coronary Supply

The anatomical connection between the IMAs and the coronary arteries via their most proximal branch (i.e., the pericardiacophrenic artery departing at the first or second intercostal space) is well documented [21,22,25] (Figures 1 and 2). Additionally, due to the connection of the IMAs with the iliac external arteries via the superior and inferior epigastric arteries, collateral supply from the caudal side amounts to approximately two thirds of the flow during IMA patency [102]. This dual blood supply along with the direct anatomical connection to the coronary circulation provided the rationale for the IMA ligation method as a surgical treatment for angina pectoris. Using a small incision between the second and third rib under local anesthesia, transthoracic surgical access and ligation of the IMAs was first performed by D. Fieschi in 1939 (i.e., before the advent of modern cardiac surgery with cardioplegia and heart-lung-bypass) [115]. Later on, the approach was tested by a series of trials carried out in the late 1950s [116–122]. The primary end point of those clinical trials was angina pectoris and, inconsistently, ECG signs of myocardial ischemia. Battezzati et al. [116], after identifying anew a connection between both IMAs and the myocardium, reported consistent improvement in terms of cardiac symptoms in a uncontrolled trial among 304 CAD patients in 1959. Notable, this improvement was sustained during a follow-up of up to four years after the surgical intervention. In a further uncontrolled trial among 50 CAD patients, Kitchell et al. [123] reported similarly favorable results with symptomatic relief in 68% of the patients undergoing bilateral IMA ligation.

The following sham-controlled trials of bilateral IMA ligation in 35 CAD patients coined the phrase "surgery as placebo" in the context of their negative results [124–126]. Although the introduction of a sham-control study design in the context of surgical trials was seminal [127], the conclusion drawn from the negative results of the IMA ligation trials at hand is questionable. In the trial by Cobb et al. [125], angina pectoris relief was found in five of eight patients (63%) after IMA ligation and in five of seven patients (71%) after IMA sham ligation. Dimond et al. [126] reported nine of 13 patients in the verum and five of five patients in the sham-operation group, respectively. Thus, the abrupt stop of bilateral transthoracic IMA ligation was mainly caused by the advent of modern cardiac surgery with bypass grafting rather than by the slim evidence against IMA ligation claimed by the controlled trials. Especially because the soft study end point of angina pectoris would have required patient numbers at one order of magnitude higher than those recruited for the sham-controlled IMA ligation trials [125,126].

Because of the slim evidence against IMA ligation and the promising surgical results in terms of symptomatic relief, this therapeutic concept was revived 75 years after the first attempt using percutaneous interventional techniques. In the context of soft study endpoints, the first observational interventional study on the function of coronary supply by the IMAs has predefined intracoronary ECG (i.c.ECG) ST-segment elevation during coronary occlusion, not angina pectoris, as the first end point for ischemia [128]. In this trial, myocardial ischemia has been induced twice with and without simultaneous IMA occlusion by proximal coronary balloon occlusion in the process of CFI measurement. Further, to eliminate the effect of coronary collateral recruitment or ischemic preconditioning occurring during the second (but not the first) occlusion on the collateral circulation, CFI measurement with simultaneous IMA occlusion was performed before the control measurement without IMA occlusion. Despite this conservative study design, the approach showed a consistently reduced i.c.ECG ST-segment elevation during ipsilateral IMA with RCA or LAD occlusion as an expression of reduced ischemia. Further, CFI has been found higher in the presence versus the absence of IMA occlusion in 68% of the measurements, and overall, this difference amounted to +0.025 compared with the absence of IMA occlusion ($p < 0.0001$) [128]. However, contralateral IMA occlusion did not cause an effect indicating the necessity of anatomic vicinity. In this trial, functional connection between the coronary arteries and the IMAs was slightly less frequent in case of LAD with left IMA occlusion (25 of 30 measurements) than in the case of RCA with right IMA occlusion (28 of 30 measurements).

Based on those functional findings, an anti-ischemic therapeutic approach consisting in distal IMA occlusion by interventional techniques could be a promising therapeutic alternative to IMA bypass grafting. In an open-label proof-of-concept study, Stoller et al. investigated a catheter-based permanent IMA occlusion in the setting of the less frequently grafted right IMA among patients with ischemia in the RCA territory [129]. In this study, 50 patients with chronic stable CAD underwent permanent device occlusion of the distal right IMA. CFI of the RCA measured immediately before and six weeks after the IMA-occlusion showed a consistent increase from 0.071 at baseline to 0.132

($p < 0.0001$). Further, this augmented coronary blood supply was reflected by the i.c.ECG as a direct measure of myocardial physiology revealing a decreased ischemia during RCA occlusion from baseline to follow-up examination ($p = 0.0015$). Figure 5 illustrates this increased collateral function along with decreased myocardial ischemia during coronary occlusion as outlined by an absent ST-deprivation in the ECG of the follow-up intervention.

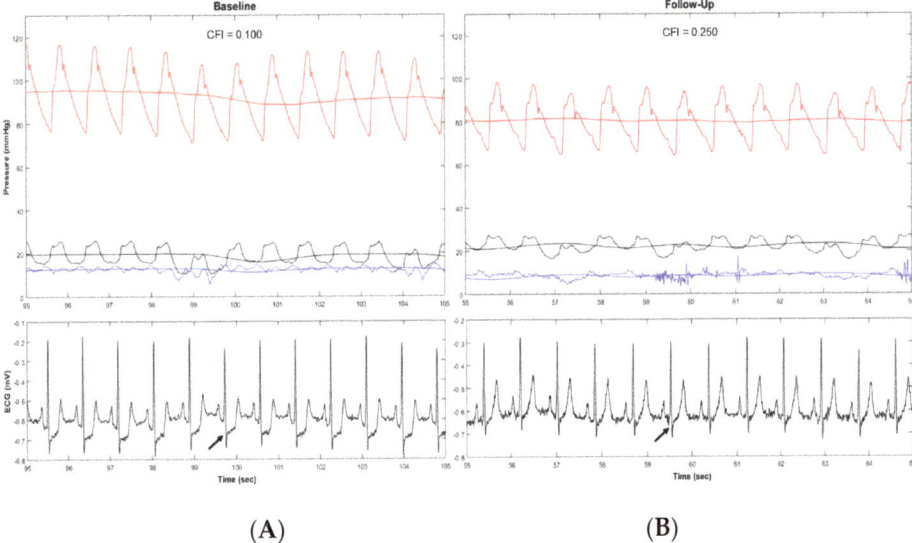

(A) (B)

Figure 5. Collateral flow index (CFI) measurements of the right coronary artery (RCA) with corresponding electrocardiograms (ECG) after a one-minute proximal coronary balloon occlusion. (**A**) CFI measured immediately before permanent right internal mammary artery occlusion showing a collateral blood supply of 0.100 and marked ST-deprivations in the ECG as a sign of ischemia (marked with an arrow). (**B**) Six weeks after the permanent occlusion, CFI increased to 0.250 (+0.150). This augmented coronary blood supply is reflected by the ECG revealing a decreased ischemia without ST-deprivations (marked with an arrow).

To conclude, augmentation of extracardiac coronary supply by permanent right IMA device occlusion is effective and feasible. However, if and how this increased collateral blood flow improves clinical outcome parameters is subject of current research. For this reason, a randomized, sham-controlled and double-blind clinical trial is currently enrolling patients (NCT03710070). It aims to include 250 patients in order to assess the clinical efficacy (measured as treadmill exercise time increment) in the next few years.

6. Conclusions

Based on the growing problem of patients with coronary artery disease and incomplete revascularization, several promising therapeutic alternatives for myocardial revascularization have been examined. Because of the known survival benefit of patients with a functional coronary collateral circulation, its promotion is a promising concept. However, until now, none of the evaluated concept could be implemented in daily clinical practice despite appealing results in clinical trials.

Biochemical concepts of angio- or arteriogenesis by growth factors seem to be prone to potentially harmful effects, since arteriogenesis shares many common mechanisms with inflammatory diseases, such as atherosclerosis. Thus, the risk benefit ratio is inappropriate and further research using growth factors was discontinued.

Biophysical concepts are based on increasing arteriogenesis via elevated tangential vascular fluid shear stress. Physical exercise training or external counterpulsation have been documented to positively affect clinical symptoms as well as coronary blood flow. The effect of both physical arteriogenic procedures is, however, transient (i.e., vanishes after its termination) and the time-consuming procedure of several hours per week limits the use to selected, highly motivated patients.

Alternative techniques such as coronary sinus reduction or promotion of extracardiac coronary supply by permanent occlusion of the distal internal mammary artery are promising approaches, since they have a permanent effect and ought to be efficacious in reducing myocardial ischemia to the effect that it is clinically relevant. Both approaches are being currently studied in ongoing clinical trials (NCT0271043 respectively NCT03710070) and the results of these investigations will clarify the clinical potential of those new therapeutic methods.

Author Contributions: Conceptualization, B.MR. and S.C.; Writing—Original Draft Preparation, B.MR. and S.C.; Writing—Review & Editing, B.MR. and S.C.; Visualization, B.MR.; Supervision, C.S.; Project Administration, C.S.; Funding Acquisition, C.S.

Funding: This research was funded by the Swiss National Science Foundation for Research (Grant #32003B_163256/1 to CS).

Acknowledgments: We thank Romy Sweda, MD, for her contribution to the revision of this manuscript.

Conflicts of Interest: The authors have no conflict of interest.

Abbreviations

CABG	Coronary Artery Bypass Grafting
CAD	Coronary Artery Disease
CCS	Canadian Cardiovascular Society-Score
CFI	Collateral Flow Index
CFR	Coronary Flow Reserve
ECG	Electrocardiogram
ECP	External Counterpulsation
FGF	Fibroblast Growth-Factor
G-CSF	Granulocyte Colony-Stimulating Factor
GM-CSF	Granulocyte-Macrophage Colony-Stimulating Factor
IMA	Internal Mammary Artery
IMR	Index of Microvascular Resistance
ISRT	Individual Shear Rate Therapy
LAD	Left Anterior Descending (Artery)
LCX	Left Circumflex Artery
MCP-1	Monocyte Chemoattractant Protein-1
NCCMBF	Noncoronary Collateral Myocardial Blood Flow
NO	Nitric oxide
PCI	Percutaneous Coronary Intervention
QCA	Quantitative Coronary Angiography
RCA	Right Coronary Artery
VEGF	Vascular Endothelial Growth-Factor

References

1. Benjamin, E.J.; Muntner, P.; Alonso, A.; Bittencourt, M.S.; Callaway, C.W.; Carson, A.P.; Chamberlain, A.M.; Chang, A.R.; Cheng, S.; Das, S.R.; et al. Heart Disease and Stroke Statistics-2019 Update: A Report From the American Heart Association. *Circulation* **2019**, *139*, e56–e528. [CrossRef] [PubMed]
2. Mehta, S.R.; Cannon, C.P.; Fox, K.A.; Wallentin, L.; Boden, W.E.; Spacek, R.; Widimsky, P.; McCullough, P.A.; Hunt, D.; Braunwald, E.; et al. Routine vs selective invasive strategies in patients with acute coronary syndromes: A collaborative meta-analysis of randomized trials. *JAMA* **2005**, *293*, 2908–2917. [CrossRef] [PubMed]

3. Epstein, S.E.; Waksman, R.; Pichard, A.D.; Kent, K.M.; Panza, J.A. Percutaneous coronary intervention versus medical therapy in stable coronary artery disease: The unresolved conundrum. *JACC Cardiovasc. Interv.* **2013**, *6*, 993–998. [CrossRef] [PubMed]
4. Al-Lamee, R.; Thompson, D.; Dehbi, H.M.; Sen, S.; Tang, K.; Davies, J.; Keeble, T.; Mielewczik, M.; Kaprielian, R.; Malik, I.S.; et al. Percutaneous coronary intervention in stable angina (ORBITA): A double-blind, randomised controlled trial. *Lancet* **2018**, *391*, 31–40. [CrossRef]
5. Bienenfeld, L.; Frishman, W.; Glasser, S.P. The placebo effect in cardiovascular disease. *Am. Heart. J.* **1996**, *132*, 1207–1221. [CrossRef]
6. Johnson, A.G. Surgery as a placebo. *Lancet* **1994**, *344*, 1140–1142. [CrossRef]
7. Leon, M.B.; Kornowski, R.; Downey, W.E.; Weisz, G.; Baim, D.S.; Bonow, R.O.; Hendel, R.C..; Cohen, D.J.; Gervino, E.; Laham, R.; et al. A blinded, randomized, placebo-controlled trial of percutaneous laser myocardial revascularization to improve angina symptoms in patients with severe coronary disease. *J. Am. Coll. Cardiol.* **2005**, *46*, 1812–1819. [CrossRef]
8. Mohr, F.W.; Morice, M.C.; Kappetein, A.P.; Feldman, T.E.; Stahle, E.; Colombo, A.; Mack, M.J.; Holmes, D.R., Jr.; Morel, M.A.; Van Dyck, N.; et al. Coronary artery bypass graft surgery versus percutaneous coronary intervention in patients with three-vessel disease and left main coronary disease: 5-year follow-up of the randomised, clinical SYNTAX trial. *Lancet* **2013**, *381*, 629–638. [CrossRef]
9. McGillion, M.; Arthur, H.M.; Cook, A.; Carroll, S.L.; Victor, J.C.; L'Allier, P.L.; Jolicoeur, E.M.; Svorkdal, N.; Niznick, J.; Teoh, K.; et al. Management of patients with refractory angina: Canadian Cardiovascular Society/Canadian Pain Society joint guidelines. *Can. J. Cardiol.* **2012**, *28* (Suppl. 2), S20–S41. [CrossRef]
10. Williams, B.; Menon, M.; Satran, D.; Hayward, D.; Hodges, J.S.; Burke, M.N.; Johnson, R.K.; Poulose, A.K.; Traverse, J.H.; Henry, T.D. Patients with coronary artery disease not amenable to traditional revascularization: Prevalence and 3-year mortality. *Catheter. Cardiovasc. Interv.* **2010**, *75*, 886–891. [CrossRef]
11. Meier, P.; Gloekler, S.; Zbinden, R.; Beckh, S.; de Marchi, S.F.; Zbinden, S.; Wustmann, K.; Billinger, M.; Vogel, R.; Cook, S.; et al. Beneficial effect of recruitable collaterals: A 10-year follow-up study in patients with stable coronary artery disease undergoing quantitative collateral measurements. *Circulation* **2007**, *116*, 975–983. [CrossRef] [PubMed]
12. Meier, P.; Hemingway, H.; Lansky, A.J.; Knapp, G.; Pitt, B.; Seiler, C. The impact of the coronary collateral circulation on mortality: A meta-analysis. *Eur. Heart J.* **2012**, *33*, 614–621. [CrossRef] [PubMed]
13. Seiler, C.; Stoller, M.; Pitt, B.; Meier, P. The human coronary collateral circulation: Development and clinical importance. *Eur. Heart J.* **2013**, *34*, 2674–2682. [CrossRef] [PubMed]
14. Bloor, C.M.; Keefe, J.F.; Browne, M.J. Intercoronary anastomoses in congenital heart disease. *Circulation* **1966**, *33*, 227–231. [CrossRef] [PubMed]
15. Reiner, L.; Molnar, J.; Jimenez, F.A.; Freudenthal, R.R. Interarterial coronary anastomoses in neonates. *Arch. Pathol.* **1961**, *71*, 103–112. [PubMed]
16. Zoll, P.M.; Wessler, S.; Schlesinger, M.J. Interarterial coronary anastomoses in the human heart, with particular reference to anemia and relative cardiac anoxia. *Circulation* **1951**, *4*, 797–815. [CrossRef]
17. Fulton, W.F. Arterial Anastomoses in the Coronary Circulation. I. Anatomical Features in Normal and Diseased Hearts Demonstrated by Stereoarteriography. *Scott. Med. J.* **1963**, *8*, 420–434. [CrossRef]
18. Scholz, D.; Ito, W.; Fleming, I.; Deindl, E.; Sauer, A.; Wiesnet, M.; Busse, R.; Schaper, J.; Schaper, W. Ultrastructure and molecular histology of rabbit hind-limb collateral artery growth (arteriogenesis). *Virchows Arch.* **2000**, *436*, 257–270. [CrossRef]
19. Piciche, M. Noncoronary Collateral Myocardial Blood Flow: The Human Heart's Forgotten Blood Supply. *Open Cardiovasc. Med. J.* **2015**, *9*, 105–113. [CrossRef]
20. Bloor, C.M.; Liebow, A.A. Coronary collateral circulation. *Am. J. Cardiol.* **1965**, *16*, 238–252. [CrossRef]
21. Hudson, C.L.; Moritz, A.R.; Wearn, J.T. The Extracardiac Anastomoses of the Coronary Arteries. *J. Exp. Med.* **1932**, *56*, 919–925. [CrossRef] [PubMed]
22. Loukas, M.; Hanna, M.; Chen, J.; Tubbs, R.S.; Anderson, R.H. Extracardiac coronary arterial anastomoses. *Clin. Anat.* **2011**, *24*, 137–142. [CrossRef] [PubMed]
23. Olinger, G.N.; Bonchek, L.I.; Geiss, D.M. Noncoronary collateral distribution in coronary artery disease. *Ann. Thorac. Surg.* **1981**, *32*, 554–557. [CrossRef]
24. Die Foramina, L.L. Thebesii im Herzen des Menschen. *Sitzungsber k Akad Wissensch Cl Wien.* **1880**, *82*, 23–25.

25. Moberg, A. Anastomoses between extracardiac vessels and coronary arteries. *Acta Med. Scand. Suppl.* **1968**, *485*, 5–26. [PubMed]
26. Bjork, L. Angiographic demonstration of extracardial anastomoses to the coronary arteries. *Radiology* **1966**, *87*, 274–277. [PubMed]
27. Shimoji, K.; Matsuno, S.; Sudo, K.; Tsuchikane, E. Coronary Chronic Total Occlusion With Collateral Channels From the Bronchial Artery. *JACC Cardiovasc. Interv.* **2019**, *25*, 406–408. [CrossRef] [PubMed]
28. Byun, S.S.; Park, J.H.; Kim, J.H.; Sung, Y.M.; Kim, Y.K.; Kim, E.Y.; Park, E.A.; Coronary, C.T. findings of coronary to bronchial arterial communication in chronic pulmonary disease. *Int. J. Cardiovasc. Imaging* **2015**, *31* (Suppl. 1), 69–75. [CrossRef]
29. Goldstein, S.M.; Nelson, R.L.; McConnell, D.H.; Buckberg, G.D. Cardiac arrest after aortic cross-clamping: Effects of conventional vs pharmacologic arrest on myocardial supply/demand balance. *Surg. Forum* **1975**, *26*, 271–273. [PubMed]
30. Baile, E.M.; Ling, H.; Heyworth, J.R.; Hogg, J.C.; Pare, P.D. Bronchopulmonary anastomotic and noncoronary collateral blood flow in humans during cardiopulmonary bypass. *Chest* **1985**, *87*, 749–754. [CrossRef] [PubMed]
31. Goldstein, R.E.; Stinson, E.B.; Scherer, J.L.; Seningen, R.P.; Grehl, T.M.; Epstein, S.E. Intraoperative coronary collateral function in patients with coronary occlusive disease. Nitroglycerin responsiveness and angiographic correlations. *Circulation* **1974**, *49*, 298–308. [CrossRef] [PubMed]
32. Rentrop, K.P.; Cohen, M.; Blanke, H.; Phillips, R.A. Changes in collateral channel filling immediately after controlled coronary artery occlusion by an angioplasty balloon in human subjects. *J. Am. Coll. Cardiol.* **1985**, *5*, 587–592. [CrossRef]
33. Seiler, C.; Fleisch, M.; Garachemani, A.; Meier, B. Coronary collateral quantitation in patients with coronary artery disease using intravascular flow velocity or pressure measurements. *J. Am. Coll. Cardiol.* **1998**, *32*, 1272–1279. [CrossRef]
34. Pijls, N.H.; van Son, J.A.; Kirkeeide, R.L.; De Bruyne, B.; Gould, K.L. Experimental basis of determining maximum coronary, myocardial, and collateral blood flow by pressure measurements for assessing functional stenosis severity before and after percutaneous transluminal coronary angioplasty. *Circulation* **1993**, *87*, 1354–1367. [CrossRef]
35. Matsuo, H.; Watanabe, S.; Kadosaki, T.; Yamaki, T.; Tanaka, S.; Miyata, S.; Segawa, T.; Matsuno, Y.; Tomita, M.; Fujiwara, H. Validation of collateral fractional flow reserve by myocardial perfusion imaging. *Circulation* **2002**, *105*, 1060–1065. [CrossRef] [PubMed]
36. Vogel, R.; Zbinden, R.; Indermuhle, A.; Windecker, S.; Meier, B.; Seiler, C. Collateral-flow measurements in humans by myocardial contrast echocardiography: Validation of coronary pressure-derived collateral-flow assessment. *Eur. Heart J.* **2006**, *27*, 157–165. [CrossRef]
37. de Marchi, S.F.; Streuli, S.; Haefeli, P.; Gloekler, S.; Traupe, T.; Warncke, C.; Rimoldi, S.F.; Stortecky, S.; Steck, H.; Seiler, C. Determinants of prognostically relevant intracoronary electrocardiogram ST-segment shift during coronary balloon occlusion. *Am. J. Cardiol.* **2012**, *110*, 1234–1239. [CrossRef] [PubMed]
38. Traupe, T.; Gloekler, S.; de Marchi, S.F.; Werner, G.S.; Seiler, C. Assessment of the human coronary collateral circulation. *Circulation* **2010**, *122*, 1210–1220. [CrossRef] [PubMed]
39. Wustmann, K.; Zbinden, S.; Windecker, S.; Meier, B.; Seiler, C. Is there functional collateral flow during vascular occlusion in angiographically normal coronary arteries? *Circulation* **2003**, *107*, 2213–2220. [CrossRef]
40. Risau, W. Mechanisms of angiogenesis. *Nature* **1997**, *386*, 671–674. [CrossRef]
41. Arras, M.; Ito, W.D.; Scholz, D.; Winkler, B.; Schaper, J.; Schaper, W. Monocyte activation in angiogenesis and collateral growth in the rabbit hindlimb. *J. Clin. Investig.* **1998**, *101*, 40–50. [CrossRef] [PubMed]
42. Carmeliet, P. Mechanisms of angiogenesis and arteriogenesis. *Nat. Med.* **2000**, *6*, 389–395. [CrossRef] [PubMed]
43. Baum, O.; Da Silva-Azevedo, L.; Willerding, G.; Wockel, A.; Planitzer, G.; Gossrau, R.; Pries, A.R.; Zakrzewicz, A. Endothelial NOS is main mediator for shear stress-dependent angiogenesis in skeletal muscle after prazosin administration. *Am. J. Physiol. Heart Circ. Physiol.* **2004**, *287*, H2300–H2308. [CrossRef] [PubMed]
44. Grundmann, S.; Piek, J.J.; Pasterkamp, G.; Hoefer, I.E. Arteriogenesis: Basic mechanisms and therapeutic stimulation. *Eur. J. Clin. Investig.* **2007**, *37*, 755–766. [CrossRef] [PubMed]

45. Hoefer, I.E.; van Royen, N.; Buschmann, I.R.; Piek, J.J.; Schaper, W. Time course of arteriogenesis following femoral artery occlusion in the rabbit. *Cardiovasc. Res.* **2001**, *49*, 609–617. [CrossRef]
46. Gloekler, S.; Meier, P.; de Marchi, S.F.; Rutz, T.; Traupe, T.; Rimoldi, S.F.; Wustmann, K.; Steck, H.; Cook, S.; Vogel, R.; et al. Coronary collateral growth by external counterpulsation: A randomised controlled trial. *Heart* **2010**, *96*, 202–207. [CrossRef] [PubMed]
47. Pipp, F.; Boehm, S.; Cai, W.J.; Adili, F.; Ziegler, B.; Karanovic, G.; Ritter, R.; Balzer, J.; Scheler, C.; Schaper, W.; et al. Elevated fluid shear stress enhances postocclusive collateral artery growth and gene expression in the pig hind limb. *Arterioscler. Thromb. Vasc. Biol.* **2004**, *24*, 1664–1668. [CrossRef] [PubMed]
48. Schaper, W. Collateral circulation: Past and present. *Basic Res. Cardiol.* **2009**, *104*, 5–21. [CrossRef] [PubMed]
49. Heil, M.; Ziegelhoeffer, T.; Pipp, F.; Kostin, S.; Martin, S.; Clauss, M.; Schaper, W. Blood monocyte concentration is critical for enhancement of collateral artery growth. *Am. J. Physiol. Heart Circ. Physiol.* **2002**, *283*, H2411–H2419. [CrossRef]
50. Ito, W.D.; Arras, M.; Winkler, B.; Scholz, D.; Schaper, J.; Schaper, W. Monocyte chemotactic protein-1 increases collateral and peripheral conductance after femoral artery occlusion. *Circ. Res.* **1997**, *80*, 829–837. [CrossRef]
51. Busse, R.; Fleming, I. Regulation and functional consequences of endothelial nitric oxide formation. *Ann. Med.* **1995**, *27*, 331–340. [CrossRef] [PubMed]
52. Seiler, C.; Kirkeeide, R.L.; Gould, K.L. Basic structure-function relations of the epicardial coronary vascular tree. Basis of quantitative coronary arteriography for diffuse coronary artery disease. *Circulation* **1992**, *85*, 1987–2003. [CrossRef] [PubMed]
53. Ito, W.D.; Arras, M.; Scholz, D.; Winkler, B.; Htun, P.; Schaper, W. Angiogenesis but not collateral growth is associated with ischemia after femoral artery occlusion. *Am. J. Physiol.* **1997**, *273 Pt 2*, H1255–H1265. [CrossRef]
54. Deindl, E.; Buschmann, I.; Hoefer, I.E.; Podzuweit, T.; Boengler, K.; Vogel, S.; van Royen, N.; Fernandez, B.; Schaper, W. Role of ischemia and of hypoxia-inducible genes in arteriogenesis after femoral artery occlusion in the rabbit. *Circ. Res.* **2001**, *89*, 779–786. [CrossRef] [PubMed]
55. Eitenmuller, I.; Volger, O.; Kluge, A.; Troidl, K.; Barancik, M.; Cai, W.J.; Heil, M.; Pipp, F.; Fischer, S.; Horrevoets, A.J.; et al. The range of adaptation by collateral vessels after femoral artery occlusion. *Circ. Res.* **2006**, *99*, 656–662. [CrossRef] [PubMed]
56. Vogel, R.; Traupe, T.; Steiger, V.S.; Seiler, C. Physical coronary arteriogenesis: A human "model" of collateral growth promotion. *Trends Cardiovasc. Med.* **2010**, *20*, 129–133. [CrossRef] [PubMed]
57. Epstein, S.E.; Stabile, E.; Kinnaird, T.; Lee, C.W.; Clavijo, L.; Burnett, M.S. Janus phenomenon: The interrelated tradeoffs inherent in therapies designed to enhance collateral formation and those designed to inhibit atherogenesis. *Circulation* **2004**, *109*, 2826–2831. [CrossRef]
58. Seiler, C.; Pohl, T.; Wustmann, K.; Hutter, D.; Nicolet, P.A.; Windecker, S.; Eberli, F.R.; Meier, B. Promotion of collateral growth by granulocyte-macrophage colony-stimulating factor in patients with coronary artery disease: A randomized, double-blind, placebo-controlled study. *Circulation* **2001**, *104*, 2012–2017. [CrossRef]
59. Zbinden, S.; Zbinden, R.; Meier, P.; Windecker, S.; Seiler, C. Safety and efficacy of subcutaneous-only granulocyte-macrophage colony-stimulating factor for collateral growth promotion in patients with coronary artery disease. *J. Am. Coll. Cardiol.* **2005**, *46*, 1636–1642. [CrossRef]
60. van Royen, N.; Schirmer, S.H.; Atasever, B.; Behrens, C.Y.; Ubbink, D.; Buschmann, E.E.; Voskuil, M.; Bot, P.; Hoefer, I.; Schlingemann, R.O.; et al. START Trial: A pilot study on STimulation of ARTeriogenesis using subcutaneous application of granulocyte-macrophage colony-stimulating factor as a new treatment for peripheral vascular disease. *Circulation* **2005**, *112*, 1040–1046. [CrossRef]
61. Buschmann, I.R.; Hoefer, I.E.; van Royen, N.; Katzer, E.; Braun-Dulleaus, R.; Heil, M.; Kostin, S.; Bode, C.; Schaper, W. GM-CSF: A strong arteriogenic factor acting by amplification of monocyte function. *Atherosclerosis* **2001**, *159*, 343–356. [CrossRef]
62. Schneeloch, E.; Mies, G.; Busch, H.J.; Buschmann, I.R.; Hossmann, K.A. Granulocyte-macrophage colony-stimulating factor-induced arteriogenesis reduces energy failure in hemodynamic stroke. *Proc. Natl. Acad. Sci. USA* **2004**, *101*, 12730–12735. [CrossRef] [PubMed]
63. Meier, P.; Gloekler, S.; de Marchi, S.F.; Indermuehle, A.; Rutz, T.; Traupe, T.; Steck, H.; Vogel, R.; Seiler, C. Myocardial salvage through coronary collateral growth by granulocyte colony-stimulating factor in chronic coronary artery disease: A controlled randomized trial. *Circulation* **2009**, *120*, 1355–1363. [CrossRef] [PubMed]

64. Hill, J.M.; Syed, M.A.; Arai, A.E.; Powell, T.M.; Paul, J.D.; Zalos, G.; Read, E.J.; Khuu, H.M.; Leitman, S.F.; Horne, M.; et al. Outcomes and risks of granulocyte colony-stimulating factor in patients with coronary artery disease. *J. Am. Coll. Cardiol.* **2005**, *46*, 1643–1648. [CrossRef] [PubMed]
65. Kang, S.; Yang, Y.; Li, C.J.; Gao, R. Effectiveness and tolerability of administration of granulocyte colony-stimulating factor on left ventricular function in patients with myocardial infarction: A meta-analysis of randomized controlled trials. *Clin. Ther.* **2007**, *29*, 2406–2418. [CrossRef] [PubMed]
66. Kang, H.J.; Kim, H.S.; Zhang, S.Y.; Park, K.W.; Cho, H.J.; Koo, B.K.; Kim, Y.J.; Lee, D.S.; Sohn, D.W.; Han, K.S.; et al. Effects of intracoronary infusion of peripheral blood stem-cells mobilised with granulocyte-colony stimulating factor on left ventricular systolic function and restenosis after coronary stenting in myocardial infarction: The MAGIC cell randomised clinical trial. *Lancet* **2004**, *363*, 751–756. [PubMed]
67. Simons, M.; Annex, B.H.; Laham, R.J.; Kleiman, N.; Henry, T.; Dauerman, H.; Udelson, J.E.; Gervino, E.V.; Pike, M.; Whitehouse, M.J.; et al. Pharmacological treatment of coronary artery disease with recombinant fibroblast growth factor-2: Double-blind, randomized, controlled clinical trial. *Circulation* **2002**, *105*, 788–793. [CrossRef] [PubMed]
68. Grines, C.L.; Watkins, M.W.; Helmer, G.; Penny, W.; Brinker, J.; Marmur, J.D.; West, A.; Rade, J.J.; Marrott, P.; Hammond, H.K.; et al. Angiogenic Gene Therapy (AGENT) trial in patients with stable angina pectoris. *Circulation* **2002**, *105*, 1291–1297. [CrossRef] [PubMed]
69. Laham, R.J.; Sellke, F.W.; Edelman, E.R.; Pearlman, J.D.; Ware, J.A.; Brown, D.L.; Gold, J.P.; Simons, M. Local perivascular delivery of basic fibroblast growth factor in patients undergoing coronary bypass surgery: Results of a phase I randomized, double-blind, placebo-controlled trial. *Circulation* **1999**, *100*, 1865–1871. [CrossRef]
70. Henry, T.D.; Annex, B.H.; McKendall, G.R.; Azrin, M.A.; Lopez, J.J.; Giordano, F.J.; Shah, P.K.; Willerson, J.T.; Benza, R.L.; Berman, D.S.; et al. The VIVA trial: Vascular endothelial growth factor in Ischemia for Vascular Angiogenesis. *Circulation* **2003**, *107*, 1359–1365. [CrossRef]
71. Simons, M.; Bonow, R.O.; Chronos, N.A.; Cohen, D.J.; Giordano, F.J.; Hammond, H.K.; Laham, R.J.; Li, W.; Pike, M.; Sellke, F.W.; et al. Clinical trials in coronary angiogenesis: Issues, problems, consensus: An expert panel summary. *Circulation* **2000**, *102*, E73–E86. [CrossRef] [PubMed]
72. Kastrup, J.; Ripa, R.S.; Wang, Y.; Jorgensen, E. Myocardial regeneration induced by granulocyte-colony stimulating factor mobilization of stem cells in patients with acute or chronic ischaemic heart disease: A non-invasive alternative for clinical stem cell therapy? *Eur. Heart J.* **2006**, *27*, 2748–2754. [CrossRef] [PubMed]
73. Zohlnhofer, D.; Dibra, A.; Koppara, T.; de Waha, A.; Ripa, R.S.; Kastrup, J.; Valgimigli, M.; Schomig, A.; Kastrati, A. Stem cell mobilization by granulocyte colony-stimulating factor for myocardial recovery after acute myocardial infarction: A meta-analysis. *J. Am. Coll. Cardiol.* **2008**, *51*, 1429–1437. [CrossRef]
74. Abdel-Latif, A.; Bolli, R.; Zuba-Surma, E.K.; Tleyjeh, I.M.; Hornung, C.A.; Dawn, B. Granulocyte colony-stimulating factor therapy for cardiac repair after acute myocardial infarction: A systematic review and meta-analysis of randomized controlled trials. *Am. Heart J.* **2008**, *156*, 216–226.e9. [CrossRef] [PubMed]
75. Deindl, E.; Zaruba, M.M.; Brunner, S.; Huber, B.; Mehl, U.; Assmann, G.; Hoefer, I.E.; Mueller-Hoecker, J.; Franz, W.M. G-CSF administration after myocardial infarction in mice attenuates late ischemic cardiomyopathy by enhanced arteriogenesis. *Faseb J.* **2006**, *20*, 956–958. [CrossRef] [PubMed]
76. Prior, B.M.; Lloyd, P.G.; Yang, H.T.; Terjung, R.L. Exercise-induced vascular remodeling. *Exerc. Sport Sci. Rev.* **2003**, *31*, 26–33. [CrossRef] [PubMed]
77. Oldridge, N.B.; Guyatt, G.H.; Fischer, M.E.; Rimm, A.A. Cardiac rehabilitation after myocardial infarction. Combined experience of randomized clinical trials. *JAMA* **1988**, *260*, 945–950. [CrossRef] [PubMed]
78. Morris, J.N.; Crawford, M.D. Coronary heart disease and physical activity of work; evidence of a national necropsy survey. *Br. Med. J.* **1958**, *2*, 1485–1496. [CrossRef]
79. Niebauer, J.; Cooke, J.P. Cardiovascular effects of exercise: Role of endothelial shear stress. *J. Am. Coll. Cardiol.* **1996**, *28*, 1652–1660. [CrossRef]
80. Bruning, R.S.; Sturek, M. Benefits of exercise training on coronary blood flow in coronary artery disease patients. *Prog. Cardiovasc. Dis.* **2015**, *57*, 443–453. [CrossRef]
81. Scheel, K.W.; Ingram, L.A.; Wilson, J.L. Effects of exercise on the coronary and collateral vasculature of beagles with and without coronary occlusion. *Circ. Res.* **1981**, *48*, 523–530. [CrossRef] [PubMed]

82. Zbinden, R.; Zbinden, S.; Windecker, S.; Meier, B.; Seiler, C. Direct demonstration of coronary collateral growth by physical endurance exercise in a healthy marathon runner. *Heart* **2004**, *90*, 1350–1351. [CrossRef] [PubMed]
83. Windecker, S.; Allemann, Y.; Billinger, M.; Pohl, T.; Hutter, D.; Orsucci, T.; Blaga, L.; Meier, B.; Seiler, C. Effect of endurance training on coronary artery size and function in healthy men: An invasive followup study. *Am. J. Physiol. Heart Circ. Physiol.* **2002**, *282*, H2216–H2223. [CrossRef] [PubMed]
84. Zbinden, R.; Zbinden, S.; Meier, P.; Hutter, D.; Billinger, M.; Wahl, A.; Schmid, J.P.; Windecker, S.; Meier, B.; Seiler, C. Coronary collateral flow in response to endurance exercise training. *Eur. J. Cardiovasc. Prev. Rehabil.* **2007**, *14*, 250–257. [CrossRef] [PubMed]
85. Hambrecht, R.; Wolf, A.; Gielen, S.; Linke, A.; Hofer, J.; Erbs, S.; Schoene, N.; Schuler, G. Effect of exercise on coronary endothelial function in patients with coronary artery disease. *N. Engl. J. Med.* **2000**, *342*, 454–460. [CrossRef]
86. Togni, M.; Gloekler, S.; Meier, P.; de Marchi, S.F.; Rutz, T.; Steck, H.; Traupe, T.; Seiler, C. Instantaneous coronary collateral function during supine bicycle exercise. *Eur. Heart J.* **2010**, *31*, 2148–2155. [CrossRef]
87. Fujita, M.; Sasayama, S. Coronary collateral growth and its therapeutic application to coronary artery disease. *Circ. J.* **2010**, *74*, 1283–1289. [CrossRef] [PubMed]
88. Belardinelli, R.; Georgiou, D.; Ginzton, L.; Cianci, G.; Purcaro, A. Effects of moderate exercise training on thallium uptake and contractile response to low-dose dobutamine of dysfunctional myocardium in patients with ischemic cardiomyopathy. *Circulation* **1998**, *97*, 553–561. [CrossRef]
89. Heaps, C.L.; Parker, J.L. Effects of exercise training on coronary collateralization and control of collateral resistance. *J. Appl. Physiol.* **2011**, *111*, 587–598. [CrossRef]
90. Niebauer, J.; Hambrecht, R.; Marburger, C.; Hauer, K.; Velich, T.; von Hodenberg, E.; Schlierf, G.; Kubler, W.; Schuler, G. Impact of intensive physical exercise and low-fat diet on collateral vessel formation in stable angina pectoris and angiographically confirmed coronary artery disease. *Am. J. Cardiol.* **1995**, *76*, 771–775. [CrossRef]
91. Möbius-Winkler, S.; Uhlemann, M.; Adams, V.; Sandri, M.; Erbs, S.; Lenk, K.; Mangner, N.; Mueller, U.; Adam, J.; Grunze, M.; et al. Coronary Collateral Growth Induced by Physical Exercise: Results of the Impact of Intensive Exercise Training on Coronary Collateral Circulation in Patients With Stable Coronary Artery Disease (EXCITE) Trial. *Circulation* **2016**, *133*, 1438–1448, discussion 48. [CrossRef] [PubMed]
92. Raza, A.; Steinberg, K.; Tartaglia, J.; Frishman, W.H.; Gupta, T. Enhanced External Counterpulsation Therapy: Past, Present, and Future. *Cardiol. Rev.* **2017**, *25*, 59–67. [CrossRef]
93. Arora, R.R.; Chou, T.M.; Jain, D.; Fleishman, B.; Crawford, L.; McKiernan, T.; Nesto, R.W. The multicenter study of enhanced external counterpulsation (MUST-EECP): Effect of EECP on exercise-induced myocardial ischemia and anginal episodes. *J. Am. Coll. Cardiol.* **1999**, *33*, 1833–1840. [CrossRef]
94. Manchanda, A.; Soran, O. Enhanced external counterpulsation and future directions: Step beyond medical management for patients with angina and heart failure. *J. Am. Coll. Cardiol.* **2007**, *50*, 1523–1531. [CrossRef]
95. Qin, X.; Deng, Y.; Wu, D.; Yu, L.; Huang, R. Does Enhanced External Counterpulsation (EECP) Significantly Affect Myocardial Perfusion? A Systematic Review & Meta-Analysis. *PLoS ONE* **2016**, *11*, e0151822.
96. Cohn, P.F. Enhanced external counterpulsation for the treatment of angina pectoris. *Prog. Cardiovasc. Dis.* **2006**, *49*, 88–97. [CrossRef] [PubMed]
97. Lawson, W.E.; Hui, J.C.; Cohn, P.F. Long-term prognosis of patients with angina treated with enhanced external counterpulsation: Five-year follow-up study. *Clin. Cardiol.* **2000**, *23*, 254–258. [CrossRef] [PubMed]
98. Buschmann, E.E.; Utz, W.; Pagonas, N.; Schulz-Menger, J.; Busjahn, A.; Monti, J.; Maerz, W.; le Noble, F.; Thierfelder, L.; Dietz, R.; et al. Improvement of fractional flow reserve and collateral flow by treatment with external counterpulsation (Art.Net.-2 Trial). *Eur. J. Clin. Investig.* **2009**, *39*, 866–875. [CrossRef]
99. Picard, F.; Panagiotidou, P.; Wolf-Putz, A.; Buschmann, I.; Buschmann, E.; Steffen, M.; Klein, R.M. Usefulness of Individual Shear Rate Therapy, New Treatment Option for Patients With Symptomatic Coronary Artery Disease. *Am. J. Cardiol.* **2018**, *121*, 416–422. [CrossRef]
100. Beck, C.S.; Leighninger, D.S. Operations for coronary artery disease. *Ann. Surg.* **1955**, *141*, 24–37. [CrossRef]
101. Verheye, S.; Jolicoeur, E.M.; Behan, M.W.; Pettersson, T.; Sainsbury, P.; Hill, J.; Vrolix, M.; Agostoni, P.; Engstrom, T.; Labinaz, M.; et al. Efficacy of a device to narrow the coronary sinus in refractory angina. *N. Engl. J. Med.* **2015**, *372*, 519–527. [CrossRef] [PubMed]

102. Stoller, M.; Traupe, T.; Khattab, A.A.; de Marchi, S.F.; Steck, H.; Seiler, C. Effects of coronary sinus occlusion on myocardial ischaemia in humans: Role of coronary collateral function. *Heart* **2013**, *99*, 548–555. [CrossRef] [PubMed]
103. Banai, S.; Ben Muvhar, S.; Parikh, K.H.; Medina, A.; Sievert, H.; Seth, A.; Tsehori, J.; Paz, Y.; Sheinfeld, A.; Keren, G. Coronary sinus reducer stent for the treatment of chronic refractory angina pectoris: A prospective, open-label, multicenter, safety feasibility first-in-man study. *J. Am. Coll. Cardiol.* **2007**, *49*, 1783–1789. [CrossRef] [PubMed]
104. Ielasi, A.; Todaro, M.C.; Grigis, G.; Tespili, M. Coronary Sinus Reducer system: A new therapeutic option in refractory angina patients unsuitable for revascularization. *Int. J. Cardiol.* **2016**, *209*, 122–130. [CrossRef] [PubMed]
105. Konigstein, M.; Giannini, F.; Banai, S. The Reducer device in patients with angina pectoris: Mechanisms, indications, and perspectives. *Eur. Heart, J.* **2018**, *39*, 925–933. [CrossRef] [PubMed]
106. Borer, J.S.; Deedwania, P.C.; Kim, J.B.; Bohm, M. Benefits of Heart Rate Slowing With Ivabradine in Patients With Systolic Heart Failure and Coronary Artery Disease. *Am. J. Cardiol.* **2016**, *118*, 1948–1953. [CrossRef] [PubMed]
107. Tardif, J.C.; Ford, I.; Tendera, M.; Bourassa, M.G.; Fox, K. Efficacy of ivabradine, a new selective I(f) inhibitor, compared with atenolol in patients with chronic stable angina. *Eur. Heart J.* **2005**, *26*, 2529–2536. [CrossRef] [PubMed]
108. Godino, C.; Colombo, A.; Margonato, A. Ivabradine in Patients with Stable Coronary Artery Disease: A Rationale for Use in Addition to and Beyond Percutaneous Coronary Intervention. *Clin. Drug Investig.* **2017**, *37*, 105–120. [CrossRef]
109. Gloekler, S.; Traupe, T.; Stoller, M.; Schild, D.; Steck, H.; Khattab, A.; Vogel, R.; Seiler, C. The effect of heart rate reduction by ivabradine on collateral function in patients with chronic stable coronary artery disease. *Heart* **2014**, *100*, 160–166. [CrossRef]
110. Patel, S.R.; Breall, J.A.; Diver, D.J.; Gersh, B.J.; Levy, A.P. Bradycardia is associated with development of coronary collateral vessels in humans. *Coron. Artery Dis.* **2000**, *11*, 467–472. [CrossRef]
111. Lamping, K.G.; Zheng, W.; Xing, D.; Christensen, L.P.; Martins, J.; Tomanek, R.J. Bradycardia stimulates vascular growth during gradual coronary occlusion. *Arterioscler. Thromb. Vasc. Biol.* **2005**, *25*, 2122–2127. [CrossRef] [PubMed]
112. Wright, A.J.; Hudlicka, O. Capillary growth and changes in heart performance induced by chronic bradycardial pacing in the rabbit. *Circ. Res.* **1981**, *49*, 469–478. [CrossRef] [PubMed]
113. Fox, K.; Ford, I.; Steg, P.G.; Tendera, M.; Ferrari, R. Ivabradine for patients with stable coronary artery disease and left-ventricular systolic dysfunction (BEAUTIFUL): A randomised, double-blind, placebo-controlled trial. *Lancet* **2008**, *372*, 807–816. [CrossRef]
114. Fox, K.; Ford, I.; Steg, P.G.; Tardif, J.C.; Tendera, M.; Ferrari, R. Ivabradine in stable coronary artery disease without clinical heart failure. *N. Engl. J. Med.* **2014**, *371*, 1091–1099. [CrossRef] [PubMed]
115. Fieschi, D. Criteri anatomo-fisiologici per intervento chirurgico liebe in malati di infarto e cuore di angina. *Arch. Ital. Chir.* **1942**, *63*, 305–310.
116. Battezzati, M.; Tagliaferro, A.; Cattaneo, A.D. Clinical evaluation of bilateral internal mammary artery ligation as treatment coronary heart disease. *Am. J. Cardiol.* **1959**, *4*, 180–183. [CrossRef]
117. Battezzati, M.; Tagliaferro, A.; Cattaneo, A.D.; Donini, I.; Bachi, V. Anastomotic relationships between the internal mammary arteries and the coronary arterial circulation. *Panminerva Med.* **1959**, *1*, 229–232. [PubMed]
118. Battezzati, M.; Tagliaferro, A.; De Marchi, G. Ligation of the two internal mammary arteries in vascular disorders of the myocardium; preventive note concerning the first experimental and clinical findings. *Minerva Med.* **1955**, *46*, 1178–1188. [PubMed]
119. Glover, R.P. A new surgical approach to the problem of myocardial revascularization in coronary artery disease. *J. Ark. Med. Soc.* **1957**, *54*, 223–234.
120. Glover, R.P.; Davila, J.C.; Kyle, R.H.; Beard, J.C., Jr.; Trout, R.G.; Kitchell, J.R. Ligation of the internal mammary arteries as a means of increasing blood supply to the myocardium. *J. Thorac. Surg.* **1957**, *34*, 661–678.
121. Glover, R.P.; Kitchell, J.R.; Davila, J.C.; Barkley, H.T., Jr. Bilateral ligation of the internal mammary artery in the treatment of angina pectoris. Experimental and clinical results. *Am. J. Cardiol.* **1960**, *6*, 937–945. [CrossRef]

122. Glover, R.P.; Kitchell, J.R.; Kyle, R.H.; Davila, J.C.; Trout, R.G. Experiences with myocardial revascularization by division of the internal mammary arteries. *Dis. Chest* **1958**, *33*, 637–657. [CrossRef] [PubMed]
123. Kitchell, J.R.; Glover, R.P.; Kyle, R.H. Bilateral internal mammary artery ligation for angina pectoris; preliminary clinical considerations. *Am. J. Cardiol.* **1958**, *1*, 46–50. [CrossRef]
124. Beecher, H.K. Surgery as placebo: A quantitative study of bias. 1961. *Int. Anesthesiol. Clin.* **2007**, *45*, 35–45. [CrossRef]
125. Cobb, L.A.; Thomas, G.I.; Dillard, D.H.; Merendino, K.A.; Bruce, R.A. An evaluation of internal-mammary-artery ligation by a double-blind technic. *N. Engl. J. Med.* **1959**, *260*, 1115–1118. [CrossRef]
126. Dimond, E.G.; Kittle, C.F.; Crockett, J.E. Comparison of internal mammary artery ligation and sham operation for angina pectoris. *Am. J. Cardiol.* **1960**, *5*, 483–486. [CrossRef]
127. Miller, F.G. The enduring legacy of sham-controlled trials of internal mammary artery ligation. *Prog. Cardiovasc. Dis.* **2012**, *55*, 246–250. [CrossRef]
128. Stoller, M.; de Marchi, S.F.; Seiler, C. Function of natural internal mammary-to-coronary artery bypasses and its effect on myocardial ischemia. *Circulation* **2014**, *129*, 2645–2652. [CrossRef]
129. Stoller, M.; Seiler, C. Effect of Permanent Right Internal Mammary Artery Closure on Coronary Collateral Function and Myocardial Ischemia. *Circ. Cardiovasc. Interv.* **2017**, *10*, e004990. [CrossRef]

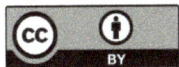

© 2019 by the authors. Licensee MDPI, Basel, Switzerland. This article is an open access article distributed under the terms and conditions of the Creative Commons Attribution (CC BY) license (http://creativecommons.org/licenses/by/4.0/).

MDPI
St. Alban-Anlage 66
4052 Basel
Switzerland
Tel. +41 61 683 77 34
Fax +41 61 302 89 18
www.mdpi.com

International Journal of Molecular Sciences Editorial Office
E-mail: ijms@mdpi.com
www.mdpi.com/journal/ijms

www.ingramcontent.com/pod-product-compliance
Lightning Source LLC
LaVergne TN
LVHW070642100526
838202LV00013B/860